Understanding Hydrolats: The Specific Hydrosols for Aromatherapy

A Guide for Health Professionals

This important book will challenge the readers and provide a good foundation for learning the art and science of distilled waters as well as their uses in aromatherapy.

Jeanne Rose
Director of the Institute of Herb and Aromatic Studies,
San Francisco, California, USA

For Churchill Livingstone:

Publishing Manager: Inta Ozols
Project Development Manager: Karen Morley, Kerry McGechie
Project Manager: Morven Dean
Design Direction: Jayne Jones

Understanding Hydrolats: The Specific Hydrosols for Aromatherapy

A Guide for Health Professionals

Len Price MIT FIFPA LIAM

Lecturer in Aromatherapy, Hinckley, Leicestershire, UK

Shirley Price FIFPA LIAM

Author, Practioner (in France) and Lecture in Aromatherapy,
Hinckley, Leicestershire, UK

Foreword by

Katja Svoboda Bsc Msc PhD

Lecture/Researcher at the Scottish Agricultural College, Auchincruive, UK

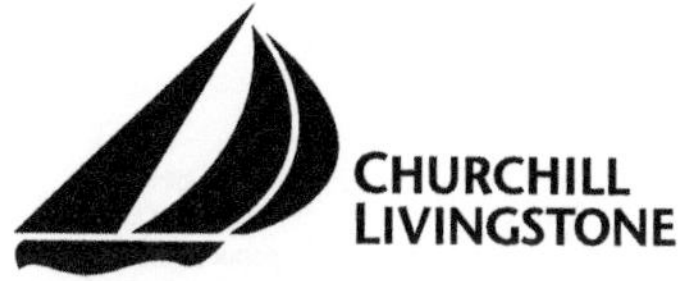

EDINBURGH LONDON NEW YORK PHILADELPHIA ST LOUIS SYDNEY TORONTO 2004

CHURCHILL LIVINGSTONE
An imprint of Elsevier Limited

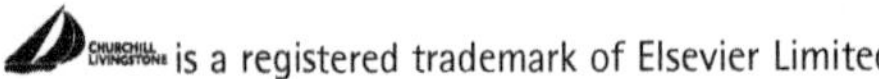

ISBN 0443 07316 3

British Library Cataloguing in Publication Data
A catalogue record for this book is available from the British Library

Library of Congress Cataloging in Publication Data
A catalog record for this book is available from the Library of Congress

Note
Knowledge and best practice in this field are constantly changing. As new research and experience broaden our knowledge, changes in practice, treatment and drug therapy may become necessary or appropriate. Readers are advised to check the most current information provided (i) on procedures featured or (ii) by the manufacturer of each product to be administered, to verify the recommended dose or formula, the method and duration of administration, and contraindications. It is the responsibility of the practitioner, relying on their own experience and knowledge of the patient, to make diagnoses, to determine dosages and the best treatment for each individual patient, and to take all appropriate safety precautions. To the fullest extent of the law, neither the publisher nor the authors assumes any liability for any injury and/or damage.

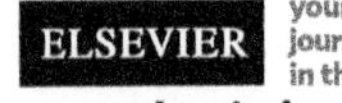

your source for books, journals and multimedia in the health sciences
www.elsevierhealth.com

The publisher's policy is to use **paper manufactured from sustainable forests**

Transferred to Digital Printing in 2008

Contents

Foreword viii
Preface x
Acknowledgements xii

Chapter 1 Introduction 1
The first aromatherapy 1
Is 'natural' necessarily safe? 2
Why are waters not used more? 3
Sourcing good materials 3
Advantages of distilled plant waters 4
What is their composition? 4
Scientific proof 5
Water-based plant extracts 7
Conclusion 8

Chapter 2 The history of aromatic medicine 9
Egypt 9
Aromatics worldwide 10
Development of medicine 10
Development of distillation 11
Arab and Spanish influences 11
The holy wars, 10th–13th centuries 13
Hungary water 13
Carmelite water 14
After the Crusades 14
Paracelsus (1493–1541) 14
New plants bring new worlds 15
Still rooms 15
Renaissance herbals 15
Eau-de-Cologne 16
Rise of science 16
Fall and resurrection of plant medicine 16
Some 20th-century pioneers 17
Conclusion 18

Chapter 3 The nature of water 19
Introduction 19
Universal distillation process 20
A basic necessity 20
Life and death 21

Physical power of water 21
Visual aspects 22
Judging by water 22
Water as a solvent and cleanser 22
Water in the body 23
Bottled water 23
Healing treatments with water 24
Scientists who investigated water 25
Structure of liquid water 26
Polar solvent – soublility in water 28
Increased dilution 30

Chapter 4 Terminology and nomenclature **31**
Introduction: what's in a name? 31
How distilled plant waters are obtained 31
Current terminology 32
Hydrosols? 34
Conclusion 34

Chapter 5 Prepared waters **35**
Identifying the product 35
Not distilled 35
Internal use 36
Fragrant waters: methods of production and uses 37
Addition of alcohol 38
Hydroessentials 38
Witch hazel 39
Eau-de-Cologne 39
Conclusion 40

Chapter 6 Extraction process and the plants used **41**
What kinds of plant yield hydrolats? 41
The plants used 42
Drying 42
Distillation 43
Water used 44
Still hardware 45
Chemical changes 45
Time of distillation 46
Yield of hydrolats 46
Volatile molecules in the distilled waters 47
Therapeutic value 48
Cohobation 49
Water oil, recovered oil 50
Are cohobated waters therapeutically useful? 51
Conclusion 54

Chapter 7 Physical aspects **55**
Introduction 55
Temperature 55
Time 56
Preservatives 57
Appearance 58

Density 58
pH 58
Odour 58
Quality 59
Cost 59
Conclusion 60

Chapter 8 Analysis 61
How do we find out what is in hydrolats? 61
Methods of extraction 61
Discussion of the molecules found in waters analysed 63
Part 1: Table of molecules found in waters 71
Part 2: Chemistry of aromatic molecules 76

Chapter 9 Alphabetical listing of hydrolats with description, properties and indications 93
Introduction 93
Arrangement of the text 94
Alphabetical list of hydrolats 95

Chapter 10 Methods, dosage and recipes 149
Reasons for using hydrolats 149
Hydrolats used in association with other therapeutic products 150
Uses of distilled waters 151
Methods: external pathways 152
Methods: internal pathways 155
Dispersants 157
Cautions 158
Conclusion 158
Recipes 160
Recipes for common ailments 160
Culinary recipes 173
Making your own hydrolats 177

Chapter 11 Case studies 181

Chapter 12 Decoctions, infusions, teas 187
Introduction 187
Infusions, teas and tisanes 188
Difference between a hydrolat and an infusion 188
Tea with added hydrolats 190
Tisanes, with and without hydrolats 190
Teas made by the authors 191
Decoctions 194
Cautions to observe when drinking medicinal teas 195

APPENDIX A Therapeutic index 197
APPENDIX B Therapeutic properties of hydrolats: quick reference 215
APPENDIX C Plant list: scientific and common names 227
APPENDIX D Analyses of distilled plant waters 231
APPENDIX E Hydrolat gas chromatographs 257

Glossary 269
References 275
Index 281

Foreword

The importance of plants, their extracts generally and essential oils specifically, has increased over the years, both as a result of changes in their uses, growing publicity, and consequently greater public awareness of the potential benefits of aromatic and medicinal plants. The mode of action of plant extracts is generally not understood by people outside the health professions. However, public awareness and concern about the use of and exposure to chemicals, drugs and additives is growing. It is clear that the science of aromatherapy has relevance to a growing number of people interested in distilled plant waters (hydrolats). There is an obvious need for an authoritative book covering their general and specific aspects, aimed at individuals of diverse backgrounds and occupations who wish to acquire an understanding of the physical and chemical aspects of these waters, their extraction from plants and their potential applications.

This book is the successful result of an earnest, scholarly effort to present an explanation of the science underlying the general concepts and principles of hydrolats. A number of specific examples are included to illustrate the application of the principles. The style of the book is straightforward and lucid and the basic format facilitates quick reference; the subject matter has been treated under several headings, used uniformly throughout. Technical terms are consistent and accurate, and a glossary is appended. The subject matter has been compiled from a very wide range of historical, medical, botanical and biochemical publications and from computer searches of appropriate databases. The paucity of scientific information on the mechanisms of actions of plant waters contrasts starkly with the more widespread knowledge in the aromatherapy profession of their effects. Although every effort has been made to clarify the nature of bioactivity, there are still many plants and their extracts in which the active principles have not been identified or whose pharmacological action has not been elucidated, despite recent advances in modern analytical techniques. This book offers a significant advance in the area of integrating the chemical, biological and therapeutic activities of distilled plant waters.

The authors of this book are well known for their contributions and pioneering work in the realm of aromatherapy. They have been dedicated in their search for scientific principles in this field, taught numerous students in the health professions and have presented lectures to non-professional groups as well. They have created a strong foundation for the responsible use of essential oils, and have provided a professional approach to their application based on the use of high-quality plants as the source material and correct distillation methods. Students and professionals in the diverse fields of science and humanities, medicine and nursing will eagerly accept this book, whose purpose is to provide a concise source of knowledge of hydrolats, including fundamental concepts of water chemistry and underlying principles of their bioactivity.

The book focuses on research discoveries and their development as therapies for use in both complementary and conventional medicines. The information will also serve researchers who are seeking new plant extracts in order to explore their potential in a variety of applications within, for example, the pharmaceutical, cosmetic, and food and drink industries. Future research on natural products will lead to more discoveries of new products, and increased access to information will empower the consumers to make choices about preventative and curative healthcare programs.

Understanding Hydrolats represents a blend of art, science and technology and it gives me great pleasure to introduce this book, which will give the reader both enjoyment and a deeper understanding of the fascinating world of plants. I am sure that it will be a great success in the scientific literature on aromatic and medicinal plants.

K. Svoboda
Auchincruive, 2004

I know a bank whereon the thyme blows,
Where oxlips and the nodding violet grows
Quite over-canopied with luscious woodbine,
With sweet musk-roses, and with eglantine . . .

A Midsummer Night's Dream
Shakespeare, Act II, Scene I

Preface

This book is not intended to be a definitive work on distilled plant waters. Rather, it is an attempt to gather together in one place a wide range of both anecdotal and scientific information in order to provide an informative survey of the current state of our knowledge, and so make it easier for others to build on this knowledge, and to expand and improve it.

While there is a great deal of information given in this book, it was found necessary to use anecdotal evidence where no scientific evidence was available – otherwise it would have been a very slim book indeed! No doubt there will be those who will criticize the lack of scientific research. The authors are already acutely aware of this and regret it, but such research evidence is simply not yet available. We would be pleased if anyone could provide us with any information which would improve this book.

When aromatherapy was first introduced as a complementary therapy, the uses of essential oils were taught in aromatherapy schools but the associated waters were seldom, if ever, mentioned. Now, about 40 years later, there is growing interest in the use of the waters produced along with the essential oils during plant distillation. For many years now almost all waters have been discarded with the exception of rose water and orange flower water, which are much used - especially in the cosmetics industry, in skin care products. Most other waters have not been generally available. This lack of availability, combined with the general lack of teaching on the subject and, until very recently, the scarcity of suitable literature, has meant that the distilled waters have been little used. As a consequence it is difficult to find case studies and even more difficult to find cases where distilled waters have been used alone, as they are often used as a complement to essential oils and other treatments, where the effects may be different. Much work – trials, projects, single case studies – is needed to determine the efficacy of these gentle and holistic healing agents.

In the beginning, and for many centuries, it was not the oils but the waters that were the most important yield from plant distillation (it is for this reason that the authors prefer to term their therapeutic use the first aromatherapy). Early forms of distillation were not as sophisticated or efficient as modern ones, though improvements were made over the centuries, for example the improvements to the cooling system credited to Avicenna (11th century). The quantity of essential oil that was available for direct collection was comparatively small, unlike today, and the waters alone were used for beauty, medicinal and other purposes. However, up to more recent times, it was the water that was discarded, usually into rivers. Recent legislation in France requires these waters to be filtered before being discarded, to prevent pollution of river water. This, coupled with the renewed interest in the use of distilled waters, may have contributed to the fact that their production and storage have now become economically more viable.

While there is no published scientific evidence to say that distilled waters are hazardous in any way, equally, there is none to say that they are not. Many of the volatile organic compounds in the waters are the same as those in the essential oils, though at much lower concentrations, and at similar levels there are other components found in the waters which are toxic. However, since 99% of a hydrolat consists of distilled water the risk factor must be a great deal smaller when compared to essential oils (account must obviously also be taken of the source of the distilled water and, as explained in this book, the plant used must be correctly identified, organically grown, and so on). Essential oils certainly call for care in use, but even there, while hazard exists, the actual risk is small if they are used by trained people.

Though there are those who consider that distilled plant waters are equally as hazardous as essential oils, the authors feel that the distilled plant waters are safe to use for anyone with the proper training. It is worthy of note that the authors have used essential oils for almost 30 years, during which time they have bottled essential oils, demonstrated and taught about them and used them for treatments, yet have suffered no adverse effects themselves; no one has reacted adversely to intensive and internal use of essential oils, and only two people have had adverse skin reactions. One of these adverse reactions proved to be due to a mental association with lavender fragranced floor-polish, which certainly contained standardized, adulterated or synthetic lavender oil, and once this association of ideas was dispelled, the student was able to use lavender essential oil without any problem. The second incident involved the use by an aromatherapist of fresh herbs grown near roses which had been treated with a pesticide. She was unable to use certain essential oils for 2 years but afterwards resumed her business without any skin problem arising.

Distilled waters have been in more or less continuous use, without any reported ill effects, for many centuries, especially during the period when all great houses had still rooms, which existed solely for the purpose of providing distilled waters for cooking and medicinal use. Scientists will no doubt, quite rightly, attempt to ascertain if their use presents risks, but at the moment they, like aromatherapists, have only anecdotal evidence. Unlike us, however, they do not have any practical experience.

The authors would like to encourage more widespread use of the distilled plant waters as being a safe and gentle means of treatment, complementary to other methods, and the purpose of this book is to present all the information currently available in a usable form, to act as a reference source and guide for the therapist.

Acknowledgements

The authors wish to thank the following people, whose understanding and practical help have been much appreciated: Claire Montesinos, an authority on and producer of hydrolats and to whom we are grateful for samples for testing and for technical information; Charles Wells and Wym Tanghe, to whom we are also grateful for samples for testing; Caroline Hoffman, Carolyn Marshall and Barbara Payne, for their generous response to our request to supply some case studies on the use of hydrolats from their own experience.

We would like to offer special thanks to Bill Morden, for carrying out the analysis of all the given waters and for reading passages of the book before publication: Dr Morden is senior mass spectrometrist at LGC Laboratories, Runcorn, Cheshire and visiting research fellow at the Department of Biochemistry, Manchester Metropolitan University. Particular thanks go to Katja Svoboda for checking the book through before publication and also for writing the foreword.

Useful Addresses

Training

Penny Price Academy of Aromatherapy
The Stables
41, Leicester Road
Hinckley
Leics LE10 1LW UK
Tel: +44 (0) 1455 25 10 20
Fax: +44 (0) 1455 25 10 65

Penny Price Academy of Aromatherapy
London centre
3 Ivory Square
Plantation Wharf
London SW11 3UE
Tel: +44 (0) 207 924 3333
Fax: +44 (0) 207 924 3330

E-mail: info@penny-price.com
Web site: www.penny-price.com

Sandra Day
School of Health Studies
Ashley House
185A Drake Street
Rochdale OL11 1EF
Tel: +44 (0) 1706 750302
Fax: +44 (0) 1706 750304
E-mail: aroma@sandraday.com
Web site: www.sandraday.com

Hydrolat & essential oil supplies
Penny Price Aromatherapy
The Stables
41, Leicester Road
Hinckley
Leics LE10 1LW UK
Tel: +44 (0) 1455 25 10 20
Fax: +44 (0) 1455 25 10 65
E-mail: info@penny-price.com
Web site: www.penny-price.com

Essentially Oils
8–10 Mount Farm
Churchill
Chipping Norton
Oxfordshire OX7 5NP UK
Tel: +44 (0) 1608 65 95 44
Fax: +44 (0) 1608 65 95 66
E-mail: essentiallyoils.com
Web-site: www.essentiallyoils.com

Aromatology/Aromatherapy Association
Institute of Aromatic Medicine
4, Woodlands Road
Hinckley
Leics LE10 1JG UK
E-mail: aromed@hotmail.com

Aromatherapy Associations
International Federation of Professional Aromatherapists
IFPA House
82 Ashby Road
Hinckley
Leics LE10 1SN UK
Tel: +44 (0) 1455 637 987
Fax: +44 (0) 1455 890 956
E-mail: admin@ifparoma.org
Web-site: ifparoma.org

Aromatherapy Consortium
PO Box 6522
Desborough
Kettering
Northants NN14 2YX
Tel: 0870 7743477
E-mail: info@aromatherapy-regulation.org.uk

1

Introduction

- The first aromatherapy 1
- Is 'natural' necessarily safe? 2
- Why are waters not used more? 3
- Sourcing good materials 3
- Advantages of distilled plant waters 4
- What is their composition? 4
- Scientific proof 5
- Water-based plant extracts 7
- Conclusion 8

The first aromatherapy

The origins of aromatic plant therapy are lost in the mists of time, going back long before written records of any kind were kept. It seems that there has always been some kind of aromatherapy and there has never been a time without it, and that plants and plant extracts have been used to improve health and well-being for countless thousands of years. We can consider their use as being probiotic, meaning *favouring* life, as opposed to the modern day antibiotic, which, if the etymology of the word is considered, has the opposite meaning – *against* life.

Aromatherapy in one form or another has been used since ancient times to promote the health and well-being of both the individual and society at large. Water itself also has a long history of universal use in healing and cleansing, including spa treatments, thalassotherapy, herbal drinks, bathing, homoeopathy, Bach flower waters. Distilled plant waters, although largely forgotten or ignored in Western Europe for the past several decades, have long been associated with healing and were in wide use long before essential oils as we know them today. In the 17th and 18th centuries, distilled waters were in common use throughout Europe, including England, where every large house had its still room. Many instances of uses for the waters given in this book are from the older herbals, yet they are nonetheless valid for that.

Distilled plant waters are the product of carefully controlled and relatively modern distillation apparatus and techniques and are obtained from (aromatic) plants. The word aromatic is put in parentheses because these plants may be those which:

1. are used for essential oil extraction
2. contain tiny, uncommercial, quantities of essential oil
3. may contain no essential oil but nevertheless yield a useful distillate containing volatile organic compounds.

In all these cases the water distillate is known as a distilled plant water – or *hydrolat* (nomenclature is discussed in Ch. 4).

The use of water distillates is sometimes considered the 'homoeopathy' of aromatherapy; it is certainly true that they are universally considered as a complement to essential oil therapy, offering an additional synergy. The American author Jeanne Rose (1999) suggests that the use of distilled plant waters is the *real* aromatherapy, while Canadian Suzanne Catty (2001) looks upon their use as the *next* aromatherapy and Frenchman Guy Roulier (1990) regards the use of waters as *dilute* aromatherapy. The authors prefer to regard their therapeutic use as being more properly described as the ***first*** aromatherapy.

Is 'natural' necessarily safe?

The beneficial effects of plants can be quite powerful and wide-ranging – there are well-identified panaceas which exist in nature (Proserpio & Dorato 1983) and there is much more to be discovered. However, just because a product is labelled 'natural' this does not in itself mean it is completely safe: many noxious and even carcinogenic substances are to be found in nature (Vevy 1989). 'Natural' is not a synonym for innocuous and it is incumbent on the users of natural products to inform themselves in the matter of their safe use. Happily, practical experience (in the absence of science-based proof) has shown that these water distillates are almost completely non-toxic.

Self-treatment with distilled plant waters is not only possible but also highly desirable, although even here one needs adequate knowledge of the waters employed and an awareness of the limitations of the lay person. If there is any doubt whatsoever, then a competent and knowledgeable practitioner should be consulted. Nevertheless, being almost entirely without unwanted secondary effects, natural aromatic waters are generally recognized as being among the safest of materials – especially when compared with essential oils, which, although very powerful in their positive effects, can have some negative secondary effects if incorrectly used. The gentle distilled plant waters are a safe alternative and a complement in almost every case.

This safety feature is a tremendous advantage when it comes to internal use. Many therapists are fearful of advocating the internal use of essential oils (although almost all practise this themselves). Several factors play a part in this:

- their training, which may have been very basic
- the warnings against internal use which are posted in practically every aromatherapy book, often stipulated by the publishers to protect themselves in case of incompetence
- the fact that inferior and unsuitable products abound on the market
- the background of the therapist, which may be in the beauty profession, whose code of conduct (in the UK) forbids internal use of essential oils.

With distilled plant waters we have a product which:

- can be recommended to counter internal problems and is used in this way by the authors and by pharmacists in France and Belgium – Baudoux (1996a, p. 109), a pharmacist, states that they may be taken for long, uninterrupted periods (1 or 2 months)
- has a long history of being used in this manner (since before the time of Nicholas Culpeper, the early 17th century astrologer and physician)
- in the authors' opinion, is as safe as any medication can be.

Why are waters not used more?

The subject of distilled plant waters is intriguing, yet not one about which much has been written. Every aromatherapist knows of them, but few know much about them, and hence most cannot reach a considered opinion about their use. Real and useful information is scarce, partly because:

1. most therapists do not understand what these waters are and – just as important – what they are not
2. there is little scientific understanding of aromatic waters
3. expert teaching of the subject is hard to find
4. writers do not always make clear whether they are discussing true distilled plant waters, other water-based products such as infusions, or the artificial 'false' waters found in most chemists' shops (e.g. 'rose' water)
5. their chemical and physical profiles are not generally available (the waters are not usually subjected to analysis by gas chromatographic methods)
6. their therapeutic properties have rarely been scientifically investigated and for many of them only a small amount of anecdotal evidence is available.

Consequently, the demand for these valuable products of the distillation process is not very high. This in turn means that suppliers have felt they can only keep low stocks of a small range of waters.

Sourcing good materials

It is the task of the therapist to seek out good quality products. Obtaining genuine natural distilled plant waters, however, may be difficult. Chapter 5, on prepared or 'false' waters, sets out some of the pitfalls awaiting the unwary buyer. The same criteria apply as for obtaining therapeutic quality essential oils. As stated earlier, even specialist aromatherapy shops and suppliers tend not to carry a large stock or wide variety of distilled plant waters. One reason is that, despite the fact that they are produced in plentiful quantities (often as a by-product of plant distillation for essential oils), they are bulky, heavy (1 kg per litre) and therefore costly to transport from place to place. The value-to-weight ratio is very low compared with essential oils, especially in view of the need to observe certain storage conditions as regards temperature and light. The situation is slightly better with the cohobated waters (explained in Ch. 6) which are more heavily charged with plant volatile compounds and so can be diluted for use.

Advantages of distilled plant waters

Everyone knows that oil and water do not mix, but it is true that distilled plant waters can advantageously be used in a combined treatment with essential oils – they work together very well. They are a great deal less aggressive than essential oils and are active on a different level. Although any treatment involving them may need to be carried out over a longer period of time than when employing essential oils, these 'potent waters' are subtle, safe and effective, being most useful in a family environment, where they may be used on babies, the frail and the very old.

The distilled plant waters have a distinct advantage over essential oils (and waters made from essential oils) when used in the bath. The latter, because of their nature, are not easily soluble in water and unless dissolved in a suitable solvent, may leave oil droplets floating on the surface of the water; with certain oils and on certain people this may cause skin irritation; also, some of the less volatile essential oils can adversely affect baths made of plastic material. Distilled plant waters, on the other hand, are completely water-soluble.

Unlike essential oils, distilled plant waters can also be used safely internally – with care, but without the need for as much specialist knowledge. Though obtained from the same plant, they are very different in nature and concentration and their chemical composition is also somewhat different from the volatile essential oils.

What is their composition?

Distilled plant waters by definition contain volatile hydrophilic compounds from the plant, but not the tannic acid and bitter substances, and make an excellent complement to their co-distillates, the powerful essential oils. Often, but certainly not always, their fragrance is reminiscent of their partner essential oils, although not as strong. Sometimes the odour is dissimilar from, and not as pleasant as, the essential oil of the same plant.

> *Their composition is different from that of the essential oil: richer in water-compatible components and free of lipophilic substances such as terpene hydrocarbons. This means highly tolerable, antiinflammative, and antiseptic substances are found in aromatic hydrosols. (Schnaubelt 1999)*

> *[Authors' note: monoterpene and even sesquiterpene hydrocarbons do in fact appear in some distilled plant waters, albeit at low levels.]*

The homoeopathic aspect of distilled plant waters is mentioned by several writers: water has the remarkable capability of picking up information relating to the vibrational energy which is found in a living plant, of storing this energy information and, under certain circumstances, of transferring it to the human body. This means that distilled aromatic waters pick up and store not only physical plant particles but possibly also subtle energy information.

Sometimes a leap of faith is asked of the reader, knowing that the make-up of oils and waters is different:

> *– Carrot seed essential oil is recommended for treating wrinkles, scar tissue, etc., so it stands to reason that the hydrosol would be recommended for the same*

uses. Very gentle, without the distinctive scent of the essential oil (actually, the hydrosol smells more like fresh carrots than the seed). (naturesgift.com/hydrosols)

Without examining the make-up of both the essential oil and the distilled plant water and making some trials it is not possible to say what effects the oil and the water would have; their effects may be the same or similar, but on the other hand they may not.

Scientific proof

In the course of writing this book, 3 or 4 years were spent searching through works on herbalism and, to a lesser extent, works on aromatherapy (where waters receive scant mention), in order to glean snippets of information on distilled plant waters. However, the quality of information found was variable and, with rare exceptions, for example recent studies by Aydin et al (1996) and Sağdiç & Özcan (2003), most would not stand up to rigorous examination. Much more information has been found in French literature, France being the country in which distilled plant waters are most used, although even there, to a lesser extent now than formerly (save for orange flower water; distilled waters last featured in the French Codex in 1965).

Therapists in the field of alternative and complementary medicine are under great pressure today to prove that what they do is valid and safe. They are in a dilemma, torn between caring for the needs of their clients and the demands from the scientific community to provide evidence of safety and efficacy.

Of course scientific proof is both desirable and necessary, but therapists are daily faced with clients who require help with their problems. There is no acceptable hard evidence that essential oil therapy can ease the pain of arthritis, but after more than 20 years' experience of treating arthritic sufferers, the authors know that it does – and without any unwanted side-effects. Clients are happy with this situation; they are content to have relief from the pain on a daily basis and are not concerned about whether a scientist has taken trouble to prove that this is the case – they know that it works for them, and are not overly concerned whether there have been trials with controls, double blinds, etc. A woman who now has a clear skin where previously she had a blotchy skin does not stop to ask if scientific trials have been carried out. In any case, double-blind trials are difficult where essential oils are concerned since we cannot say to someone that they are not being treated with (say) eucalyptus oil if they are, because it is obvious to all concerned.

Empirically derived knowledge, by the very basis of its method of building evidence, must be taken seriously, and distilled plant waters and essential oils have a long history. Beneficial experiences have been repeated time and time again, over a long period, and thus the empirical basis of the healing properties of these plant extracts cannot and must not be lightly dismissed. In our science-based society it is necessary to demonstrate the proof of how these agents work, but until the necessary proof is forthcoming it would be foolish to discontinue the traditional practices of using healing plant extracts (Price 1990). 'We must be receptive to possibilities that science has not yet grasped. It is absurd not to use treatments that work, just because we do not yet understand them' (Siegel 1988).

What is scientific proof?

There are two fields of science:

1. hard science – chemistry and physics, which, after experimentation, can express things in numbers and can be proved
2. soft science – social science and medicine, which, after experimentation, is never actually proved beyond doubt.

How does one prove such an experiment? One cannot – but it can be *dis*proved. Science is made up of what has been disproved, and current science is what we cannot refute at the moment – in fact, everything in science is provisional information.

'Scientific proof' is referred to in almost every television advert and the concept is in danger of being devalued. It is dragged out to support the whiteness of wash, the efficacy of wrinkle creams, the shampoo that 'repairs' broken hair, etc.

Scientists rely a lot on animal testing, yet what really is the relevance to the human body of massive doses imposed on small animals (whose physiology is different from humans) or putting essential oils onto the entrails of sacrificed animals? In the opinion of Drs Andre Menache and Ray Greek, of the London-based organization Doctors and Lawyers for Responsible Medicine:

> *The use of animals in research is as much a scientific issue as it is an ethical one. Animal experimentation is bad science. It continues to mislead scientists and holds back real medical progress. The sooner the scientific community realises this, the better for both people and animals. (Menache & Greek 1999)*

> *They [scientists] also rely on literature searches, but then it all depends on how selective you are when carrying out the search. (Fowler & Wall 1997)*

Perhaps the best and most succinct description of the scientific method was given 30 years ago by John Ziman (1968) in his book *Public Knowledge*. Pennington (1999) quotes him as follows:

> *Science is public knowledge . . . not merely published knowledge or information. Anyone can make an observation or conceive a hypothesis and, if he has financial means, can get it printed and distributed for other persons to read. Scientific knowledge is more than this. Its facts and theories must survive a period of critical study and testing by other competent and disinterested individuals and must have been found so persuasive that they are almost universally accepted. The . . . goal is a consensus of rational opinion over the widest possible field.*

The role of scientists in policy making and the reasons why scientists rarely determine policy directly, but rather inform and guide, were issues addressed by Don K. Price in his 1962 classic *Government and Science*. He gave three reasons why governmental executives cannot use science alone to get answers to problems created by new technology:

1. Some problems which need more research call for an immediate answer, but these are often problems for which inaction is itself an answer – and possibly a wrong one.

2. One question often leads to another: Price tells us that it is a matter of infinite regression. You cannot get anywhere if you first
   (a) make a complete study of what you ought to study; and then
   (b) make a complete study of the methods you ought to use, and then
   (c) make a complete study of the way in which the results should be applied.
   By that time, he says, you would need to study the extent to which changes in the situation had made the original question obsolete.
3. Non-scientific issues cannot be ignored. For example, the public uses a rather sophisticated formula in assessing health risks. Scientific data only partly come into it. In addition to the possible number of harmful factors (quantitative probabilities of harm), additional 'fright factors' play an influential role. Thus, 'risks are seen as more worrying if they are perceived to be poorly understood by science and are subject to contradictory statements from responsible sources'.

The authors are acutely aware that much – indeed most – of the information given in this book regarding the properties and therapeutic effects of distilled waters is open to just criticism. What is intended is not a strict scientific exposition, but rather a gathering under one 'roof' of all relevant information on the use of waters with, wherever possible, the source, so that the reader may judge for him- or herself and ascribe whatever value is thought appropriate. This is not a definitive work, but an attempt to lay out, for all to see, the methods and possible and probable merits of using distilled plant waters in a constructive way. It is hoped that both therapists and lay people will view the information given in a positive manner, and use it as a springboard to try them, perhaps for the first time, or, for the person already acquainted with them, in new ways and in new situations. To advance knowledge, any case studies with either good or bad outcomes should be written down and communicated to other therapists; perhaps this useful information may even find its way into a future edition of this book.

Water-based plant extracts

There are several kinds of water-based aromatic products used in therapies, including two or three types of aromatic waters which vary in nature according to the method of production. They fall into the following categories:

- infusions, teas, tisanes
- wines
- vinegars
- aromatic waters
  - distilled
  - prepared
  - concentrated
- Bach flower remedies.

Some plants, whether containing essential oils or not, are distilled specifically for the plant water and not for the essential oil: when this is the case the quality of the water used for distillation is of great importance. Although there may not be a commercial quantity of essential oil within a plant (e.g. plantain), some volatile organic molecules appear in the distilled plant water. Thus the distilled plant waters stand intermediate between, and represent to some extent a fusion of, aromatherapy and herbalism, containing as they do some of the useful plant molecules from both worlds. These waters are used in conjunction with both essential oil treatments and herbalism, as well as on their own.

Conclusion

It is hoped that the reader will find the information in this book both interesting and informative and will be spurred on to try distilled plant waters, either on their own or as a gentle complement to essential oils, so that a large number of case studies and information may be accumulated. Distilled plant waters are safe to use, in practical terms totally without aggression, and should be valued by aromatherapists and phytotherapists alike as a complement to both disciplines. These valuable products of the distillation process deserve to be much better known and far more widely used; they are only now becoming the subject of research.

The use of distilled plant waters will increase in the near future because of probable changes in the rules governing the production and manufacture of products bearing an organic label. Some licensing authorities (e.g. Ecocert) are intending to tighten up the regulations concerning the use of aromatic waters in cosmetic and therapeutic products, so that in future firms will not be able to use prepared waters in recipes which currently have an organic certificate. To gain the recognition and status conferred by the award of an organic certificate, natural distilled waters will have to be used. Thus these stricter regulations will improve the availability of true distilled plant waters for the therapist. Nevertheless, though distilled plant waters are used more and more and the demand for them is increasing, there is still a shortage generally of natural ones. This may in part be due to the widespread use of the solvent extraction process (used for perfumes), which uses the bulk of the flower material available.

2
The history of aromatic medicine

- Egypt 9
- Aromatics worldwide 10
- Development of medicine 10
- Development of distillation 11
- Arab and Spanish influences 11
- The holy wars, 10th–13th centuries 13
- Hungary water 13
- Carmelite water 14
- After the Crusades 14
- Paracelsus (1493–1541) 14
- New plants bring new worlds 15
- Still rooms 15
- Renaissance herbals 15
- Eau-de-Cologne 16
- Rise of science 16
- Fall and resurrection of plant medicine 16
- Some 20th-century pioneers 17
- Conclusion 18

Egypt

Timeless mists and mystical times

Aromatic plant medicine has part of its beginnings perhaps 5000 or 6000 years ago, in the incense-filled temples of Egypt, where pharmacy and doctoring took their first feeble steps. Over many years the River Nile had been the centre of the known world for medicinal plants which were imported to the botanic gardens on its fertile banks, and consequently Egypt and the Nile became a focus for learning. Among the plants imported were myrrh, cedarwood, frankincense, cinnamon, spikenard and labdanum, which were brought from Yemen, Lebanon, Syria, Persia, India and other lands.

Egyptian learning in respect of bactericides and hygiene, and their effectiveness, so uniquely demonstrated in the art of mummification, meant that the influence of these ancients remained potent until modern times. Egyptian understanding of these powerful antiseptic natural substances must indicate that they realized the implications for the health of the living body too, and indeed they had many healing recipes: one Kyphi recipe, for example, found engraved on the wall of a laboratory at Edfu and identified by Victor Loret in 1887, included 16 plant extracts. Kyphi was used as a perfume, an antiseptic and an anti-inflammatory agent when taken internally (Lee & Lee 1992). It was later adopted by the Greeks and Romans as a medicine – it was said by Plutarch to calm anxiety and induce sleep.

In the hot Egyptian climate and the state of sanitation then current, the use of aromatics made daily life both safer and more pleasant. The royal barges of the pharaohs were sprinkled with flower-scented waters, and the flamboyant queen, Cleopatra, had the sails sprayed with perfumes for her meeting with Mark Antony. Cleopatra also had the habit of sleeping on a pillow of rose petals for its sedative effect. Many types of aromatics were in general use including scented barks, perfumed oils, flower waters, balsams, resins, aromatic vinegars and spices.

Aromatics worldwide

Egypt was not the only land to develop the use of aromas for religion and medicine, and every civilization discovered and adapted aromatics to their own use. Assyrians, Babylonians, Phoenicians, Jews, Chinese, Indians, Greeks, Romans and Christians all burnt resins in religious, mystic and purification ceremonies.

In ancient China, Emperor Huang Ti wrote a treatise about 3000 BC entitled *The Yellow Emperor's Classic of Internal Medicine*, which included herbal medicine; and, since time immemorial, Chios mastic or Lentisk resin has been used in the Orient to treat stomach problems, to staunch bleeding, to detoxify, and to strengthen the gums (Gattefossé 1993, p. 31).

About 2000 BC Babylonian writings described the use of such herbs as bay, caraway, coriander, thyme, with methods of preparation and use of herbal cures. An inscribed tablet dated *circa* 1800 BC tells us that cedar, cypress and myrrh were imported from Egypt at that time.

Development of medicine

About 500–400 BC Greek and Cretan doctors visited the medical places of learning along the Nile and as a result the famous medical school was set up on the island of Cos. The presence of Hippocrates (460–370 BC), known as the 'father of medicine', added considerable stature to this establishment. Using their capacity for organization, the Greeks were able to classify and index the knowledge that they had gained from the Egyptians and so present it in a more scientific way. Hippocrates described the effects of 300 plants and Diodes of Carystus wrote a treatise on *Herbal Medicine*, a classic in its time. A perfume invented by Megallus – therefore called Megaleion – was well known to the Greeks and had the dual purpose of being both a perfume and a healing medium, with the properties of healing wounds and reducing inflammation. The knowledge built up by the Egyptians and the Greeks in turn influenced the Romans who, up until then, had not been great users of perfumes and spices. However, as the Roman empire spread, the knowledge of the healing properties and uses of herbs spread with it. In fact

Roman soldiers took with them seeds and plants to ensure their availability. Many of the 200 plants (including borage, fennel, parsley, rosemary, sage, thyme) brought to Britain by the Romans became naturalized and now grow wild.

A Roman, Dioscorides, in AD 50, wrote *De Materia Medica*, in which were listed in detail the healing properties of around 500 herbs. Together with the distillation knowledge gained by this time, the book proved to be very influential and was translated into many languages including Persian, Hebrew, Arabic and Anglo-Saxon.

Development of distillation

Extraction by distillation

It is hard to believe, as some authors insist, that a simple process of distillation did not already exist before the time of the Arab philospher and physician Avicenna (*b.* AD 980) to whom credit is sometimes given for the discovery of the distillation process, as there is ample evidence that the necessary equipment and knowledge had been available for many years before this period. Indeed, an Italian, Dr Rovesti, discovered in 1975 at Taxila (a town in the foothills of the Himalayas) a terracotta still subsequently estimated to be about 5000 years old.

There exist drawings of Greek laboratory equipment dating between AD 200 and 500 which show equipment that could clearly be used for distillation (Sherwood Taylor 1938, p. 63). Distilled plant waters were known to the Egyptians before the 4th century BC according to the writings of Synesius of Ptolomais and of Zosymos of Panapolis (Egypt, 3rd century BC), both of whom described in detail the distillation apparatus of the Egyptians.

The early 'stills', like the one at Tepi Gawra in the Indus Valley, were little more than boiling pots which allowed the fragrant steam to condense and run into an outer shell. While this might seem simple compared to modern methods, it was a great step forward. When cabbage, for example, is boiled, the steam smells of the cabbage and this 'water' is like a toilet water. If, instead of cabbage, you use a fragrant oil-producing plant such as melissa or eucalyptus, the end water will contain some of the fragrant, water-soluble parts of the plant – in other words it will be an elementary, distilled plant water (Hephrun 2000a, p. 18).

In the beginning, up until the early Middle Ages, the process of distillation was used almost exclusively for obtaining distilled plant waters; even after this time it was the chief aim of distillation for several centuries. When the distillation process produced not only an aromatic water but also an essential oil, for example the crystallization of rose oil on the surface of the distilled rose water, then probably the essential oil was looked upon as an unwanted by-product (Urdang 1948).

Arab and Spanish influences

With the fall of the Roman Empire, a long period of darkness and barbarity settled over Europe: the old learning was forgotten and no new knowledge was forthcoming. Light dawned in the East with the rise of Islam. The Arabs were not only warriors and merchants of the caravan, but were also masters of alchemy (which was attributed to the Egyptian god Tehuti) and medicine. The Berbers of North Africa had an aromatic which was known to the Arabs as *bokhour el Berber*, ('the perfume of the Berbers'). Its many beneficial properties included weight gain, and it acted as a tonic and was helpful for stomach pains. It is possible that the water from distilled orange flowers was included in this medicine, as many women in North Africa to this day follow time-honoured tradition and use simple distillation equipment in their kitchen to produce distilled plant waters which are used as a panacea (Price 1990). On a visit to Tunisia one of the authors was given the traditional remedy for the inevitable stomach upset – orange flower water, distilled in the kitchen of our host from the blossom in their orange grove. Many drugs and methods of Arab origin, such as distillation and sublimation, are still in use today.

For a time between AD 800 and 1300 the Arabs developed many chemical techniques, some to do with distillation, thus enabling higher-quality essential oils and distilled plant waters to be extracted from plants. Perfumes and medicines held a notable place in the resurgent Islamic civilization, and from the 9th century Baghdad was the chief centre for rose oil and rose water from Persia, a perfume industry developed in Damascus.

Prominent scholars of this period, at the height of Arab science, included Ibn Sina (the Arabic name of the philosopher, astronomer, physicist and physician better known to us as Avicenna) who was born in AD 980 in Afshana near Bokhara, Persia, and Geber from Córdoba (Geber is the Latin form of Jabir) who was the 14th-century author of several books that were among the most influential works on alchemy and metallurgy. Although the still itself had already been discovered in its earlier form of the Kerotakis or Ambix (alembic), the Arabs much improved it – principally Avicenna, who introduced the idea of lengthening the cooling pipe by coiling it, which greatly increased the overall efficiency of the distillation process. The development of the art of glass blowing in Greece and Venice was also a contributory factor in providing some of the hardware for technical achievements in chemistry.

The industrial development of steam distillation and the procedure to make high-grade alcohol (*al kohol* in Arabic) by the Arabs were the seeds from which the modern production of odorants began. During his lifetime, Avicenna (who also wrote the *Book of Healing* and the *Canon of Medicine*, used by many medical schools – remarkably, up to as late as 1650 at Montpelier) introduced rose oil and rose water, obtained from *Rosa centifolia*, a rose highly prized by the Arabs. These extracts were soon produced on a large scale and exported around the world. Using this technology, other essential oils and essences were produced in quantity, although the grade or quality of the materials was still an unknown quantity (Ohloff 1994).

The renowned Spanish surgeon Abu al-Qasim (Albucasis) gives a detailed description of distillation in his work on pharmacy, *Liber servitoris*, and did much to raise the status of surgery in Córdoba, an important centre of commerce and culture with a hospital and medical school equal to those of Cairo and Baghdad. He wrote the first illustrated surgical text, which was widely influential in Europe for several centuries.

Some distilled plant waters have long been known and valued for their therapeutic properties: in *De medecinis universalibus et particularibus*, Mesue (Yahya ibn Măsanwaih al-Mărdĭnĭ) described the distilled waters of rose and wormwood (Mesue 1471), and Nonus Theophanes, Byzantine doctor to the Emperor Michael VIII of Constantinople, recommended rose water for its remedial qualities.

Avenzoar (Abu Marwan 'Abd Al-Malik ibn Abi Al-'Ala 'Zuhr!), also called Abumeron (1090–1162), of Seville, was one of medieval Islam's foremost thinkers and the greatest medical clinician of the western caliphate. He was physician to the caliph Ebn Attafin of Morocco and used rose water as an eye lotion. He wrote the *Practical Manual of Treatments and Diet.* In the 10th century, Abn Jafar Ahmed described rose water, essential oil of rose and camphor as everyday medicaments.

Although plant essential oils had been produced in some form for thousands of years, the first description of a distillation process that yielded essential oils and distilled plant waters close to those we know today was by a Catalan physician named Arnald de Villanova who lived between about 1235 and 1311. It has to be remembered that in ancient and medieval texts the meaning of distilled was not as precise and specific as that conveyed today; rather it was a 'collective term' covering the preparation of animal as well as vegetable extracts. Whether de Villanova prepared genuine distilled essential oils or not is of little significance for the purpose of this text; what he did do of great importance was to praise the therapeutic qualities of distilled waters, with the result that valuable remedies were introduced into the pharmacies of medieval and later periods throughout Europe (Urdang 1948, p. 4).

The holy wars, 10th–13th centuries

The uncouth crusaders from Europe who went to war in the East to teach the comparatively highly civilized infidel a lesson, suffered wounds (and of course digestive upsets) which were healed with Arab medicine. They returned home with stories to tell and gifts of rose water for their wives, and so news of successful Arab plant medicines began to be disseminated throughout Christian Europe.

Happily, the monasteries cultivated aromatic plants; Benedictine monks brought thyme and melissa from Italy to grow and flourish in monastery gardens and Abbess Hildegard of Bingen cultivated lavender at her convent in the 12th century. Her interest was not only in the aroma but also in the therapeutic properties of the plant extracts.

Hungary water

Royal Hungarian water was produced by distilling alcohol and fresh rosemary blossoms: it was first used in the 14th century by the Countess of Hainault. She thought it worthwhile to send the recipe to her daughter, the wife of Edward III, and it has been in use ever since. The ingredients of Hungary water, with the exception of the otto of lemon peel, may be obtained from ordinary garden plants. It is made of 1 gallon of grape spirit; 2 ounces of otto of rosemary; 1 ounce each of otto of balm and lemon peel; $\frac{1}{2}$ drachm of otto of mint; and 1 pint each of extract of rose and orange flower. Should the orange flower extract prove difficult to obtain, it can be omitted and the extract of rose increased to 2 pints. Hungary water may be applied to the handkerchief and will refresh a tired mind, but its primary use is as a face wash or to add to bath water, when it will act as an invigorating tonic (Genders 1972, p. 122).

Carmelite water

In 1379, when Charles V, King of France, was in advanced senility (shortly after the people of Brittany had risen against him), a toilet water was prepared by the nuns of the Carmelite abbey of St Just, who took care of him. He apparently used this water in his daily bath and inhaled it to refresh his once vigorous intellect during his declining years. So renowned did the water become that the nuns were requested to send samples to all parts of Europe, and their monastery achieved wide fame, the water continuing in use for three and a half centuries.

The distillation became known as Carmelite water and was an important addition to the toilet preparations of cultured men and women of medieval Europe. Its principal ingredient is balm, *Melissa officinalis*, which grows wild in central and southern Europe and which has become naturalized in the hedgerows of southern England. Carmelite water is made by taking 2 lb of fresh balm leaves; $\frac{1}{4}$ lb of lemon peel; 2 oz each of nutmeg, cloves and coriander seed, and some cinnamon and angelica root. These are placed in a still with $\frac{1}{2}$ gallon of orange flower water and 1 gallon of alcohol and slowly distilled until a gallon of the celebrated water is obtained (Genders 1972, pp. 122–123).

After the Crusades

The contemporary view, at a time when the alchemists were still pursuing the Holy Grail of turning base metals into gold, was that the distilled plant water was the principal goal of the distillation process; the essential oil floating on the distilled water was looked upon as being of little or no use.

During this period there was a change in emphasis from alchemy to pharmacy, together with further improvements in technique. Distilled plant waters appeared for the first time in pharmaceutical texts – the *Dispensatorium Noricum* of 1543, 1552 and 1563 and the work on distilled plant waters by Peter Mathiolus (1554) and Adam Lonicer (1578) are worthy of note.

Paracelsus (1493–1541)

The physician and alchemist Paracelsus was born in Einsiedeln, in the country now known as Switzerland. He taught the doctrine of signatures (if the plant was heart shaped it was beneficial for the heart; if kidney shaped, it benefited the kidneys, and so on), showing that he was persuaded by other than purely scientific reasoning. He felt that distillation separated the non-essential from the highly desirable essential part with the aid of fire, and this should be the goal of the alchemist. This view encouraged others to seek new essential oils and by the year 1500 oils, including benzoin, cedarwood, calamus, cinnamon, frankincense, myrrh, rose, rosemary, sage, spikenard and turpentine, were well known to the pharmacist.

New plants bring new worlds

Voyages of discovery during the adventurous times of the 15th and 16th centuries by such great explorers and navigators as Bartholomew Diaz, Vasco da Gama and Christopher Columbus, and the conquistadors Cortés and Pizarro, brought many new plants back to Europe (Lautié & Passebecq 1979, p. 10). This search for spices and plants had interesting side-effects – for example the discovery of America! Spices such as pepper helped to initiate trading on a global scale.

During this time, many gardens with medicinal plants were established in monasteries in France. At Oxford, in England, in 1621, some apothecaries created a garden for teaching their students, calling it a 'physic garden'; another such garden, destroyed in the Great Fire of London, was later re-established at Chelsea and is well known today.

Still rooms

For a period from the 16th century onwards a household task in the still rooms of the grand houses was the distillation of herbs and flowers. The household of the fifth Earl of Northumberland kept books containing the names of 'herbes to stylle' for the production of sweet waters (Genders 1972, p. 158). Plants such as rosemary, lavender, lemon balm, sage, marigold and tansy were grown in the garden and either dried in a special room or distilled in the still room to gain the sweet waters to be used in personal hygiene, as medicines and to flavour cooking. It was common for more than one plant to be distilled together, and one recipe for lavender water in a manuscript dated 1615 says that the lavender flowers, together with canella bark, wallflowers and grains of paradise, should be placed in the still to achieve a good lavender water. Many people had their own recipes for distilled waters; for example, Queen Henrietta Maria grew rosemary, rue and white lavender to yield the most pleasing of all lavender waters (Genders 1972, p. 159).

The still room was the domain of women and it was they who developed the manuscripts which became known as the still room books. In this kind of book were recorded the herbs and combinations of herbs (sometimes as many as 20) found suitable for foods such as soups, salads or sweets, and perhaps for medicine (Clarkson 1972).

Renaissance herbals

During this time many herbal books were written, William Turner's being one of the first. He described the plants in the vernacular, English, instead of in the Latin more traditionally used for works of scholarship, making this knowledge available to a wider section of the population. The fact that printing presses were now in existence also made the books more affordable. Essential oils and their waters were first mentioned in an official pharmacopoeia around the year 1600 in Germany, and in 1653 Nicholas Culpeper wrote his famous *Complete Herbal*.

The Renaissance saw essential oils much more widely used as a result of the improved methods of distillation and the steady progress of chemistry. There was a whole new range of products for medicine, perfumery, skin care (where the floral waters were mostly employed), balsams, ointments, aromatic oils and so on. The physician to Louis XIV, Nicolas Lémery, describes many of these in his *Dictionnaire des drogues simples.*

Eau-de-Cologne

In 1665, a former Franciscan monk, Paul Feminis, a dealer in essences, came from northern Italy to live in Cologne. The recipe for his '*Aqua mirabilis*' (wonderful water) became world famous through his nephew J. M. Farina and is still known today under the name eau-de-Cologne. This preparation contains bergamot, orange and lemon essential oils as well as lavender, rosemary, thyme, neroli water and strong ethanol, and used to be widely used as a health promoting lotion.

Rise of science

At the beginning of the 18th century there appeared the small beginnings of the commercial exploitation of essential oils which was to grow into the large industry that we know today. Concurrent with this increasing importance of the essential oils was a diminishing regard for the distilled plant waters. From this time onwards more attention began to be paid to the essential oils produced, which had previously been regarded as undesirable by-products in the procuring of aromatic waters. Other improvements to distillation were made and new lotions and ointments were formulated. Production and use of distilled plant waters reached its height during the 18th century.

Salmon's *Dispensary* of 1896 contains numerous aromatic remedies, but by this time all forms of plant-based therapies were in serious decline due to the increasing importance of chemical science. Even rose water, so popular as a skin tonic, was made synthetically. There was little sympathy for the 'Vital Force' point of view and generally it was thought better to isolate the active therapeutic principles from plants and use them alone – better still to synthesize them in laboratories cheaply and in quantity. Thus numerous serious side-effects were introduced into healing, but the drugs produced are extremely powerful and have a place in modern medicine, for example penicillin and aspirin, which are synthetic copies of naturally occurring materials.

Synthetic copies do not, however, seem to have the same respect for living human tissues and tend to be more toxic. The natural materials are not subject to the ever increasing dosage that the synthetics are, as germs tend to change and adapt and become resistant to synthetics. Many synthetic drugs are addictive, which is unknown with essential oils and distilled plant waters. Moreover, the latter two leave the human system in a stronger condition after a course of treatment.

Fall and resurrection of plant medicine

There has been a gradual diminution of the numbers of distilled plant waters listed in the French Codex and consequently their therapeutic use has also faded away.

In 1837 the number of distilled plant waters listed was down to 42; in 1884 there were 22, and by 1908 only seven remained. Their last appearance in the Codex was in 1965, since when they have not made an appearance (Montesinos 1991), with the exception of orange flower water.

Paradoxically, the early years of the 20th century also saw signs of a new realization of the merits of plants and their extracts. A few scientists began seriously to investigate and research the healing properties of essential oils – and, to a lesser degree, distilled plant waters.

The last 30–40 years have seen a cautious and informed return to aromatic remedies, which were, after all, a mainstay of medicine until the first half of the 20th century. At that time knowledge which had been painstakingly gathered by caring observation over the centuries was largely cast aside and had it not been for the dedicated work, chiefly of a few people in France and Italy, this invaluable knowledge might have been lost forever. Griggs (1997) quotes the observation by Dr Jean-Claude Lapraz that when he was a boy everybody used plants:

> *– they drank them in infusions, they made an oil to treat burns – oh yes, plants worked, I saw that clearly. But later, in all the years I spent in medical school, nobody ever mentioned plants. Not a single one.*

There was more than one reason for this state of affairs: the recently developed synthetic drugs were introduced following the 1939–1945 war; they were quick in effect and easy to use, requiring no effort or responsibility on the part of the sufferer, as opposed to the traditional plant remedies which took time and effort in the preparation, were slower in effect and took time and trouble to apply. However, the willing participation and cooperation of the invalid is an important factor in the recovery process. This changeover from natural to synthetic is echoed by Bonnelle (1993) who surveyed the older peasant population in the south of France and reported their views: 'Nowadays plants are not strong enough; I used nothing else before but now you have to get the doctor's medicines. When they discovered the new drugs, everyone forgot about the plants.' The other main cause of change was the introduction in this same period of state medicine in Western Europe, making the new synthetic drugs easily available and cheap to the individual: 'Before social security, when people had to pay, they didn't call the doctor out. That's why people then used to treat themselves with plants. The doctor never came to our house in those days' (Bonnelle 1993).

The long-term effects of synthetic drugs were then unknown, so the seemingly miraculous results achieved by the drugs overshadowed the pale effects of plant cures. Today, because of the often inevitable side-effects of synthetic drugs, opinion has begun to change.

Some 20th-century pioneers

In France the use of not only essential oils (in compresses and internal use), but also *hydrolats* (distilled plant waters, medicated waters) has been taken seriously by the establishment – some notable people include Belaiche, Girault and Pradal – so that both essential oils and *hydrolats* are prescribed by doctors and stocked by pharmacists, and their purchase price can usually be reclaimed from health insurance. At the same time much work on plant extracts has been, and is being, carried out by the complementary movement (e.g. Lautié, Passebecq, Lamblin).

Grieve

First published in 1931, Maud Grieve's *A Modern Herbal* was the first comprehensive encyclopedia of herbs and herbalism since the days of Culpeper. It incorporates some of the wisdom of the old herbalists, adds some of the discoveries of more modern times, and also gives much botanical information and many interesting recipes, using essential oils, distilled plant waters, syrups, infusions, decoctions, etc. It lists in detail over 1000 plants.

Valnet

Against the background of rediscovery and research of the first part of the 20th century when progress was slow, the impact on a much wider audience of the publication of Dr Jean Valnet's excellent book *Aromathérapie* in 1964 was tremendous. Subsequent translation into English (1982) further widened the appeal of aromatherapy in a world that was just waking up to the inherent dangers of some of the synthetic drugs being used. This work treats aromatherapy in its very broadest sense and includes not only essential oil therapy and distilled plant waters, but also use of the plants in food and various extracts, including infusions, syrups, tinctures, inhalations and decoctions.

Conclusion

Empirically derived knowledge, by the very basis of its method of building evidence, must be taken seriously. Beneficial experiences are repeated time and again over a long period, and the evident empirical basis of the healing properties of herb extracts – including volatile oils and distilled plant waters – cannot and must not be lightly dismissed. In our science-based society it is necessary to continue to attempt to demonstrate how they work, but until the necessary proof is forthcoming it would be foolish to discontinue the traditional practices of using these healing materials. This is especially true in the case of the distilled plant waters, which are so innocuous in use yet at the same time so beneficial.

3

The nature of water

- Introduction 19
- Universal distillation process 20
- A basic necessity 20
- Life and death 21
- Physical power of water 21
- Visual aspects 22
- Judging by water 22
- Water as a solvent and cleanser 22
- Water in the body 23
- Bottled water 23
- Healing treatments with water 24
- Scientists who investigated water 25
- Structure of liquid water 26
- Polar solvent – solublity in water 28
- Increased dilution 30

Introduction

Water (H_2O) is a unique substance, and, despite the fact that it is the most abundant liquid on earth, difficult to understand. It can exist in solid form, as a liquid, vapour or gas (when superheated). When liquid it is odourless, tasteless, colourless and transparent; it may exhibit a bluish tinge in large quantities. When solid it takes the form of ice. The solid and liquid forms together cover about 70% of the earth's surface. When gaseous, it may be water vapour, or wet or dry steam. Water has a great capacity to do things without itself being altered and the addition of salt to water changes its behaviour only slightly.

As water is such an important part of the distilled plant waters, being composed as they are almost entirely of water, it is worthwhile exploring the nature of water itself and looking into the special relationship which exists between human society and this life-sustaining liquid. We should be aware not only of its nature but also of its character and the connotations of its social, religious and cultural uses which have existed for millennia and are part of our collective unconscious.

Universal distillation process

The aromatherapist studies distillation during training, so it is interesting to realize that a natural system exists uniquely on the earth – a massive natural thermal machine – to distill our water. Thanks to the heat energy derived from the sun, about 577 000 km^3 (cubic kilometres) of water are changed into vapour each year. The bulk of the water comes by evaporation from the sea (about 505 000 km^3 each year) and the rest from lakes, rivers and the transpiration of plants. Once in the air this water falls as rain or snow, mainly back into the sea – but fortunately the wind carries some of the rain clouds over the land to transfer 47 000 km^3 to the earth, where the rivers eventually return it to the sea. There is also an evaporation/precipitation cycle over the land itself amounting to 72 000 km^3. This is made up of evaporation from lakes and transpiration from vegetation, plus the water from the sea. In the biosphere water is in perpetual motion, rising and falling (Fig. 3.1).

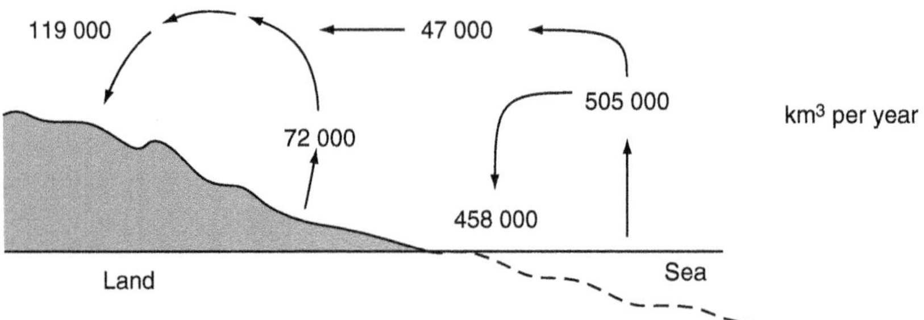

Figure 3.1 Movement of water in the biosphere.

A basic necessity

Distilled plant waters have their beneficial properties, but when they are used, particularly in a therapeutic context, their 'background' has to be considered, as they consist almost entirely of H_2O.

Water is a basic necessity of life and since prehistoric times mankind has always given priority to having a source of fresh water. This meant initially that settlements grew up alongside rivers, by lakes and waterholes; later man began to manage the water supply required for everyday needs by building aqueducts, digging wells, creating artificial pools as reservoirs and using natural springs. Very often a tremendous amount of time and energy was put into the task of finding a suitable and sufficient supply of water to maintain life and then transporting it to the home; this is still true in many parts of the world and not everyone has the luxury of water on tap inside the home.

Tap water itself is not without its problems and its quality varies in different areas of the country. London water, for example, is recycled many times on its passage across the city and contains residues, not least of which are synthetic female hormones which come from the large number of women taking the contraceptive pill: these hormones are recycled after urination. In rural farming areas chemical sprays seep into the water system. Pure water is rare and it is difficult to avoid some sort of pollution (Davies 1985, p. 47).

Life and death

The public fountains and wells provided for community use in villages and towns years ago were a source not only of life but, on occasion when they became infected, also of disease and sometimes death. Water, with the power of life and death, has traditionally been an object of veneration. It is easy to understand how this liquid, in the form of rain, springs, sea, lakes or rivers has been – and still is – regarded by various societies with awe, worship and veneration, and has a strong place in myth and religion.

Life giving, supporting and affecting the emotions

Water is not only universally regarded as life supporting, but often also as life *giving*, and is equated with the flowing liquid life forces in the body – blood, sweat, and semen. In some languages the same word is used for both water and semen; for example the Ashanti in Africa designate their patrilinear groups as *ntoro*, which means water, river and semen, while Papuans call their patrilinear clans *dan*, meaning water and semen.

In the same sense, there was a belief that raindrops were heaven's seed which caused the earth to bear fruit, and it used to be believed that springs and rivers likewise brought fertility. According to Aeschines (4th century BC), Greek girls bathed in the Scamander river before marrying, asking the river to take their virginity; magical rites in which water serves as a substitute for semen are numerous.

Water gives the impression of having life itself, of being alive, because it is very often moving and makes noises, from rippling brooks to roaring storms at sea; thus it provokes our emotions, varying from calmness and peace in the first case to fear and anxiety in the latter.

More practically, water is viewed as life-giving because of the rainwater from heaven that moistens the earth, and the spring in an oasis which brings forth life out of the desert, refreshing both animals and plants: 'For the earth which drinketh in the rain that cometh oft upon it, and bringeth forth herbs meet for them by whom it is dressed, receiveth blessing from God' Hebrews 6: 7.

Physical power of water

Water can provoke in people a sense of awe because of its great power, which can show itself in many ways. It is a force capable of destroying man-made structures as, for example, when tidal waves occur or when an avalanche is created by water in the form of snow, and misery and death can be caused to whole populations by flooding. This power of water can also show itself in another significant way by its effect on the physical environment we live in. It changes the shape and form of the earth's surface owing to the sculpting action of glaciers and rivers, which, together with the rivers and oceans, transport all sorts of materials great distances.

Visual aspects

Water changes its appearance and colouring according to the ambient light of the sun, moon or stars falling upon it. Its mirror-like quality reflects the local surroundings, giving reflections of the people and animals who look into it. These reflections in water gave rise to oracles claiming to have prophetic or divinatory powers to foretell the future and reveal the past. In modern times shamans use metal mirrors in place of water for divination.

Judging by water

Water has ever been widely regarded as a means of judgment, from ducking stools to testing whether alleged witches would float or sink. Perhaps the greatest judgment ever was the Deluge (myths of this great flood are widespread over Eurasia and America) which destroyed the sinful, disobedient people, with only a few chosen people being preserved. This was an expiation by water on a grand scale, giving rise to the creation of a new type of world: 'Whereby the world that then was, being overflowed with water, perished' 2 Peter 3: 6.

Water as a solvent and cleanser

Water is a general solvent – a polar solvent - because it has small negative and positive charges, with the ability to dissolve ionic and polar substances to form aqueous solutions in which the hundreds of chemical reactions that occur continuously to keep organisms alive all take place. It is universally used for washing and cleaning clothes, as a cleanser for the body to wash away dirt and also to cleanse the spirit to wash away sin. Thus it is used as a means of purification and for forgiveness; this is especially so in arid areas where water is very precious.

Lustration (ceremonial purification), sprinkling, or immersion in water is a common requirement for entry into new communities and to welcome new life, as, for example, in baptism, where the use of water is the only common factor in the baptismal ceremony of all traditions. Water lustration is widely observed after touching the dead, after menstruation and childbirth, and also as part of the ceremonial washing and purification of priests and kings: 'When Pilate saw that he could prevail nothing, but that rather a tumult was made, he took water, and washed his hands before the multitude, saying, I am innocent of the blood of this just person' Matthew 27: 24.

It is owing to the solubility in water of such substances as sugar and salt that foods may be flavoured and made more palatable. The hydration of its ions tends to cause a salt to break apart (dissolve) in the water. In the dissolving process the strong forces present between the positive and negative ions of the solid are replaced by strong water–ion interactions. Hydration occurs when an ionic solid such as salt dissolves in water, and the positive ends of the water molecules are attracted to the anions while the negative ends of the water molecules are attracted to the cations.

Water in the body

A living organism could be regarded as a kind of aqueous solution when we consider that certain parts of plants, such as leaves and flowers, are composed of up to 97% water. Between 70 and 90% of the total weight of the animal kingdom is water, and from 65 to 75% of humans.

The proportion of water in our bodies lessens throughout our life, beginning with 94% in an embryo of 1 month, 80% in a new-born baby, 75% at age 1–2 years, 70% at 10–15 years and 65% for an adult of 50 years; this remains fairly constant until the onset of old age when there is a tendency to dehydration (Luu & Luu 1993, p. 4). Not that all parts of our bodies are the same in this respect; adipose tissue consists of about 30% water, with the organs, including the skin, having between 70% and 80%; our bones are 22% water and even tooth enamel is 2%. Our body fluids obviously have a much higher water content, somewhere between 90% and 98.5%. The average adult loses about 1 litre of fluid per day through sweat and other bodily processes.

Movement of water in the body

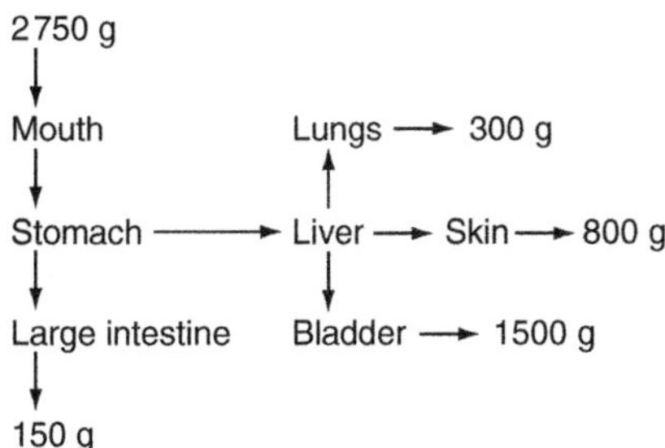

Bottled water

Some spring waters may contain high levels of bacteria, especially as they may be bottled and stored for a considerable number of months before reaching the customer; sparkling bottled waters tend to have the lowest levels of bacteria because the carbon dioxide inhibits their growth. Those waters labelled simply as 'spring' or 'table' water have to conform to the same standards as tap water and may be obtained from any source, varying from natural springs to mains water, or they may be blended from any of these sources (unlike natural mineral waters which cannot be disinfected and nothing may be added or taken away). Bottled waters may be filtered, irradiated with ultraviolet light to kill bacteria – and then supplied at an extremely elevated cost (Ryrie 1998, p. 102).

Bottled waters are now sold at high prices – up to £9 per litre – and despite the fact that water is heralded as a means of improving the appearance of skin, eyes and hair and for boosting energy levels and detoxifying the body, these purported benefits are unsubstantiated, the minimum of eight glasses per day recommended by the World Health Organization and the British Dietetic Association being questioned (nutrition.org.uk). People do not have to drink water – the daily fluid necessary can be gained by a sufficient intake of drinks such as beer, tea, coffee, soft drinks and watery foods such as vegetables, salads, fruit, soups – but no doubt there are differing opinions.

Healing treatments with water

Water brings refreshment to the weary and to invalids and it has healing qualities. Hindus believe that water has a soul and that bathing in it is a spiritual ceremony to restore balance and harmony between body, mind and spirit and to connect with the divine. Water cults still exist and many wells used to be 'dressed' with flowers in thanks; this continues at Tissington in Derbyshire. Steam baths (Turkish baths) are still much used for relaxation and stress reduction, as are saunas. Each year about 6 million people visit Lourdes in the hope of healing physical and mental problems, following the instruction given by the apparition to Saint Bernadette to 'Go drink at the fountain and cleanse yourself there' (Liébaert 1975). In Jerusalem there was a pool known as Bethesda where many people came to be cured of their ailments (Youth Bible 1993):

> *In the porches lay a great multitude of impotent folk, of blind, halt, withered, waiting for the moving of the water. For sometimes an angel went down at a certain season into the pool, and troubled the water: whosoever then first after the troubling of the water stepped in was made whole of whatsoever disease he had. John 5: 3–4 plus note to v.3*

Thalassotherapy

As some of our body tissues are composed of 90% water, the suitability of mineral-rich sea water for bodily treatments has for long been recognized. This treatment combines the benefits of the actual sea water itself with the accrued benefits from the sun (vitamin D) and the seaside atmosphere. It can of course be rather cool at the seaside, and while this is bracing to convalescents who are run down, a temperature of less than 20°C can be contraindicated for those suffering from rheumatism, arthritis, broken bones, etc. Consequently it has become the practice in northern climes to use heated sea water in such treatments, often also associated with the use of seaweed.

Thalassotherapy is an ancient form of treatment: in 480 BC Euripides and Plato agreed that 'the sea cures maladies of men' and that 'the sea cleanses all the hurts of man'. At this time thalassotherapy became a separate therapy, with organized centres offering a wide variety of treatments based on sea water. Treatments are said to be balancing to the body, thanks to the skin permeability, which allows negative ions and the trace elements in sea water to enter it. Sea water contains sulphur, cobalt, fluorine, phosphorus, magnesium and potassium and at the same time it has antibiotic and antibacterial properties (Mise en Scène 2002a, p. 20). Luu & Luu (1993, p. 7) report the composition of sea water as follows: chlorine 19, sulphate 2.6, bicarbonate 0.14, bromine 0.06, iodine traces, sodium 10.6, magnesium 1.3, potassium 0.4, calcium 0.4, strontium 0.01 g/l.

Spa treatments

The beneficial effects of many spa waters and thermal cures have long been recognized, and the Romans had many cure and hygiene centres based around naturally hot and artificially heated springs. These centres were mainly for relaxation, but in the Middle Ages therapeutic spas were instigated to cure the maladies of the crusaders returning from Palestine (Luu & Luu 1993, p. 106). In modern times these 'cures' last about 3 weeks and are used chiefly for convalescents and those suffering from chronic complaints for which classic treatments have had little effect. Treatments at various stations are offered for a range of conditions including chronic pain, rheumatism, nerve pain, digestive troubles, digestive tract spasm, gynaecological problems, problems due to obesity, respiratory infections, osteoarthritis, skin diseases, sports injuries, re-education. These sessions may perhaps allow a reduction in aggressive orthodox treatments, which is an advantage to the well-being of the person, even though it may be just a temporary respite.

This is borne out by the experience of the author's mother, who was a chronic arthritic. The numerous drugs she was taking (mostly because of the side-effects of the cortisone which, it has to be said, enabled her to walk after several years of poor mobility) left her in a very debilitated state. This was alleviated every time she was able to spend a few weeks at spa centres such as Harrogate and Buxton – unfortunately too expensive to take advantage of often enough. Her improved state lasted a mere 6 or 7 weeks, but the high cost meant she had to wait almost a year for her next visit.

Scientists who investigated water

In ancient Greece it was generally believed (for example, by Aristotle) that water was an element, an indivisible body, and this belief persisted for almost two millennia. It was not until the early 1780s that almost simultaneous discoveries in France and England showed that water is, in fact, made up of two different molecules in the proportion of one oxygen atom to two of hydrogen.

Henry Cavendish (1731–1810), an English physicist and chemist who did experiments in many fields, discovered the composition of air, the nature of hydrogen, the specific heat of certain substances, the composition of water and some important properties of electricity. Cavendish's experiments on air, described in 1784–1788 and based on earlier work by Joseph Priestley (also an English scientist), led to the discovery that water is not an element but a compound. Joseph Priestley had noted (but did not think it significant) that when a mixture of hydrogen and air is exploded by means of an electric spark, a method that had been proposed a few years before, the walls of the vessel are covered with moisture.

By a careful repetition of Priestley's experiment, Cavendish concluded that this moisture was mainly water. A similar conclusion was reached at about the same time by James Watt, the Scottish engineer, and communicated to Priestley and to the Royal Society. Meanwhile in France, in 1783, Antoine Laurent Lavoisier and Pierre Simon de Laplace succeeded in synthesizing a few grams of water from a mixture of oxygen and hydrogen. The reverse action was found to be possible by passing a red hot piece of iron through water. About 20 years afterwards, following the invention of the battery, the decomposition of water by electrolysis was achieved, where the volume of hydrogen obtained was double that of the oxygen. Thus, chemically, water is a compound of hydrogen and oxygen whose formula is H_2O.

Structure of liquid water

The liquid state of water has a very complex structure, which certainly involves high association of the molecules. Water appears sometimes as a true solution and sometimes as a colloidal system where the water dissolves, ionizes, disperses, stabilizes, breaks down and reconstructs very diverse molecular structures.

Hydrogen bonding

Hydrogen bonding is a special kind of bonding resulting from weak electrostatic bonds. This bonding (i.e. attraction between the molecules present in liquid water) produces very different values for the properties of water, such as viscosity, surface tension and boiling point, than could be expected for a liquid containing such tiny molecules.

Electronegativity

Of the three main types of atom (see pp. 76–78) (carbon, hydrogen and oxygen) found in essential oils and waters, some have a stronger tendency to attract electrons than others. The oxygen atom, with its eight protons, has a large positive charge compared to that of a hydrogen atom, which has only one proton. Because of this, when oxygen and hydrogen bond together to share a pair of electrons, this shared pair of electrons locate themselves rather nearer to the oxygen because of its larger positive charge.

This tendency displayed by the oxygen atom to attract the shared electrons is known as electronegativity, and oxygen shows this property to a greater degree than carbon and hydrogen. Thus, oxygen is said to be more electronegative than these other two atoms.

In a covalent bond between two atoms of different electronegativities the bonding electrons will be located closer to the more electronegative atom.

Within the water molecule the effect of this electronegativity is that the shared hydrogen electrons are attracted to orbit nearer to the oxygen atom, which becomes slightly electronegative. Consequently, with the hydrogen electrons in orbit further away from the hydrogen nuclei, the two hydrogen atoms become slightly electropositive. The result of this is that the complete water molecule has an oxygen end which is slightly negatively charged, and hydrogen ends which are slightly positive.

Due to this phenomenon the complete water molecule is a dipole with positive and negative poles. Thus water is a polar molecule and will either be attracted to or repelled by other polar molecules (Figs. 3.2–3.4).

The two H-O bonds form an angle of about 105 degrees (Fig. 3.3) – an arrangement that results in a polar molecule, because there is a net negative charge toward the oxygen end (the apex) of the V-shaped molecule and a net positive charge at the hydrogen ends.

Consequently, each oxygen atom is able to attract two nearby hydrogen atoms from two other water molecules. This electrostatic attraction is known as hydrogen bonding. Hydrogen bonding is always found where there is an oxygen-hydrogen group (—OH). Hydrogen bonds in water are strong enough to bind, yet weak enough to break easily. Every water molecule wants to form a three-dimensional structure

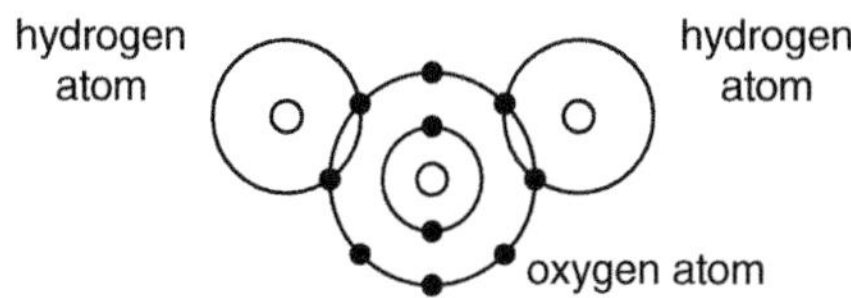

Figure 3.2 Water molecule.

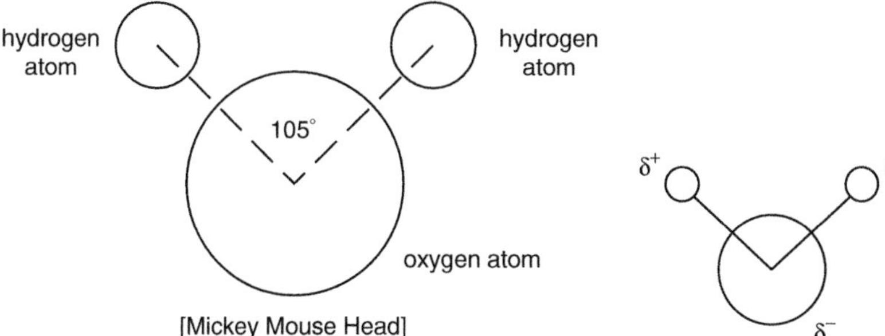

Figure 3.3 The two H-O bonds form an angle of about 105 degrees.

Figure 3.4 The polarity of a water molecule.

with its neighbours, with the oxygen end of the molecule losing electrons to other molecules and the hydrogen end gaining electrons, so that water molecules bond easily with others (Fig. 3.5).

These hydrogen bondings give water its surface tension, keeping water liquid at ordinary temperatures – made possible because of the polar nature of water. The water molecules attract one another sufficiently to increase the molecular weight, which has the effect of raising the boiling point so that water exists as a liquid rather than the gas that would normally be expected for such a tiny lightweight molecule. Based on the size of its molecules, water should have a boiling point lower than its actual boiling point, by about 200°C (360°F).

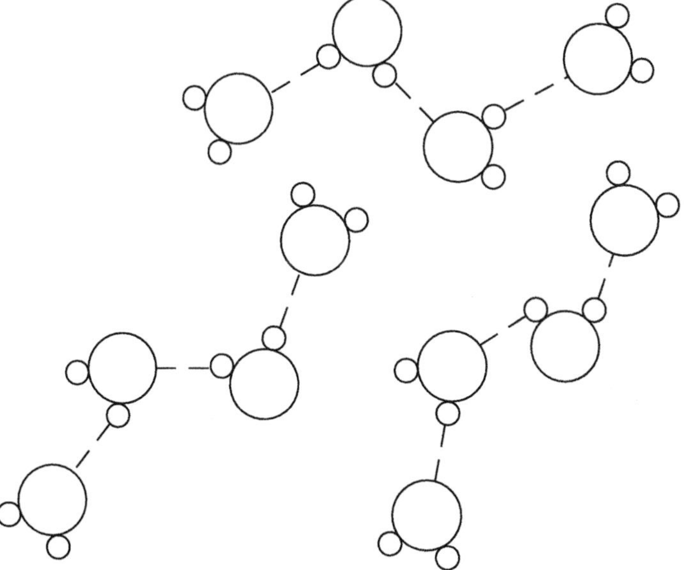

Figure 3.5 Boiling of water molecules.

Thanks also to the hydrogen bonding, water is able to build structures in three dimensions in the freezing process where each molecule of water bonds to three other molecules – creating empty space. When freezing, the water increases in volume (due to these spaces), so that the ice takes up more space than water, and because it is therefore less dense, it floats on the unfrozen water.

Due to these hydrogen bondings between molecules, the latent heats of fusion and of evaporation and the heat capacity of water are all unusually high, so water serves both as a heat-transfer medium (for example as ice for cooling and steam for heating) and as a temperature regulator (the water in lakes and oceans helps regulate the climate).

The gas-like vapour phase is made up of independent water molecules relatively distant from each other because, as the water comes to boiling point, the hydrogen bonds are broken and the molecules are set free. There is no linking between the molecules in the gaseous state of water, in contrast to the solid and liquid states which exhibit extensive linking among the water molecules.

Polar solvent – solubility in water

Water is a polar compound and is known as a polar solvent, due to the small negative and positive charges. As a solvent, it is very good at dissolving ionic (electrovalent) compounds such as common salt, which is made up of negatively charged chlorine ions and positively charged sodium. When dry, salt is quite stable but in water the chlorine is instantly attracted to the electropositive hydrogen and the sodium to the negatively charged oxygen. Any molecule which dissolves in water is described as being hydrophilic (having an affinity for water – from the Greek *hydro* meaning water and *philos* meaning love).

The terpenes, which consist only of hydrocarbons, do not have opposite poles – they are apolar – because the electronegativity of carbon and hydrogen atoms is the same, so polarization cannot take place. Therefore, because they are not polarized and do not possess any strongly electronegative atoms, they are unable to join in the electrostatic interlacing of the water molecules, and so are excluded from the molecular network (Bowles 1995, p. 54). In other words they will not dissolve in water and are termed hydrophobic (repelling water – from the Greek *hydro* meaning water and *phobos* meaning fear, dislike).

Many non-ionic compounds are soluble in water, for example, ethanol (C_2H_5OH), the non-terpenoid alcohol found in wine and beer, dissolves in water very easily. Ethanol has two carbon atoms but is partially soluble in water because its structure contains a polar –OH bond similar to that in water, and this allows hydrogen bonding and facilitates interaction between the two (Figs 3.6 and 3.7).

The insoluble non-polar carbons are dragged into solution by the hydrophilic strength of the polar–OH bond. The longer carbon chains of the terpenoid alcohols will be slightly soluble in water, but the solubility of these depends on the proportion of polar to non-polar sections of the molecule, so the monoterpenols with their 10 carbon chains will thus be more soluble in water than the sesquiterpenols with their longer 15 carbon chains.

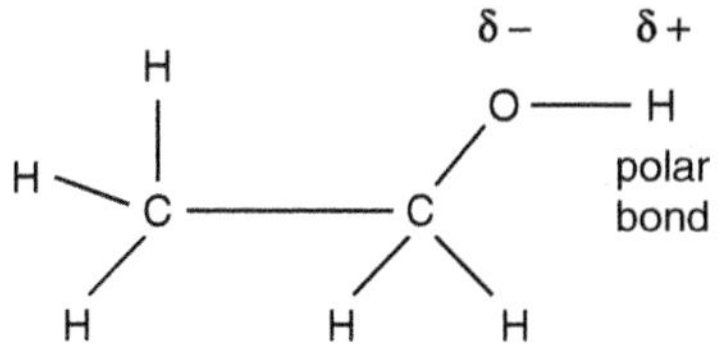

Figure 3.6 Ethanol.

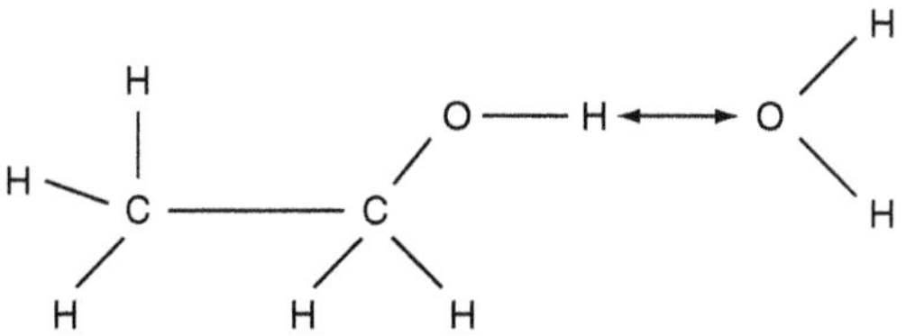

Figure 3.7 Ethanol–water interaction.

Phenols are a special case due to the acidic nature of the -OH group: the delocalization of the electrons in the aromatic ring makes the -OH group behave differently from the -OH in alcohols (W. Morden, personal communication, 2003).

The short carbon chain (2-5C) acids are quite soluble in water as they contain both the C=O radical and the -OH group on the same carbon, which strengthens the hydrogen bonding, and having short carbon chains there is less 'resistance' to solubility. These acids tend to occur rather more in the distilled plant waters than in the non-polar essential oils.

Aldehydes, ketones, esters, ethers and oxides also contain an oxygen atom, but there is no hydrogen atom attached to it, as the oxygen is either double bonded to carbon or is bonded either side to two carbons. As the oxygen atom is so electronegative, there is some polarization and an attraction between the hydrogen atom in the water and the lone pair of electrons in the C–O–H or C=O bonds and so ketones and aldehydes are frequently found in the distilled plant waters, for example thujone, pulegone, butanal, butenal.

Bowles (1995, p. 54) says that the hydrocarbon mono- and sesquiterpenes are non-polar and incompatible with water, because there is no difference between the electronegativity of the carbon and hydrogen atoms and thus no polarization. However, our experience has shown that mono- and sesquiterpene hydrocarbons are found in distilled plant waters, viz. caryophyllene in marjoram, peppermint and catnip, germacrene D in marjoram, melissa and hyssop, pinene in horsetail, sabinene in carrot and geranium, and so on.

In general, polar and ionic substances are soluble in water. In the triangular structural relationship between the two hydrogen and the single oxygen atoms, the electron of each hydrogen atom is attracted by the oxygen atom and a dipole is created. There is a negative pole at the oxygen atom and a positive pole at the hydrogen position. This polarity influences both the chemical and the physical properties of the water.

Although completely pure water is a poor conductor of electricity, it is a much better conductor than most pure liquids because of its self-ionization, i.e. the ability of two water molecules to react together to form a hydroxyl ion OH^- and a hydronium ion (H_3O^+) (Concise Columbia Encyclopedia 1991). Water is also chemically active, reacting with certain metals and metal oxides to form bases, and with certain oxides of non-metals to form acids.

Increased dilution

Understanding the nature of water is not easy. It would seem obvious to assume, when any substance is dissolved in water, that as more and more water is added, the dissolved molecules in the water would 'float' further apart from each other in the greater volume available as the solution became increasingly dilute. Such seems not to be the case, as reported by Samal et al (2001) who discovered that some molecules act in quite another way and instead of becoming more scattered and isolated tend to seek each other's company, forming small groups; then as the solution becomes more dilute they group together in larger clusters. This effect was tested with a variety of substances; dilution typically made the molecules cluster into aggregates five to ten times as big as those in the original solutions. The growth was not linear and it depended on the concentration and history of the original – the more dilute at the start, the larger the aggregates. This seemingly nonsensical behaviour occurs only when one end of the dissolved molecules is positive and the other end negative and the surrounding medium, water, is a polar solvent.

Controversially, it is said that this finding may possibly give a clue to solving the mystery of how successive dilutions of homoeopathic remedies, with their increasing potencies, are effective. In the extreme, no active ingredient is present and only the 'memory imprint' is left, thought by some to be more effective than the active part itself. The French immunologist Jacques Benveniste (1988, p. 816-818) made the debatable statement that a solution that had once contained antibodies still worked because it bore information 'imprints'. Ryrie (1998, p. 58) gives an example of a snowflake, which is made up of a billion billion water molecules in a specific arrangement, saying that no two snowflakes are exactly alike, yet if a snowflake is melted it will refreeze into precisely the same arrangement; it seems to remember its previous pattern. This is as yet unproven.

This subject of dilution is recognized as being important with regard to essential oil therapy; with melissa oil, skin allergies and respiratory problems are often made worse if not treated with a suitably low concentration (Price & Price 1999, p. 333). When dissolved in pure water, many essential oils have great bactericidal power in doses between 0.2 and 2%, and Lautié & Passebecq (1979, p. 92) state that in a concentration of 0.18%, essence of cloves kills the tubercle bacillus in a few minutes, without damaging the tissues and without poisoning the organism – a risk run by many pharmaceutical preparations and many antibiotics.

It may be that some of the above may relate to the distilled plant waters, perhaps accounting for their effectiveness.

4

Terminology and nomenclature

- Introduction: what's in a name? 31
- How distilled plant waters are obtained 31
- Current terminology 32
- Hydrosols? 34
- Conclusion 34

Introduction: what's in a name?

Why is it that so few aromatherapists consider distilled essential waters for use in the treatments they give? One reason may, surprisingly, be because there is no single commonly accepted name for them. Essential oils are called essential oils by all English-speaking people and there is a common understanding of what is meant by the term; but the waters issuing from the distillation process have several names in common use, all used in different ways by different people. Thus therapists when communicating with each other use different words (e.g. hydrosol, hydrolat, aromatic water, floral water) for the same product – the aqueous distillate – and sometimes the same words to describe different products (e.g. prepared water, water with essential oils added, fragrant water).

It is little wonder that the number of names in common use – floral water, hydrosol, hydrolat, prepared water, aromatic water, water distillate – for this one product causes confusion in the minds of aromatherapists (although in some countries, for example Germany and France, no confusion exists because the word hydrolat is commonly used). These names may or may not accurately describe the products under discussion. The various names in use will be examined, but first a brief description of these waters will give an understanding of what is being discussed.

How distilled plant waters are obtained

Distilled plant waters, (*hydrolats*, as they are known in France) are a product of distillation and can be considered as true partial extracts of the plant material from which they are derived. They may be by-products of distillation for volatile oils, for example chamomile water and lavender water, or distillation of plant material which has no (or an insignificant amount of) volatile oil, for example elderflower, cornflower, plantain. Their method of preparation, by definition, necessitates that they be totally natural products with no added synthetic fragrance components. During the process of distillation the volatile components of the plant are carried over by the steam and after condensation are found in the hydrolat.

With some essential oils having a relatively high proportion of water-soluble compounds, much of the essential oil can be lost to the hydrolat during the distillation process; in such cases it is imperative to have cohobation (see Ch. 6). This is a system whereby the water/steam in contact with the biomass during distillation is recirculated, giving maximum opportunity for the water-soluble elements of the essential oil and the plant to pass into the water. Eventually this water reaches saturation point, when no more of the essential oil components can pass into solution, and it is at this stage that the complete essential oil is gained. Thus a water is produced that is rich in hydrophilic essential oil molecules from the plant.

Distilled plant waters may have, in certain cases, generally similar properties to the parent oils depending upon their composition, but not of course to the same degree, and can be used as gentle therapeutic agents. Their mild action, which is without toxicity, makes them ideal for use as skin tonics or in healing baths and they have long been used in these ways. They have a subtle effect without the risk of irritation and are suitable for sensitive skins, babies, children, and even eye care as their action is mild compared to that of the essential oils, and because of their non-aggressive quality they can be used on open wounds for disinfection and on mucous surfaces.

> *Distilled aromatic waters, as with other partial plant extracts, will only possess the claimed activity of the plant if the active constituents of the plant are contained within that fraction of the plant which forms the partial plant extract. Many partial plant extracts, particularly distillates, have the advantage of being virtually colourless, making for ease of incorporation into a range of products. Unfortunately, this has led over the years to the production of distillates from a wide range of plant materials which are not suitable to this form of processing, and therefore little credence can be given to any claimed activity of the plant material or its extract. (Helliwell 1989)*
> [Here distillate = hydrolat]

As Rose (1999, p. 164) very sensibly argues:

> *These hydrosols are not simply misters (i.e. perfumed sprays), nor are they water to which droplets of essential oil have been added. They are a separate and natural product of the distillation process and can be termed 100% non-alcoholic distillates. They cannot be manufactured synthetically in the laboratory. A hydrosol has to be produced during the distillation process.*
> [Here hydrosol = hydrolat]

Current terminology

Aromatic water: This is inappropriate because it does not exclude laboratory-made synthesized waters.

Floral water: (Sometimes called *eau florale*.) This is inaccurate as by no means all distilled waters are from flowers.

Fragrant water: This is inappropriate as a description of distilled plant water because it does not exclude laboratory-made synthesized waters.

Prepared water: This is an assembly of products to simulate a natural product, often designed to fulfil a particular requirement of the customer. Prepared waters vary considerably in quality, ranging from filtered products cleaned up and 'improved' for food use, waters with added parabens as bacteriostats, others not only with bacteriostats but also fungicides incorporated, plus sometimes with up to 14% alcohol added because of legislative requirements, to even more questionable compounds. Some waters are produced from plants which give no therapeutic benefit at all, but possibly look good when listed on the label. All these waters are used in the cosmetics industry, but for therapeutic use the genuine, unadulterated, distilled plant water is required.

Essential water: An ancient name which aptly describes the distilled plant water but which has now gone out of use; pharmacologists once described distilled plant water as a rarefaction and an exaltation of the purest and most essential hydrophilic parts of the plant, calling them essential waters and distilled waters (Montesinos 1991, p. 5).

Hydrolat: In France the word *hydrolat* is used to describe the condensed steam which has passed through the plant material. Guérain (1886) defined hydrolat – a pharmaceutical term – as 'a colourless liquid which is obtained by distilling water with odorous flowers or with some other aromatic substances'. A hydrolat is a product of distillation.

Hydrosol: The word 'hydrosol' is often used in the English language, especially in the USA, when referring to distilled plant waters. This word is not appropriate, as it is a generic term, and not sufficiently specific, being applied to a wide range of products. The definition of hydrosol is given in *Chambers Science and Technology Dictionary* as a colloidal solution in water (Walker 1991), the word hydrosol being actually from the Greek *hydro* (water) and the Latin *solvere* (to loosen; see also Glossary). A colloidal solution (i.e. dispersion of material in a liquid) is characterized by particles of very small size (between 0.2 and 0.002 microns) where water is the dispersant medium (Montesinos 1991, p. 3). Grosjean (n.d., p. 12) claims to have given the name hydrosol for natural flower water or *hydrolat* and another (aromatherapy) source gives the derivation of hydrosol as coming from *hydro* (water) and *sol* (sun's energy); this is imaginative but suspect. By definition, distilled plant waters must be the product of a distillation process, and distillation does not form part of the definition of a hydrosol. A hydrolat is obtained by recovering, after condensation, the distillation water (Roulier 1990, p. 17), while a hydrosol may be obtained by prolonged impregnation of essential oil in pure water.

Medicated water: One translation of *hydrolat* is given as medicated water (Mansion 1971).

Hydrosols?

All of this leaves us with the problem of how properly to designate waters containing plant compounds as a result of extraction by distillation. As can be seen, 'fragrant', 'aromatic' and 'floral' are not appropriate for the subject of this book on distilled plant waters and there appears to be no dedicated word in the English language. Nor is the term hydrosol appropriate, since:

1. The word hydrosol may, depending on background and context, signify different things to different people, including: a water soluble fertilizer, a reducing agent for bleaching wool, an agent for cleaning machinery, a trade name for white spirit, an anaesthetic medicated ointment, starch, ink and similar substances; and some mushrooms contain monomethyl hydrosol (also found in rocket fuel).
2. The chief objection is that **distillation** is not essential to a hydrosol, while it is the key feature in obtaining true distilled plant waters.
3. Hydrosol is a generic term and is not specific to distilled plant waters.
4. Some of the organic particles in distilled plant waters are of molecular size, some are in solution, which, by definition, argues against the hydrosol description.
5. A prepared water (i.e. essential oils or synthetics in water) is also a hydrosol – but it is *not* a hydrolat.
6. There is confusion among aromatherapists concerning the word hydrosol, enfleurage.com (2001) describing the product of plant distillation as a hydrosol and at the same time, stating that floral waters are made by adding essential oils to distilled water and that these are not hydrosols. They are, in fact, hydrosols also.

Conclusion

The authors feel that in anglicizing the pronunciation of the French word *hydrolat* we have at our disposal a useful and specific word in English which can be dedicated precisely to the distilled product used in aromatherapy.

5

Prepared waters

- Identifying the product 35
- Not distilled 35
- Internal use 36
- Fragrant waters: methods of production and uses 37
- Addition of alcohol 38
- Hydroessentials 38
- Witch hazel 39
- Eau-de-Cologne 39
- Conclusion 40

Identifying the product

Every aromatherapist should be – and is surely – aware of the potential pitfalls in buying essential oils. The quality of these healing oils is very variable and a diligent search is often needed to find a reliable source of therapeutic-quality essential oils. As with essential oils, so it is with distilled plant waters; the quality and nature of waters available ranges from the genuine distilled article (see Ch. 6) to synthesized products which do not have the same therapeutic qualities. As Battaglia (1995, p. 425) writes: 'some are water and alcohol mixes, some are distilled water with a little oil or perfume added, some are glycerine and water with essential oils.' There are other variants too. Part of the problem is, once again, the question of nomenclature, which is confusing, as these products also are commonly known by several different names, for example artificial waters, prepared aromatic waters, false medicated waters, simulated waters, toilet waters, fragrant waters, false hydrolats, etc. The name fragrant water (used by Keville & Green 1995, p. 90) has a certain appeal, as these made products are always formulated to have a pleasant smell, which is not always the case with the natural distilled waters. As with essential oils, hydrolats (distilled waters) should be purchased only with an analytical report as a certificate of authenticity.

Not distilled

Whatever their name, prepared waters are not produced by the distillation process but are put together in a laboratory and consist of water with the addition of one or more essential oils, which may or may not themselves be genuine plant essential oils – they may even be absolutes or concretes and any of them may be partially or wholly artificial (synthetic).

Distilled plant waters are simulated by the use of more than one method, but the simplest is by means of dissolving essential oils in water, sometimes spring water, often distilled water. This is achieved by purely physical means – a vigorous shaking of the essential oils together with water, with no other substances being involved. The simulated aromatic waters produced by this method can lack the top fresh notes of their distilled counterparts, and any water-soluble plant compounds which may be present in the plant, but which do not form part of the essential oil, are missing too.

Essential oils are not generally soluble in water – probably on average 20% of the oil – but many of the oils can be 'knocked' into solution by shaking to produce a saturated solution. For each litre of distilled water, in a glass container, 2–3 grams (40–60 drops) of essential oil can be added; this must be shaken frequently and vigorously for 2 or 3 days and then stored in a cool place. Essential oils suitable for this method are anise, basil, borneol, chamomile, caraway, centaury, cinnamon, citron, coriander, cypress, eucalyptus, fennel, garlic, gentian, geranium, goosefoot, hyssop, juniper, laurel, lavender, lemon, marjoram, melissa, niaouli, nutmeg, onion, orange (Seville), origanum, peppermint, rosemary, sage, santolina, sassafras, savory, tangerine, tarragon, turmeric, verbena and ylang ylang (Lautié & Passebecq 1979, p. 91). Such waters are expected to have the properties of the essential oils; it is merely another means of diluting them for use and can be compared with diluting them in vegetable oil for massage. Prepared waters, which can be stored successfully at 10–15°C for several months, do not have the same make-up as hydrolats (distilled plant waters) and therefore cannot have exactly the same therapeutic properties.

Internal use

Waters prepared as above may be used for gargles and mouthwashes, for bathing wounds and for ingestion, where 20 ml of the made water contains one drop of essential oil and therefore one teaspoonful contains about a quarter of a drop. The purpose of ingestion is not, as some aromatherapists think, to administer a large dose but to deliver an appropriate dose to the target area. Some prepared waters are made with the use of alcohol and these are not recommended for use alongside some treatments. Those not containing alcohol are suitable for children, especially as they may be sweetened with sugar. Many essential oils exhibit significant bactericidal power at a concentration of 0.25% as found in prepared waters, for example, in a concentration of 0.18%, clove essential oil kills the tubercle bacillus in a few minutes without causing any tissue damage or risk of toxicity, in contrast to some other preparations and antibiotics (Lautié & Passebecq 1979, p. 92). Whether introduced into the human body via the skin (alcohol preparations, aromatized oils, cold cream, ointments), via the mouth, or via the nose (inhalations, perfumes), essential oils spread throughout the whole body before being at least partly expelled by the lungs, sweat and urine.

Fragrant waters: methods of production and uses

Sale of prepared waters is mainly to skin care product manufacturers for use in 'natural' skin toners, refreshers and washes, and this is the use for which Keville & Green (1995, p. 90) recommend them, in a pleasant, lighter way, calling them 'fragrant waters' to distinguish them from 'true aromatic hydrosols' (i.e. hydrolats). They say that they are inexpensive, easy to make, but less effective as moisturizing agents because they do not contain the same hydrophilic compounds as hydrolats, but comment that adding aloe vera juice to 'fragrant waters' can boost the moisturizing properties if they are to be used as toners or as cosmetic body sprays. These fragrant waters have many uses, depending on the essential oils chosen, and allow the application of diluted essential oils onto the skin without the use of a vegetable oil. Spray or splash on fragrant water after your daily shower, to cool down on a hot day, or whenever you are in the mood for instant aromatherapy. They can also be refreshing to the face and to the mind on long journeys.

As early as 1907 the Swiss pharmacopoeia (4th edn) listed a prepared water, 'concentrated distilled water' (elder, lime), with the instruction to macerate the dry plant material with alcohol for 24 hours followed by steam distillation. This was followed by redistillation, and the final product was used at a dilution of one in ten. In the pharmacopoeias of many countries distilled waters were gradually replaced by prepared waters made up of essential oils dissolved in water, with or without the addition of alcohol, for example the German pharmacopoeia (6th edn, 1926) and the US pharmacopoeia set aside the process of distillation. The Swiss pharmacopoeia of 1934 (5th edn) laid down the regulations for the preparation of certain waters (rose, orange flower, cherry laurel, mint and fennel).

Generally waters were prepared quite simply using the appropriate essential oils, water and a medium for trituration. They were made either by saturating distilled water with essential oil, achieved either by the use of a vehicle such as alcohol (see below) or by increasing the even distribution of the essential oil by trituration using a neat powder (e.g. talcum, kaolin, sugar, magnesium carbonate), also calcium phosphate, silica, paper pulp, followed by a means of filtration in order to obtain a clear or slightly opalescent liquid. Alternatively, they may be made by distilling water with the same oils, or by making strong alcoholic extracts and adding to water in specific quantities. Normally a bacteriostat is added to prevent fungus and bacteria proliferation.

Grieve (1998, pp. 20–21) mentions a prepared and concentrated pimento water (not a true hydrolat) of the British Pharmacopoeia Codex, which is made as follows:

Oil of pimento	1 fl oz
Alcohol	12 fl oz
Purified talc	1 oz
Distilled water	up to 20 fl oz

Dissolve the oil in the alcohol; add the water gradually, shaking after each addition; add the talc, shake; allow to stand for a few hours, occasionally shaking; and filter.

It is recognized that these various methods do not achieve a genuine distilled water and that distillation is the only true method of obtaining a hydrolat. True distilled waters, hydrolats, have not in the past been available on a commercial scale, and most waters available today are made to BP quality, thus we may expect to find their make-up something like the following:

Lavender flower water BP = 3% lavender oil + bergamot oil + traces of other natural materials in alcohol and distilled water.
Rose water BP = rose absolute + alcohol + distilled water.
Orange flower water BP = neroli essential oil + alcohol + distilled water.

Addition of alcohol

It is not unusual for alcohol to be added to both genuine distilled waters and prepared waters. This can be effected in more than one way. Sometimes alcohol is added to the genuine distilled water collected from the distillation process, or it may even be put into the still and distilled together with the plant. This technique was never authorized in France, but was nevertheless used in some other countries and listed in their pharmacopoeias (AGORA 2001).

The addition of alcohol to the still, or to the distillate, could help non-polar molecules dissolve in the water. If added to the still, it would fractionate over into the receiving flask quite early in the distillation run since its boiling point is below that of water. If added to the biomass it may assist in the 'extraction' of the volatiles from the plant material. (W. Morden, personal communication, 2003)

The addition of alcohol to distilled plant waters prolongs shelf-life because it acts as a preservative. If the water is to be used as an invigorating skin rub (e.g. in sport), then perhaps this is no bad thing; however, for therapeutic use, especially for the eyes and for internal use, waters with alcohol added are to be avoided.

Some 'fragrant' waters are supplied with the appellation 'triple distilled' but this is a misnomer because it means concentrated, i.e. not let down with the full quantity of distilled water. The higher alcohol percentage (usually 15%) helps preserve the product and give it a long shelf-life; it is also cheaper to transport, being less bulky and less heavy.

Concentrated waters invariably contain alcohol to maintain in solution high levels of volatile oils and/or absolutes, which may again be wholly or partially synthetic. Concentrated waters are often diluted on the basis of one part of the concentrate to 39 parts of water to produce an aromatic water, but this cannot be compared in either strength, aroma or effect to the similar prepared water made by dissolving the volatile oil, absolute or concrete in water to produce a saturated solution.

Hydroessentials

One kind of commercially produced simulated water contains the natural fractions present in essential oils which are spontaneously water soluble. These compounds are extracted from the essential oils and have a low presence, approximately the same as in the waters obtained by steam distillation of the aromatic plant material yielding the essential oil (Vevy 1989). Usually this water soluble portion is between 0.01/1000 and 0.5/1000. During the preparation of these fragrant waters the water itself is carefully prepared by dispersing parabens (preservative) using propylene glycol, then the temperature is kept above 37°C while mechanical dispersion goes on.

The end product is designated as a *natural aromatic water* and it is claimed that there is no difference between this product and a water obtained by steam distillation. The products are aqueous and for good shelf-life the product is first filtered then either alcohol and/or a solubilizer is added at very low levels to ensure clarity. The main volume of sales of these waters is to skin care manufacturers for use as natural skin toners and refreshing sprays but they may also be suitable for the food industry. These products possess an aroma similar to the plant and the essential oil; they are colourless (or nearly so) thin liquids and have a shelf-life of 6 months minimum when properly stored.

The waters on offer include orange flower, rose, elder flower, chamomile, peppermint, honeysuckle, jasmin, lemon, sweet orange and lavender. The relative density at 20°C is 0.98–1.02 with the exception of rose (1.042–1.052) and elder flower (0.950–1.010). Preservatives added are denatured ethanol and sodium benzoate and the residual alcohol level is 1% V/V max.

The authors feel that although these hydroessentials cannot in any way be called hydrolats, their composition is such that they could possibly be used for some aromatherapeutic purposes, bearing in mind that the alcohol content is extremely low and they are already used by the food industry.

Witch hazel

Witch hazel water is a clear, colourless distillate prepared from recently cut and partially dried leaves and/or twigs of *Hamamelis virginiana* and is a genuine distilled water; however, it differs from others in that it is always sold with a high ethanol content.

Witch hazel is neutral or slightly acid to litmus solution with a pH of between 3.0 and 5.0. and the relative density is 0.976–0.982. It has an ethanol content of 70–80% and a tannin content of 2–9%, but the witch hazel water bought over the counter contains 15% ethanol (Winter 1999, p. 458) and 0.03 mg/ml tannin.

Eau-de-Cologne

Perhaps the most famous of the toilet waters is eau-de-Cologne (*Kölnisches Wasser*). It is not a water in the true sense as it contains alcohol to a very large extent. However, since it is relatively easy to make we can include some ideas on the various forms of cologne. Traditional cologne was made from a mixture of bergamot oil, lemon oil, neroli oil and perhaps a touch of rose oil. Having said that, eau-de-Cologne is a water with 101 variations so that you can add almost any aromatic material as part of its recipe. Petitgrain, of course, resembles neroli and is very much cheaper; rosemary is another possible ingredient and was one of the original ingredients for the famous 'Elizabeth of Hungary' water. Palmarosa is another oil which resembles the effect of the honey note of rose oil and can be used in oriental types.

A typical formulation would be at the rate of about 3% of oil dissolved in alcohol. There is a problem if you wish to make 'normal' eau-de-Cologne because you would have to add 70% alcohol and about 30% water. However, it is possible to experiment with all the ingredients until you have something which is both acceptable and pleasing (Hephrun 2000b, p. 19).

Conclusion

Water which has had essential oil(s), synthetics or alcohol added to it has its uses but it is not a distilled plant water and should not be confused with the genuine article. To achieve a genuine plant water suitable for all therapeutic purposes **distillation** is the only true method. Prepared waters – 'fragrant waters' – whatever their method of production, do not have the same make-up as distilled plant waters, and therefore will not have exactly the same therapeutic properties. Floral waters purchased from a chemist's shop are almost always synthesized and standardized with regard to the aroma. It should be noted that preservative is often added to natural hydrolats to improve the shelf-life and the therapist should be aware of this.

The distilled water of any particular plant may have a different make-up from the essential oil from the same plant and so the action of the water may be different from that of the essential oil. Water which has had essential oil added is, therefore, not necessarily a substitute for a distilled plant water, and much work will have to be carried out in the future to clarify the situation and to determine the properties of both hydrolats and fragrant (prepared) waters.

6

Extraction process and the plants used

- What kinds of plant yield hydrolats? 41
- The plants used 42
- Drying 42
- Distillation 43
- Water used 44
- Still hardware 45
- Chemical changes 45
- Time of distillation 46
- Yield of hydrolats 46
- Volatile molecules in the distilled waters 47
- Therapeutic value 48
- Cohobation 49
- Water oil, recovered oil 50
- Are cohobated waters therapeutically useful? 51
- Conclusion 54

What kinds of plant yield hydrolats?

Hydrolats are obtained by steam distillation of plant material, in the same way as essential oils, and although some aromatherapists may think that only plants containing essential oil molecules are distilled, this is not so. Some plants which contain volatile organic components are not commercially distilled and therefore are not normally used in aromatherapy, yet they yield useful hydrolats when distilled (e.g. cornflower, oak, plantain, box, ferns). These plants are processed primarily for the hydrolats, as are some plants whose essential oils may be hazardous but which can nevertheless safely be included in the aromatic armoury of hydrolats.

In the French literature, a nominal distinction is made between waters obtained from oil-bearing plants and those obtained from non-oil-bearing plants:

- hydrolat is the name given to the product from steam distillation of aromatic plants
- distillate is the name given to the steam distilled product of medicinal plants not containing essential oil.

In general, the distillates are as odorous as the hydrolats (Montesinos 1991, p. 34).

Plants distilled mainly for their essential oil can be steam or water distilled; plants distilled for their water alone are usually water distilled, and the quality of the water used for this is of great importance.

Hydrolats are potentially therapeutic both on their own and used in synergistic conjunction with both essential oil treatments and herbalism. They are not as powerful as undiluted essential oils (which can be aggressive) and therefore can be used safely, usually without their needing to be diluted. Essential oils, on the other hand, are almost always diluted to some degree in some medium to obtain a solution which can be used safely.

The water from each plant, like the essential oil, is unique and acts according to its constituents. *Hypericum perforatum* is an example of a plant containing an essential oil, but it is rarely distilled for this because of the extremely small yield, which would make its extraction prohibitively expensive. It is, however, distilled for the hydrolat alone (which therefore contains a minute percentage of essential oil) and is also macerated in vegetable oil, where those molecules soluble in vegetable oil are taken into solution by exposure to strong sunlight over a period of time.

Plantago lanceolata (plantain) is an example of a non-aromatic plant (containing no essential oil) which is distilled for its hydrolat alone and illustrates that water-soluble molecules other than volatile essential oil molecules can be taken into the steam, yielding a therapeutic hydrolat at the end of the process (Montesinos 1991). Montesinos also says that analysis of the distillates of *Urtica dioica*, *Equisetum arvense* and *Plantago lanceolata* shows that they contain electrolytes from the plants, that they contain few or no acids, and that their oxydo-reduction potential is virtually the same as that of a distilled water.

The plants used

Plants used for the distillation of hydrolats must be selected with the same care as is taken when selecting plants for the production of essential oils, namely the correct variety harvested at the optimum time. A wide variety of plants and parts of plants may be used, roots, wood, bark, leaves, flowers, fruits and seeds, and these must be carefully harvested at the right moment: leaves at the beginning of flowering; flowers after full flowering; fruits and seeds when fully matured. Plant waters can be distilled both from odorous plants (such as juniper berry, fennel, lavender, chamomile, oregano, sage, thyme) and inodorous plants (blessed thistle, poppy, lettuce, mallow, purslane).

All parts of a plant can be put into a still to obtain a hydrolat which contains the volatile hydrophilic and polar molecules. Seeds, stalks and roots are often comminuted (crushed or chopped) to allow the steam to access the oil cells and volatile molecules deep in their structure in glands and canals, while flowers, leaves and non-fibrous parts do not need comminution because the volatiles are more accessible in sacs and glandular hairs.

Drying

Some plants whose plant material would lose some of its aromatic properties on drying should be freshly harvested and processed fresh. Others may be dried (under good conditions) if their properties are known not to be lost to any great degree during the drying process (or even enhanced, such as elder, melilot, coriander; Baudoux 1996a, p. 106); dried plants can be stored until a convenient time, when they are macerated before distillation. Sometimes plants are dried before distillation in order to improve the yield per charge of plant in the still, as the dried plant takes up less space than the fresh.

Lavender is a plant that traditionally is dried for 2–3 days before being distilled in order to reduce its bulk. Because oil cannot evaporate directly through the wall of the plant tissue, evaporation does not account for a loss of oil such as might be expected. Once dried out, the plant suffers only a slight loss of volatile molecules through hydrodiffusion or evaporation because of the lack of moisture in the cells, although the material may deteriorate when exposed to air and light. Lavender provides up to 10% less of the essential oil when dried, but for peppermint the yield from the fresh and dried plant material is practically the same; the effect on the hydrolat of drying the plant has not been determined.

The physical and chemical properties of the oil change during plant drying. Aqueous distillates from fresh and air-dried plants can differ considerably. This is especially true of flowers, leaves and herbs which, in their fresh state, contain a lot of moisture. During drying, cell membranes break down and liquids are free to penetrate from cell to cell, which gives rise to the formation of new volatile compounds by (for example) glycoside splitting. For instance, fresh patchouli leaves are virtually odourless – the well-known patchouli scent comes only after curing and drying. On the other hand, certain plants must be macerated for a while before distillation (e.g. valerian), but melissa must be distilled immediately after harvesting, otherwise the small percentage of volatile organic compounds present would be lost. The precise effects of plant drying on the resultant waters will have to be established individually for each species.

Distillation

The general principle of distillation can be seen in the domestic setting, when a kettle is boiled for some time with the spout pointing towards a tiled wall. On contact with the cold tiles, the steam from the spout is suddenly cooled. The condensed water that trickles down the tiles is now distilled pure water and has a different composition from the water remaining in the kettle, which is a mixture of pure water with salts of calcium, magnesium, other salts and solid impurities. These could not evaporate so remained in the kettle as a solid deposit, while the pure water which left the kettle is recovered by condensation. Much the same happens in the distillation of essential oils, but this time it is the plant material – flowers, leaves and stalks – which is left behind in the still and the vaporized oils and steam pass through a pipe to be condensed.

Distillation is a combination of science and art. A good distillation process involves careful preparation of the plant material for distillation, the use of as little water as possible, the maintenance of a low temperature and following the appropriate time of distillation. Successful distillation involves judgement and experience, but it is not possible to extract an essential oil that is identical to that present in the living plant.

The distillation methods used to extract essential oils and distilled plant waters are:

- Water distillation, where the plant material and the water come into direct contact.
- Water and steam distillation, where the plant material is in direct contact only with the steam and not the water (although there is water present separated from the plant material by a perforated grid, the steam is fully saturated and is never superheated – i.e. heated above its boiling point by increasing operating pressure).
- Steam distillation, where no liquid water is used and live steam, saturated or perhaps superheated (at increased pressure), is fed through perforated coils to make contact with the plant material supported on a grid. The pressure in the system is approximately 2 bar and the temperature at this pressure should not exceed 100°C.

The boiling water or steam penetrates the substance of the plants, breaks down cell walls, and reaches the tiny droplets of essential oil secreted in the vegetable matter, causing them to vaporize and mingle with the water vapour. The two vapours rise from the still, pass into a condenser which is cooled by cold water, causing the mixed vapours to condense; the cooling should be gradual and arranged so as to avoid thermal shock to the hydrolat which might cause damage to the volatile molecules, affecting their therapeutic value. The condensed liquids settle in a 'flask' (essencier/Florentine vase) and the water and direct essential oil separate spontaneously due to having different densities.

Water used

Quality of water used

When distilling for hydrolats, it is important that the water used in the distillation process should be of good quality, preferably from a non-polluted spring, where the water is low in minerals. The water should also be free of any of the chemical cleansers that are commonly used to clean the still when changing from one plant to another.

pH of the water used for distillation

The nature of the water used for distillation has an effect on the quality of the end product, including the pH value. Pure water (e.g. freshly distilled) stands midway on the acid/alkaline scale, having a pH of 7. Should this water be left exposed to the air, then the pH will decrease (i.e. it will become more acid) due to dissolved carbon dioxide from air. The relationship between pH and the water characteristics, mainly hardness and dissolved material, is rather complicated; generally very hard water will tend to be alkaline while soft water tends to be acidic. This can be changed by various acids from distilled plants, particularly in soft water, which would be normally be used for distillation, otherwise the build up of calcium/magnesium carbonate stone would make distillation difficult (I. Svoboda, personal communication, 2002). In a hard water area it has been found that the distillation of some conifers (e.g. pine, cedar) will clean the still of limescale while the opposite effect is found when distilling melissa (M. Maneuvrier, personal communication, 2003).

This variation in pH does lead to variation in the composition of hydrolats. When the water used in the distillation process is alkaline (high pH) then the analysis of the collected water will be different from the composition of a water collected from a process using acidic (low pH) water. Thus two hydrolats of the same plant material may have different compositions if they have been distilled in different areas using water with different pH values (K. Svoboda, personal communication, 2002): this factor is taken into consideration for some essential oils, specifically those which are used under standard conditions for the food or pharmaceutical industries.

Still hardware

As for essential oils, the still itself should be made of stainless steel in preference to copper or iron; some plants attack mild steel, such as cypress, juniper and thyme, and others attack copper, such as those rich in azulene (Montesinos 1991, p. 10). The essencier (Florentine vase) is often made from galvanized iron or aluminium but this is not good enough when waters are being collected – it should be of stainless steel or glass. To ensure that the hydrolat will have a reasonably long life, all the distillation hardware must be scrupulously cleaned before the process is begun. Similarly the containers in which the hydrolats are to be stored must be sterilized with steam, the hydrolat itself being filtered before being put into the storage containers. Rose distillation in Turkey takes place in 40-year-old seasoned copper stills (Watt 2000, p. 12).

Chemical changes

In theory all the above methods of distillation should give similar results, but in the heat and moisture inside the still various changes can occur, such as hydrodiffusion, hydrolysis and decomposition, all of which can affect one another.

Hydrodiffusion is the movement of molecules across permeable plant membranes by osmosis, allowing volatile molecules from within the plant to join with the steam. Distillation offers good conditions for osmosis of oils because the steam furnishes moisture to the cell walls and there is a raised temperature. Hydrolysis is a chemical reaction which occurs between the distillation water and some essential oil compounds such as esters, possibly leading to their breakdown, so at any one time esters, water, acid and alcohol are all present (the use of superheated, dry steam minimizes hydrolysis). Heat is always present during the distillation process and as all constituents of an essential oil are unstable at elevated temperatures they will tend to change and decompose with heat. Just like essential oils, the hydrolats have a 'still note' – an odour due to artefacts – which quickly disappears.

Cohobation (see below) is an important factor in the quality of both essential oils (it is imperative for some) and distilled plant waters.

Time of distillation

The time of distillation is important for a variety of reasons. It must be adjusted for the particular plant being processed and should be long enough for all the desired components which contribute to the therapeutic quality of the hydrolat to be drawn from the biomass: to allow this extraction to be as complete as possible the plant should not be too compressed in the still. A short distillation time is economically desirable to keep down costs, although too short a time produces an essential oil which may be incomplete. The longer the distillation time the more expensive it is, but more of the heavier molecules are extracted; however, there is more chance of some molecules being broken down and degraded. Artefacts – molecules not found in the plant – are produced during the distillation process and also appear in the final oil and water.

The compounds which pass into the hydrolat at different phases of the distillation process are not always of the same composition and the final hydrolat is a blend of these various fractions. It is up to the distiller to use his or her judgement to achieve the product most suitable for the purposes of the customer.

In the production of Turkish rose water, the first distillation takes about an hour and three-quarters and then the distillation water is pumped to the second distillation units with fresh flowers, where cohobation occurs for about half an hour (Watt 2000, p. 12). This results in rose hydrolat (and a second rose oil, which is then blended with the first to produce rose otto). The hot rose water is immediately stored in stainless steel tanks which reduces the possibility of atmospheric microbial contamination. The quality of Turkish rose oil and rose water is state controlled.

Yield of hydrolats

It is thought by some that large, or even unlimited, quantities of hydrolats can be produced from a small amount of plant material but this is not true; when distilling a plant to obtain hydrolats the process must be controlled so that, for example, there is a strict relationship between the quantity of biomass (plant material) being processed and the amount of hydrolat made. In other words, the quantity of hydrolat collected must be proportionate to the plant weight and to the type of plant.

Yields of hydrolats are usually between 1 and 5 litres per kilogram of plant, varying according to the particular plant. The hydrolats of thyme, savory and rosemary require a smaller quantity of plant than those of lettuce, hawthorn, yarrow or hemp agrimony. Some are known as 'weight for weight' products, for example 100 lb of roses are distilled with sufficient water to yield 100 lb of fragrant rose water (Poucher 1936). Viaud (1983, p. 23) says roughly the same – i.e. usually between 1 and 4 litres of hydrolat per kilogram of plant material, with thyme and savory, for example, yielding more hydrolat than, say, hawthorn leaves or yarrow. Paris (2000) considers that the weight of hydrolat taken from the condensed steam should be equal to that of the original plant material.

Other authors have different ideas on this subject. Grosjean (1993a) agrees that the quality of the hydrolat depends on the water used (spring water) and on the use of wild plants which have not been chemically treated, or plants grown biologically or biodynamically. She also writes that she only collects the first 20 litres of distilled water (Grosjean 1993a, p. 113), as these contain micro particles of essential oil in suspension at 4–6% and at the end of the distillation time the waters contain 1–3% of essential oil particles in suspension. It is difficult to make sense of these statements since no details are provided about the weight of plant material used or the duration of the distillation process.

Essential oils are capable of dissolving slightly in water – in the region of 0.03% to 0.05%. Montesinos (1991, p. 5) states that the water received at the end of the distillation process contains a dilution of 1/2000 of essential oil. There is also some undissolved oil present and it is good practice to separate the excess volatile oil from the distilled waters; this can be achieved by use of a Florentine vase or by filtering the waters through a filter suitably damped to separate the non-dissolved essences. It is helpful to shake the water distillate thoroughly to ensure maximum content of the essential oil molecules extracted before filtration. In some circumstances this filtration procedure is necessary – as in the case of laurel water, for example, in order to prevent an unwanted side-effect; laurel leaf oil obtained by steam distillation is moderately toxic if ingested and an irritant on the skin (Winter 1999, p. 273).

Volatile molecules in the distilled waters

Essential oils are made up of many different types of volatile molecules which may be soluble (i.e. hydrophilic), partially soluble, or completely insoluble (hydrophobic) in water, and thus dissolve to a greater or lesser degree in the hydrolat. Water oil collected at the still is different from the primary essential oil since although a particular compound may be present as a significant proportion of the primary essential, if the compound is hydrophobic then it will not be present at all (or perhaps only slightly) in the hydrolat. Thus the proportion of soluble and partially soluble compounds in the hydrolat will be different when it is compared to the essential oil and the general profile of the essential oil found in the hydrolat (i.e. the volatile molecules found there) may be quite similar to – or may be quite different from – that of the direct essential oil (which separates spontaneously and is collected at the end of the distillation process).

Hydrolats, which contain only volatile compounds with a maximum molecular weight of 250, are different from infusions and decoctions which contain molecules of a heavier nature and fewer aromatic compounds.

Owing to this somewhat limited solubility in water of essential oil molecules, hydrolats contain only a very small quantity of volatile components, though this obviously varies from plant to plant, since some essential oils contain a greater proportion of water-soluble compounds than others, although none is very high. A *Rosa damascena* steam-distilled water of French origin that was tested (hexane extracted) showed that it contained less than 0.02% essential oil compounds (Fiche Technique 1996; unfortunately this sample was polluted by thyme and so is not included in the analyses in Appendix D). Generally it can be assumed that the approximate content of water-soluble parts of the essential oil freely dispersed in an ionized form in the water is somewhere around 0.01–0.02%, although typical solubility can be up to 0.04% (i.e. a range of 0.1–0.4 g/l).

According to Lautié & Passebecq (1979), essential oils have greater bactericidal power when dissolved in pure water at between 0.2% and 2%, which is interesting with respect to hydrolats, where some of the dissolved molecules are present at very low concentrations.

The essential oil constituents which are to some extent soluble in water are partially dissolved, thus forming an aqueous solution of the oil, and these water-soluble compounds are mainly the oxygenated compounds such as alcohols and aldehydes, which are heavier than the hydrocarbon compounds (monoterpenes, sesquiterpenes). The distillate contains oil not only in solution but also suspended in minute droplets and in emulsified form (Guenther 1948, vol. 1, p. 154). Alcohols and phenols are hydrophilic to a certain extent because of their polar nature; certain of the alcohols found in plants are water soluble to such an extent that they are almost absent from the essential oil and are to be found only in the hydrolat, for example lavandulol in *Lavandula angustifolia.* Solubility of alcohols is of the order of 0.1–0.4 g/l and the phenols more so, at 0.2–1 g/l (Montesinos 1991, p. 4); however, this is not our experience, as no phenols appear in the analyses in Appendix D, while there are many instances of alcohols.

Nasr (2000, p. 24) writes that the hydrolats contain polar molecules such as acids, phenols, alcohols and aldehydes from the plant material and adds that the possibly more problematic components of essential oils, such as ketones, terpene hydrocarbons and ethers, are not likely to be present. However, both ketones and hydrocarbons were found in the some of the waters tested.

Streicher (1996) writes that hydrolats contain the water-soluble components of plant life, but not the tannic acid and bitter substances, and complement the oil-soluble component of plant life. They retain in solution during distillation not only the hydrophilic components but also some hydrophobic components.

The water oils (i.e. any essential oils which may be present in the hydrolat) generally have a much smaller amount of terpene hydrocarbons and no sesquiterpene hydrocarbons, while there is usually a higher proportion of the alcohols. In fact it is impossible to forecast composition of the water oil in relation to the direct oil with any degree of certainly – with many plants there are similarities while with others there are distinct differences. For example, with thyme, particularly the carvacrol chemotype, we can expect to find a lower proportion of phenolic compounds in the direct oil compared with the water oil. The linalool chemotype has been said to have the same proportion of linalool in the hydrolat as in the oil (about 70%).

Therapeutic value

A GC (see glossary) analysis can give us a very good idea of the chemical composition of a particular substance, but gives no idea of its therapeutic properties. Nasr (2000, p. 26) writes that essentially the actions and uses of hydrolats are similar to those of the essential oils of the plants in question. However, as seen above, this may not always be the case (except in prepared waters – see Ch. 5); also there may be some hydrophilic parts of the plant present in the hydrolat which may not be identified and which never appear in the essential oil.

Streicher (1996) writes that the less volatile odorous molecules are integrally dispersed in the water in ionized form, which avoids all irritation of the skin and mucous surfaces; this is useful in cases of eczema, ulcers, colitis and burns.

Cohobation

Almost every essential oil contains – to a greater or lesser degree – molecules which are soluble or partially soluble in water. During the water or steam distillation process to obtain essential oils, some of the water-soluble parts of the essential oil are taken into the water used in the distillation process. These compounds are retained in solution and perhaps in suspension in the distillation water in the Florentine vase; they do not separate out and so do not form part of the essential oil which normally floats on top and can be collected directly. The essential oil which is collected directly is known as 'primary' or 'decanted' essential oil.

That proportion of the essential oil present in the plant which finds its way into the condensate water is often discarded, and thus is lost. This loss may be significant, perhaps as high as 25% (Fleisher & Fleisher 1985) showing that the hydrolats can have useful properties. When the main aim of distillation is the essential oil attempts are made to recover the retained essential oil from the condensate water; this is known as 'water oil' or sometimes as 'recovered' or 'secondary' essential oil. This can be done by either of two methods of cohobation, explained below.

The quantity of the dissolved essential oil components depends upon the solubility of the volatile oil compounds in the plant which is being distilled. These water-soluble components are part of almost every essential oil to a greater or lesser degree and are taken into the water used, which becomes completely saturated at the prevailing temperature (Guenther 1948, vol. 1, p. 154) and thus they do not form part of the essential oil directly collected (see Water oil, below).

The essential oil constituents which are to some extent soluble in water are partially dissolved, thus forming an aqueous solution of the oil. These water-soluble constituents are mainly the oxygenated compounds (alcohols, aldehydes, etc.) which are heavier than the hydrocarbon compounds (monoterpenes, sesquiterpenes). For essential oils which have a relatively high proportion of water-soluble compounds (e.g. the high monetary value oils of melissa and rose) much of the precious essential oil would be lost in each fresh lot of water used. A system for the recovery of these 'lost' parts of the essential oil is imperative, and cohobation is just such a system.

Cohobation, in the original meaning of the word, is a system whereby the water in contact with the plant material (biomass) during the distillation process may be recirculated after condensation, thus increasing the opportunity for the water-soluble elements of the essential oil and the plant to pass into the water, which eventually reaches saturation point. At this stage no more of the essential oil hydrophilic components can be taken into solution/suspension by the water and all further essential oil molecules separate out from the water in the Florentine vase so that the complete essential oil is gained, usually floating on the now saturated hydrolat: 'Every aromatic substance has a maximum solubility in water and only after this point is reached will these aromatic compounds, the essential oils, start to separate into a distinct layer on top of the distillation water' (Schnaubelt 1999, p. xvi).

Cohobation by recirculating the water during the distillation process yields a water that is rich in some of the essential oil molecules. The quantity of distillation water collected is limited according to the kind of plant and the weight of plant material so that optimum quality is obtained (see distillation, above). For some plants, previously cohobated saturated water is used for the distillation of fresh plant material so that a complete essential oil can be obtained immediately.

To obtain a high therapeutic quality distilled water, the spring water used for the distillation passes through the selected plants several times, collecting water-soluble substances, and this makes it possible to obtain particularly concentrated floral waters, charged with active principles (Sanoflore 2000). Mojay (1996, p. 12) agrees that when the hydrolat is used to form the new distillation steam it becomes more concentrated in the process.

Water oil, recovered oil

The essential oil parts 'trapped' in the water during the distillation process can be extracted. This is known as 'water oil', to distinguish it from the essential oil collected from the Florentine vase directly. The hydrophilic oxygenated compounds retained in the distillation water tend to be heavier than the hydrocarbons and so the water oil generally has a higher relative density than direct essential oil. Distillation water contains not only oil in actual solution but also minute droplets in suspension and in emulsified form (Guenther 1948, p. 154). This can give the water a slightly milky appearance, confirming the presence of a small proportion of the oil. Hence the suggested derivation for the French word *hydrolat* as coming from water (*hydro*) and milk (*lait*).

To recover this water oil, the distillation water may in certain circumstances be pumped to a separate still with indirect heating, to be redistilled separately (for most distilled waters only 15% needs to be distilled off to recover most of the dissolved or suspended oil). This process of recovering the water oil from the aqueous distillate is, confusingly, also referred to as cohobation.

Rajeswara Rao et al (2002) cite the methods used to extract the dissolved essential oil from the aqueous distillate, yielding the water oil:

- cohobation (Gokhale 1959, Bohra et al 1994)
- extraction with diethyl ether (Bouzid et al 1997)
- adsorbing oil constituents on to an adsorbent followed by ethanol extraction (Bohra et al 1994, Machale et al 1997)
- poroplast technique (Fleisher 1991)
- hexane extraction followed by distillation of the hexane (Rajeswara Rao et al 2002).

Sometimes, to obtain a complete essential oil, it is more convenient to return the water to the still via a connecting system of pipework while the distillation process (described above) is going on; this is cohobation in its original sense.

Thus there are two quite distinct and different processes which, unfortunately, are both called cohobation:

1. The original method whereby the water is recirculated during the distillation process. This yields a complete direct essential oil plus a saturated hydrolat.
2. The second method involves the separate redistillation of the aqueous distillate. This yields the water oil and leaves a water devoid of any therapeutic value. The complete oil is achieved by adding the water oil which has been recovered from the hydrolat to the essential oil which has been directly collected.

Guenther (1948, p. 155) cites the work of Fölsch (1930a) to give an indication of the quantities of water oils which may be recovered by cohobation of some distilled waters (Table 6.1). This gives us some insight into the nature and possibilities of distilled plant waters.

Table 6.2 also indicates the average oil content, by weight percentage, in completed distillates, as established by von Rechenberg in 1910.

Various studies show that the oil lost to the water may be up to 30% of the total essential oil extracted from the plant. This amply demonstrates the fact that the condensate water following steam or water and steam distillation of plant biomass may be rich in plant compounds and therefore of practical use in therapy. Comparatively, the primary oil tends to be richer in hydrocarbons due to their low solubility in the distillation water (Machale et al 1997), whereas the secondary oil is relatively richer in oxygenated compounds. Oxygenated components contribute to the richness and fullness of the organoleptic profile of an essential oil (Fleisher 1991). In rose-scented geranium the 7% loss (mostly of oxygenated constituents) in the distillation water renders the primary oil incomplete in terms of organoleptic richness and fullness (Rajeswara Rao et al 2002).

Are cohobated waters therapeutically useful?

Opinion on this question is broadly split between the New World and the Old. A body of opinion in the USA holds that cohobated distilled waters are of no real

Table 6.1 Quantities of water oils recovered by cohobation

Plant material	*Quantity of water oil recovered from 1000 kg of distillation water (g)*	*% by weight*
Chamomile flowers	100–120	0.01–0.012
Coriander seed	625–650	0.062–0.065
Dill seed	360–450	0.04–0.045
Fennel seed	175–200	0.018–0.02
Lavender flowers	150–200	0.015–0.02
Peppermint	400–500	0.04–0.05
Sage	300	0.03
Tansy	540	0.054

Table 6.2 Average oil content of distillates (von Rechenberg 1910)

Plant material	*% Water oil (volatile oil in the water distillate)*
Ajowan seed	0.77
Angelica root, fresh	0.03
Angelica seed	0.19
Aniseed	0.81–1.16
Arnica flowers	0.001
Arnica root, dry	0.06
Bay leaves	0.75–0.77
Calamus root, dry	0.23–0.24
Calamus root, fresh	0.12
Caraway seed	2.22–3.04
Cedar wood	0.97–1.41
Celery seed	0.17
Chamomile flowers, dry	0.004–0.007
Cinnamon Ceylon	0.31–0.34
Cloves	0.60–0.86
Clove stems	1.03–1.52
Coriander seed	0.56–0.57
Costus root, dry	0.01
Cubebs	1.2
Cypress	0.12–0.2
Elecampane root	0.05
Fennel seed	1.42–2.08
Galangal root	0.05–0.08
Ginger root	0.28
Juniper berries	0.20
Lovage herb, fresh	0.02
Lovage root, dry	0.05
Lovage root, fresh	0.02
Patchouli leaves	0.12–0.13
Peppermint herb, fresh	0.11
Pimento berries	0.18
Sandalwood, East Indian	0.05–0.16
Sandalwood, West Indian	0.23–0.34
Savin	0.25–0.31
Vetiver root	0.015–0.02

therapeutic value while the belief in Europe is that they are indeed of great value. There is no research available at this time to support either view.

If cohobation is achieved by the method which involves recycling the hydrolat during the distillation process there is the possibility of artefacts being formed, since, when distilling aromatic plant material, there may be some decomposition of the non-volatile plant compounds which then find their way into the distillation water. These would produce dissolved impurities in the form of alcohols, aldehydes, ketones, short chain fatty acids, phenols and nitrogenous compounds and may be exacerbated by repetition of the heating and cooling cycle, leading not only to artefacts but also to polymerization.

For some oils, cohobation (by recirculation of the hydrolat) is regarded as a necessity and the distilled plant waters produced are not only of high quality but, because of their increased strength, are usually used diluted in some degree for therapeutic use. The cohobated waters must be obtained from a process where the recirculation of the water is controlled, for the reasons given above. If conditions are carefully monitored, cohobation during distillation does not make distilled waters therapeutically of no value, as some have claimed (e.g. Rose 1997, Catty 2001), otherwise that would rule out rose water (probably the most widely used distilled water) as being therapeutic; this is always produced using cohobation – method 1.

The following statements by Catty would hold true if the cohobation referred to were separate redistillation – method 2: 'The downside of cohobation is that the resulting hydrosol is nearly useless from a therapeutic point of view, as it contains almost no dissolved essential oil' (Catty 2001, pp. 28–29). She also says: 'Hydrosols are of better quality when essential oil is also produced in the distillation process. . . . If you want your hydrosol to have maximum therapeutic value, you should not cohobate' (Catty 2001, p. 63).

The reason put forward for this assertion is as follows:

> *The essential oils found in hydrosols are frequently in solution, meaning that they are not visible on the surface and do not separate out of the water. It is for this reason that a cohobated hydrosol is undesirable, since in cohobation the majority of the essential oil micro drops will bind together and become big enough to separate from the hydrosol, improving oil yield but reducing the therapeutic ingredients in the water. (Catty 2001, p. 13)*

However, the whole point of cohobation by recycling during the distillation process is to saturate the distillation water with the water-soluble molecules so that eventually a complete essential oil will be produced and can be directly collected in the Florentine vase. The distillation of plant material where the hydrolat is not recycled, not cohobated, produces a lot of water described as 'soft' and which contains some elements of essential oils which can be dissolved in water. This type of distillation unit is not very common as such units are not efficient and allow some of the essential oil to escape. Efficient stills cohobate, where the water is recycled and smells strongly of the original material, producing such wonderful water as rose water (Hephrun 2000a, p. 18).

Cohobation can improve the distillation process for plants which have little essential oil or an essential oil which has a high percentage of water-soluble compounds. For rose, melissa and orange flower, cohobation (method 1) is almost always used, producing very good quality distilled aromatic waters, so good in fact that for therapeutic use these particular waters are usually diluted to some degree. If cohobated waters are therapeutically useless, as claimed by Rose and Catty, then these three popular and widely used waters would be ruled out for therapeutic use simply because they are almost invariably produced using cohobation.

It is the authors' experience that with *Melissa officinalis*, it is certainly not possible to produce a whole melissa essential oil without cohobation because of the high percentage of water-soluble compounds in the essential oil. When cohobation is used some of the cohobated water is retained from one season to the next so that as soon as distillation begins a complete essential oil is produced the first and each time the still is charged with fresh plant material. Clearly in this case the distilled essential water remains saturated and therefore of good therapeutic quality and the above quoted statements do not hold good.

> *– From the theory of cohobation it should be clear that the cohobate should contain a higher concentration of volatile oil molecules, either dissolved or in the form of colloids (hydrosols). The reason for cohobation is to minimise the losses of oil from low yielding operations, particularly where the oil is very expensive, for example yarrow. Although the solubility of oils in water is relatively low, the amount of distillate is large and oil losses through it could be significant. Thus in stills which use water, not steam, cohobation is possible, and the distillate can be returned for further distillation. Since it is saturated with oil, no more oil is going to dissolve in it and the losses are thus cut to minimum. (I. Svoboda, personal communication, 2002)*

This means that the cohobated (by recycling) aromatic water is more strongly charged with volatile molecules than uncohobated water and so is therapeutically superior. On the other hand, were the separate redistillation method of cohobation used to extract the volatile molecules in a separate still (method 2), then the water would therapeutically be quite useless and the above statements by Catty and Rose would be true.

Conclusion

The water used in distillation retains in solution the volatile water-soluble molecules from the plant material. Therefore, to achieve a more concentrated hydrolat, the system should incorporate cohobation, where the water is recirculated during the distillation process and eventually becomes saturated with the volatile hydrophilic (polar) parts of the plant.

To sum up, it can be said that the introduction of controlled cohobation into the distillation process (i.e. recycling the water during the process) enriches and enhances, rather than detracts from, the therapeutic quality of the distilled plant waters. On the other hand, cohobation by redistillation results in a therapeutically useless hydrolat.

7

Physical aspects

- Introduction 55
- Temperature 55
- Time 56
- Preservatives 57
- Appearance 58
- Density 58
- pH 58
- Odour 58
- Quality 59
- Cost 59
- Conclusion 60

Introduction

The keeping qualities and shelf-life of hydrolats depend on the particular plant source and the conditions under which they are stored. General conditions of storage of hydrolats are that they must be stored in a cool place, in the dark (or at least out of sunlight), in suitably sterilized containers made of appropriate material (such as coloured glass or lined aluminium – some companies supply them in blue plastic bottles), protected from oxidation and kept at a constant temperature. If the proper storage conditions are not maintained some hydrolats tend to produce a mould, especially if they have not been well filtered; juniper berry, for example, is prone to mould, as is elderflower. As a general rule, hydrolats should be used up within 6 months to 1 year maximum; for example, the producers of Bulgarian rose water recommend that it be used within 1 year when it is stored in a coated steel barrel in cool conditions.

Temperature

Hydrolats need to be stored at a temperature of less than 14°C and in the shade, according to Viaud (1983, p. 24). Catty (2000) says that the life of hydrolats should be regarded as being similar to that of carrier oils; she gives similar limits on the storage temperature, giving a constant temperature of 12°C plus or minus 3°C without sudden fluctuations.

Some hydrolats are inclined to display flocculation (separation of suspended particles) when the storage temperature is somewhat higher than these limits, for example mistletoe and linden (lime). Such hydrolats gradually precipitate a whitish or greenish flocculation which is formed by microscopic particles of vegetal matter which sometimes multiply and form filaments like egg white (Montesinos 1991, p. 5). These vegetal particles belong to algae (*Protococcus, Haematococcus*), to fungi (*Hygrococcis*) and to bacteria (*Leptothrix, Micrococcus*), etc. The presence of bacteria in a normally slightly acid hydrolat indicates an advanced change; in a hydrolat which is normally neutral or alkaline their presence is proof of age only if the bacteria are abundant. It has been observed that, in certain hydrolats, the microorganisms produce some soluble colouring matter.

Flocculation may be got rid of by filtering or by the addition of a drop of lavender essential oil (Viaud 1983, p. 24). Another suggestion to correct these 'stringy' distilled waters is to add two or three drops of bismuth subnitrate, shake and filter; after this treatment the appearance of the hydrolats returns to normal and their quality is not affected. Montesinos (1991) advocates filtration from time to time during storage, preferably using 'glass cotton' instead of paper. Another source recommends storing hydrolats in 1 litre bottles, corked and laid in racks in a cellar so that the liquid covers the cork.

Time

In general the maximum period hydrolats should be stored, under the conditions given, must not exceed 1 year, since some are fragile and break down relatively quickly. They are therefore best purchased in small quantities. Rouvière & Meyer (1989, pp. 82–83), however, say that, while hydrolats from plants which do not contain any essential oil last only for a short time, those resulting from the distillation of plants for essential oils last for 2–3 years (echoing the authors' own experience); this is due to the presence of soluble compounds from the essential oils, which inhibit bacterial growth. As with the essential oils, not all hydrolats have the same useful life; those which keep best are the ones containing antiseptic phenols, for example the hydrolats of *Satureia hortensis, Thymus vulgaris* ct. thujanol-4 and *Origanum vulgare* can be kept for more than 2 years with no discernible change (Montesinos 1991, p. 7).

The authors have stored hyssop hydrolat for more than 4 years in their barn in the south of France (in the dark, the temperature fluctuating slowly with the seasons) and it is still of good appearance and aroma. This accords with the experience of Catty (1998a), that a constant temperature with little fluctuation is even more important than the constant nominal 14°C level, and temperatures as high as 18°C (65°F) seem to be acceptable provided they are constant. When storage conditions are such that the ambient temperature varies, especially on a short time scale, condensation can occur inside the storage containers and may cause deterioration of the hydrolats. Nasr (2000, p. 26) writes from personal experience that orange flower water used to be stocked in glass bottles and exposed to the strong rays of the sun for a whole day, changing the colourless hydrolat to a pale orange yellow colour. This was done to improve the keeping quality, and the hydrolat could then be stored for up to a year.

It is a well known fact, culled from the distillation of whisky, that during distillation copper is dissolved from stills made from that material. Copper is therefore likely to be present in waters distilled in copper stills and the amount will depend on the acidity of the water used for the distillation process and the time the water remains in contact with the still. Copper ions are known to be bacteriostatic (I. Svoboda, personal communication, 2002) and it is therefore true that the aqueous distillate from a copper still will stay fresh for longer than that from a still made of mild or stainless steel. If the pH of the water is quite low then organo-metallic ions will be present which will drag more ions from the plant into the water (P. A. Whitton, personal communication, 2003). However, copper is not always a suitable material for stills (see Ch. 6) as it is attacked by some plants containing azulenes. As well as copper, silver also is an antibacterial element and is currently used in some water filtration systems (Ryrie 1998, p. 68). The ancient Romans used to put a silver coin into a vessel which contained drinking water to keep it fresh. Before the 1940s and the introduction of newly discovered antibiotics, silver colloid was known and used worldwide as an antiseptic (Higher Nature 2002).

Preservatives

Essential oils can have a very long shelf-life, partly due to the types of chemical compounds that they contain. However, aqueous products are notoriously prone to go off as they have less 'natural' preservative than the essential oils. Therefore the handling and storage of hydrolats has to be undertaken with great care. They can undergo physicochemical changes, bringing about fluctuations in appearance, such as changes in colour and flocculation (appearing as cloudiness), and there may be an alteration in pH (due perhaps to biological changes involving the growth of microorganisms, e.g. bacteria, moulds, even algae) and the presence of an 'off' odour.

To minimize the chance of these unwelcome occurrences, some simple precautionary measures can be taken, as outlined above – i.e. protect the hydrolats from light, heat and moisture in sealed containers and ensure that they are used within 1 year of the container being opened. If hydrolats are handled under sterile conditions and stored in glass containers (also sterilized), this will favour optimum shelf-life. A spray top bottle minimizes contact with the ambient air and fingers. The conditions under which hydrolats are distilled can also have an influence (see Ch. 6, on distillation).

Ideally, hydrolats should not contain preservatives or stabilizers, as these could affect their therapeutic qualities. Many companies, however, for purely commercial reasons such as longer shelf-life and less stringent (therefore cheaper) storage conditions, add some sort of preservative. EEC regulations decree that hydrolats, which come under the regulation governing cosmetics, can no longer be sold commercially unless a preservative is added; as a result, most companies now supply aromatic waters (which may or may not be true hydrolats) with up to 14% ethanol incorporated. This means that such waters should not be used on or around the eyes or indeed on the skin, except with care, as alcohol is very drying to the skin.

Sometimes, it is at the request of particular customers that hydrolats are adulterated in this way, and preservatives such as potassium sorbate (a mould and yeast inhibitor), methyl iodide (a poison and a carcinogen) and propyl iodide are often incorporated at their behest. So far it seems that there is no natural preservative available which fulfils the exacting requirements of stabilizing and prolonging the shelf-life of hydrolats.

Appearance

Very few hydrolats possess a strong colour; most are clear and almost colourless, with only a slight, delicate coloration. An exception is cinnamon hydrolat, which is always opalescent. The following true colours were noted by Viaud (1983, p. 23) 1 month after distillation of the fresh plants:

Rosemary	Very pale grey-pink
Sage	Pale green-yellow
Gentian	Very pale violet becoming greenish-yellow
Soapwort	Strong carmine pink
Savoury	Very pale red
Tansy	Orange pink
Meadowsweet	Pale mauve
Eucalyptus	Light orange
Everlasting	Pale pink
Cornflower	Violet pink
Pine	Very pale violet
Melilot	Pale violet

Density

As hydrolats have a very low content of plant constituents the relative density is very close to 1.0.

pH

Hydrolats are usually neutral to slightly acid; sometimes they have a weak acid reaction owing to the volatiles contained in them, with a pH of between 5 and 6 (Montesinos 1991, p. 5). The lower the pH the more there is a tendency for the oil to emulsify into the water. A pH of 5.5 is considered to be optimum for use in face creams and lotions because it reduces the amount of preservatives needed. The acidity of the hydrolat is a useful indicator of its quality and periodic monitoring will bear witness to any change and possible deterioration.

Odour

It is not reasonable to expect that all hydrolats will have exactly the same aroma as the essential oils obtained from the same plants, since the two products contain a molecular mix which may differ markedly. The olfactive characteristics are peculiar either to the oil or to the hydrolat. The same plant molecules are unlikely to be present in the same proportions in both the hydrolat and the essential oil (see composition, Ch. 8), and so the odour of the hydrolat may well be very different from that of the essential oil. As with an essential oil, it is difficult to judge the quality of a hydrolat from the smell; as noted, a true distilled water does not necessarily smell the same as the oil from the same plant because it has a different chemical make-up – it contains some different molecules. The oxygenated compounds (alcohols, phenols, aldehydes, acids) especially are hydrophilic (partially or wholly water soluble) and will be present rather more in the water oil than in the direct essential oil. Their smell may be generally reminiscent of the original plant material, but this is not always the case – distilled lavender water, for example, often disappoints those who anticipate the typical lavender aroma.

When freshly distilled, essential oils usually have an odour and taste of the still due to the formation of artefacts, but this disappears fairly quickly, usually within 3 or 4 days. The same is true of freshly distilled hydrolats, and again the still note fades away in a short space of time. The hydrolat does not develop its typical aroma until after about 1 month of careful storage. If a distilled water becomes bad after a period of storage, then this is usually easily recognized by its malodorousness, even though it may appear normal.

Quality

The basic requirements for obtaining a good quality hydrolat are the same as those for procuring a genuine essential oil, i.e.: a known botanical species, grown organically or wild, with a known chemical make-up; the distillation must be of sufficient duration and at low pressure; and the resulting hydrolat must have had nothing added and nothing extracted. The ratio of weight of hydrolat to plant weight must be observed.

It is advisable that the only products used therapeutically should be those obtained during steam distillation and without colouring matter and alcohol. Products procured from a high street chemist's shop do not usually conform to this particular standard: they often contain synthetics to achieve a desired aroma or may even be entirely artificial. Natural hydrolats are sold with stabilizers and preservatives added and it would be interesting to see research done on the therapeutic value of hydrolats containing these antioxidants and free radical scavengers.

Cost

Unfortunately, the majority of hydrolats from plants distilled for their essential oils are discarded – most are allowed to run back into the earth/river beside the still, though in France legislation now requires the water to be treated before being discarded. Often hydrolats are saved only if they have been already ordered by a customer, because of the difficulties with storage explained above.

It is generally thought that because hydrolats are often thrown away, they should be inexpensive; this is not the case, as the costs associated with transporting the bulk, volume and weight of the product are reflected in the final cost to the customer.

Conclusion

The plant, or part of the plant, to be distilled, should be properly identified and preferably of known origin and the equipment used must be absolutely clean. The water used in the still influences the quality of the aqueous distillate, which should be collected in a container sterilized by steam before being transferred to smaller sterile containers, the smaller the better.

Conditions for storage must conform to good practice, and if this is done, some hydrolats will keep in good condition for 3 years; however, most last for a shorter time than this, even under good conditions. After opening the container, a life of 1 year at most can be expected.

8

Analysis

- How do we find out what is in hydrolats? 61
- Methods of extraction 61
- Discussion of the molecules found in waters analysed 63
- Part 1: Table of molecules found in waters 71 (analyses can be found in Appendix D)
- Part 2: Chemistry of aromatic molecules 76

How do we find out what is in hydrolats?

The basic task of monitoring hydrolats involves the detection of the organic components in the water, elucidating their identity and, if required, measuring their concentration.

Hydrolats can be injected directly into a gas chromatography (GC) column but this is not the preferred method. Some deactivation of the column can occur and water does not behave as an 'ideal' solvent. If the concentration of the components in the water were at the 2–3% level then direct injection might produce satisfactory results, but this is not the case with hydrolats.

Apart from the redistillation of the waters in a cohobation still, there are other methods of extracting the components gained during the distillation of the plant material. Usually it is necessary to 'concentrate' the components of interest by some method of enrichment or extraction prior to analysis by GC or GC-MS (gas chromatography-mass spectrometry).

Methods of extraction

Dr Bill Morden, a senior mass spectrometrist with the LGC at their laboratories in Runcorn, Cheshire, UK, describes some of the methods of extracting the water oil from the distillation water prior to analysis.

Liquid–liquid extraction

This is the most commonly used method of extraction. In its simplest form extraction may be performed by shaking the hydrolat with an organic solvent such as hexane, in a separating tunnel. Once the water and solvent have separated, the solvent containing the organic components may be run off, concentrated and analysed by gas chromatography-mass spectrometry (GC-MS). Liquid–liquid extraction can be time-consuming and often involves the use of toxic solvents. Moreover, the separation of the aqueous and organic phases can be prone to emulsion formation, a common problem in manual separation methods. Because the success of liquid–liquid extraction depends on the organic compounds in the aqueous phase being more soluble in the solvent, the choice of solvent can be problematic.

Solid phase extraction

Solid phase extraction can be used to remove organic compounds from waters. The principle is based on partitioning. The hydrolat is passed through a sorbent bed or membrane to retain the organic compounds, which are simply removed by washing with an organic solvent such as dichloromethane. Large volumes can be handled by relatively small amounts of sorbent, which in turn require only small amounts of solvents for extraction, obviating the need for solvent concentration. The method is suitable for components with low, medium or high polarities depending on the sorbent used, so it may be necessary to pass the hydrolat through different sorbent beds to extract the components of different polarities. The resultant solvent washings are combined, concentrated if necessary and analysed by GC-MS.

Liquid–solid partitioning

Liquid–solid partitioning, also known as solid phase partitioning, is particularly suited to hydrolats rich in polar components. The hydrolats are passed through specially treated resin beads which 'trap' the organic components. The resin is dried and the trapped components are eluted with an organic solvent, concentrated and analysed by GC-MS. More recently, the technique has been adapted so that the trapped components can be eluted by thermal desorption directly into a special inlet on the GC-MS system thus ensuring the highest degree of sample enrichment.

Purge and trap

This technique is of particular use in the extraction of non-polar components from a hydrolat. An inert gas, such as helium, is bubbled from a fine sinter through the hydrolat in a sealed system causing the purgeable organics to move from the aqueous phase into the gas phase. The helium and organic vapours are passed through a tube containing an adsorbent which traps out the organic compounds. The tube containing the trapped compounds is subjected to rapid heating which desorbs them from the adsorbent. Since the desorption takes between 1 and 5 minutes, the compounds are recondensed by cryogenics before being flash-heated into the inlet of the GC-MS for analysis. Purge and trap is suitable for the extraction of compounds with a wide range of polarities but is particularly useful for non-polar compounds.

Static and dynamic head space extraction

In static head space extraction the hydrolat is placed in a sealed vial and heated. The heating drives the organics out of the water and into the 'head space' where they can be sampled by a gas syringe for introduction into the GC-MS system for analysis. Static head space by its very nature implies that the sample is taken from one-phase equilibrium. In other words, the components that enter the head space do so depending on their vapour pressures. If the hydrolat is rich in volatile organics then they will predominate the head space. In order to overcome this limitation dynamic head space has been developed whereby the phase equilibrium is continuously displaced by purging the head space with helium. The eluents are trapped in the same manner as described in purge and trap.

Discussion of the molecules found in waters analysed

There appeared to be a significant difference in the concentration level of components in some of the waters compared with others; cornflower and viola water proved to be fairly low in organic compounds, whereas the waters of helichrysum and sage appeared to be highly charged.

Of the 33 waters analysed, the molecules eucalyptol (1,8-cineole) and linalool were the commonest and were each found in 30 of the waters under scrutiny. Others were acetone (found in 27 waters), α-terpineol (26), camphor (20) and dimethyl sulphide (17). A summary of molecules found in the waters tested is shown in Table 8.1, pp. 71–75.

The distilled plant waters differ in composition from the direct essential oils in many ways, for example the hydrolats contain a lot fewer hydrocarbons. Some monoterpene hydrocarbons were found, although in small amounts, such as sabinene (carrot, marjoram, geranium), alpha- and beta-pinene (carrot, geranium), alpha- and beta-phellandrene (angelica, geranium). Theoretically, no sesquiterpene hydrocarbons should be found in the waters, but some small amounts of caryophyllene (hyssop, melissa, clary sage) and germacrene D (hyssop, melissa, marjoram) were present.

A few ketones were found, such as pinocamphone and isopinocamphone (hyssop, marjoram), with acetone in abundance in addition to camphor; also there was a significant presence of carvone in costmary water, and a small amount in Roman chamomile. Thujone may also be found; according to Tyman (1990), thujone is not to be treated lightly, but there are four thujones, which may differ in their effects.

An analysis of a peppermint hydrolat which was the product of a specific distillation of the fresh plant, rather than the dried plant usually used, showed the chromatographic profile to be similar to that of an essential oil, particularly with respect to menthone and menthol (AGORA 2001).

Generally the waters tend to be more acidic than the oils because of the water solubility of plant acids, although practically no free acids were found in the waters analysed. Some of the acids which may be found in hydrolats are: geranic and acetic acids in rose water, cinnamic acid in cinnamon and isovaleranic acid in valerian (the direct essential oil of valerian – acid value 275 – is said to be less acid than that of the water oil – acid value 543). If during the analytical process dichloromethane is used to extract the volatiles from the hydrolat, then the free acids will be left in the water and so will not appear in the analysis (P. A. Whitton, personal communication, 2003).

Alkali

Ammonia is to be found in pepper water, producing an alkaline water.
Amines (water of *Chenopodium vulvaria* L.).

Alcohols

Linalool was the most commonly found compound in the three dozen waters tested, and others found were: lavandulol, methyl alcohol, ethanol, fenchyl alcohol, geraniol, α-terpineol, terpinen-4-ol (present in tea tree water oil at 86% compared with approximately 37% in the direct essential oil).

Ethanol

Properties:
allergenic (Mitchell & Rook 1979), anaesthetic (Borchard et al 1991), anhidrotic (Reynolds 1993, p. 784), pruritic (Reynolds 1993, p. 783), antiseptic (Reynolds 1993, p. 784; Winter 1984, p. 107), astringent (Reynolds 1993, p. 784), CNS-depressant (Winter 1984, p. 107; Reynolds 1993, p. 783), haemostatic (Reynolds 1993, p. 784), hepatotoxic (Reynolds 1993, p. 783), rubefacient (Winter 1984, p. 107; Reynolds 1993, p. 784), sclerosant (Reynolds 1993, p. 783), skin disinfectant (Reynolds 1993, p. 784), ulcerogenic (Reynolds 1993, p. 783).

Used in mouthwashes (Winter 1984, p. 107).

Fenchyl alcohol

Flavour (Beckstrom-Sternberg & Duke 1996, p. 395).

Geraniol

trans-3,7-dimethylocta-2,6-dien-1-ol
$(CH_3)_2C{=}CHCH_2{-}CH_2C(CH_3){=}CHCH_2OH$
Boiling point 230°C
Specific gravity 0.883
Molecular weight 154.25
Flash point 217°F

Colourless liquid of rose type odour. Widely distributed in essential oils, in both free state and esterified; isomeric with linalool. This alcohol is found in rose, gingergrass, palmarosa. It is separated from palmarosa, citronella and geranium oils. It has a sweet, floral, rosy, fruity aroma and is used as a base for many artificial floral aromas, and used together with phenylethyl alcohol in rose compounds for use in soaps.

Properties:
allergenic (Mitchell & Rook 1979), anticarcinogenic (Muroi & Kubo 1993, p. 1103), antiseptic (7 × phenol) (Wagner & Wolf 1977), antitumour (Yu et al 1995, p. 2144), bactericide (Muroi & Kubo 1993, p. 1103), cancer-preventative (Stitt 1990), candidicide (Beckstrom-Sternberg & Duke 1996, p. 397), embryotoxic (Beckstrom-Sternberg & Duke 1996, p. 397), emetic (3 × ipecac) (Beckstrom-Sternberg & Duke 1996, p. 397), flavour (Beckstrom-Sternberg & Duke 1996, p. 397), fungicide (Keeler & Tu 1991), herbicide (Keeler & Tu 1991), insectifuge (JSPR 1986), insectiphile, nematicide (Nigg & Seigler 1992), sedative (Wagner & Wolf 1977), spasmolytic (Buchbauer et al 1990).

Linalool

$(CH_3)_2C{=}CHCH_2CH_2\text{-}C(CH_3)(OH)CH{=}CH_2$
3,7-dimethylocta-1,6-dien-3-ol
Old name = Licareol
Boiling point 195–199°C
Specific gravity 0.859–0.867
Molecular weight 154.25
Flash point 175°F

Occurs in the free state in cayenne, Brazilian and Mexican linaloe, coriander and Ho oils and in the form of esters in numerous essential oils (see esters below). It is isomeric with geraniol and nerol. A colourless liquid with a soft, sweet odour, it is used in floral perfumes (e.g. lily, lilac, honeysuckle, sweet pea, rose, neroli).

Properties:
allergenic (Beckstrom-Sternberg & Duke 1996, p. 402), antiallergic (Huang 1993), anticarcinogenic (Muroi & Kubo 1993, p. 1103), antihistamine (Huang 1993), antiseptic (5 × phenol) (Wagner & Wolf 1977), antishock (Huang 1993), antiviral (Spring 1988, p. 65), bactericide (Muroi & Kubo 1993, p. 1103; Spring 1988, p. 65), bronchorelaxant (Huang 1993), cancer-preventative (Stitt 1990), candistat (Kang et al 1992, p. 2328), expectorant (Huang 1993), flavour (Beckstrom-Sternberg & Duke 1996, p. 402), fungicide (Acta Botanica, p. 49), insectifuge (Jacobson 1990, p. 213), motor-depressant (Beckstrom-Sternberg & Duke 1996, p. 402), nematicide (Shoyakugaku Zasshi, p. 183), sedative (Wagner & Wolf 1977), spasmolytic (Beckstrom-Sternberg & Duke 1996, p. 402), termitifuge (Jacobson 1990), viricide (Spring 1988, p. 65).

α-Terpineol

p-menth-1-en-8-ol
$C_{10}H_{17}OH$
Boiling point 218°C
Specific gravity 0.9364
Molecular weight 154.25
Flash point 195°C

Occurs in the essential oils of linaloe, geranium, bergamot, magnolia, gardenia, petitgrain, neroli and others. Prepared artificially on a large scale from turpentine. Used as the basis for lilac perfumes and in soaps. Found in the distilled water of *Pelargonium graveolens* 0–1.4%, it is given as being antiseptic (Winter 1984, p. 262).

Aldehydes

Hexanal

Used as flavouring.

Esters

Esters found in the waters tested were: linalyl acetate, bornyl acetate, lavandulyl acetate.

Linalyl acetate

$CH_3COOC_{10}H_{17}$
Boiling point 108-110°C
Specific gravity 0.908–0.920
Molecular weight 196.29
Flash point 85°C

Found in numerous essential oils including lavender, bergamot, petitgrain, clary sage, neroli, basil, rose, also in jasmin and gardenia. This is the most important ester. Linalyl acetate is a colourless liquid which has an aroma similar to deterpenated bergamot and is used in many perfumes – jasmin, lime blossom, ylang ylang and cologne. It has no known toxicity (Winter 1984, p. 161).

Properties:
flavour (Beckstrom-Sternberg & Duke 1996, p. 402), motor-depressant (Beckstrom-Sternberg & Duke 1996, p. 402), sedative (Beckstrom-Sternberg & Duke 1996, p. 402), spasmolytic (Taddei et al 1988, p. 465).

Myrtenyl acetate

Used in perfumery.

Bornyl acetate

Bornyl acetate has a strong pine odour (found in pine needles) and so is used in perfumery and flavouring (Winter 1999, p. 92); it can cause nausea if swallowed (Winter 1984, p. 206).

Properties:
antifeedant (Jacobson 1990 p. 213), bactericide (Harborne & Baxter 1983), expectorant (Harborne & Baxter 1983), insectifuge (Beckstrom-Sternberg & Duke 1996, p. 385); sedative (Beckstrom-Sternberg & Duke 1996, p. 385), spasmolytic (Taddei et al 1988, p. 465), viricide (Beckstrom-Sternberg & Duke 1996, p. 385).

Hydrocarbons

Sabinene: only one of the three carrot waters analysed contained sabinene, and then it was present at 50%, which is curious. The sabinene presence in geranium water is significantly higher than in the essential oil and in marjoram it was 27%. Other hydrocarbons found were:

monoterpenes: α-pinene, β-pinene, α-phellandrene, β-phellandrene
sesquiterpenes: caryophyllene, germacrene-D.

Pinene

Properties:
antiseptic (Spring 1988, p. 65), bactericide (Spring 1988, p. 65), expectorant (Spring 1988, p. 65), fungicide (Lydon & Duke 1989), herbicide (Lydon & Duke 1989), spasmogenic (Taddei et al 1988, p. 465), spasmolytic (Taddei et al 1988, p. 465).

α-Pinene

Properties:
allelochemic, allergenic (Mitchell & Rook 1979), antiflu (Economic and Medicinal Plant Research, p. 195), antiinflammatory (International Journal of Oriental

Medicine 1990, p. 194), antiviral (Economic and Medicinal Plant Research, p. 195), bactericide (Rivista Italiana Eppos 1994, p. 5), cancer-preventative (Stitt 1990), expectorant (Castleman 1991), herbicide (Keeler & Tu 1991), insectifuge (Jacobson 1990, p. 213), irritant (Harborne & Baxter 1983), sedative (Beckstrom-Sternberg & Duke 1996, p. 379), tranquillizer (Beckstrom-Sternberg & Duke 1996, p. 379).

β-Pinene

Properties:
allergenic (Mitchell & Rook 1979), herbicide (Keeler & Tu 1991), insectifuge (Jacobson 1990); also used as a flavour and in perfumery.

Sabinene

Used in perfumery.

Caryophyllene

Properties:
anticarcinogenic (Muroi & Kubo 1993, p. 1103), antioedemic (Shimizu et al 1990, p. 2283), antifeedant (Keeler & Tu 1991), antiinflammatory (Shimizu et al 1990, p. 2283), antitumour (Zheng et al 1992, p. 999), bactericide (Kang et al 1992, p. 2328), flavour, insectifuge (Jacobson 1990), spasmolytic (Jacobson 1990), termitifuge (Jacobson 1990).

Germacrene-D

Pheromonal (Beckstrom-Sternberg & Duke 1996, p. 397).

Ketones

Ketones found were:

Acetone (found in the majority of the waters analysed).
Camphone: *iso*pinocamphone and pinocamphone.
Camphor was found in two-thirds of the waters tested.
Carvone which is present in the distilled water at almost double the level in the direct essential oil. Pinocarvone and pinocamphone tend to co-elute during the analytical process and so are difficult to discriminate. The combined figure for them in *Chamaemelum nobile* (Roman chamomile) water is 6.5% (in the essential oil the figure is 1.6%).
Thujones: *cis*-thujone, *trans*-thujone; *alpha*- and *beta*-thujone were found in yarrow and costmary waters.

Acetone

Properties:
allergenic (Mitchell & Rook 1979), CNS-depressant (Reynolds 1993, p. 1099), narcotic (Reynolds 1993, p. 1099).

Used as a solvent in nail polish removers, fats, oils and waxes. It can cause splitting of the nails, skin rashes; inhalation may irritate the lungs (Winter 1984, p. 16). It is said that acetone is not normally present in sufficient quantity in distilled waters to cause any problem: it is present at more than 10% in lavender water oil, almost 20% in angelica, melissa and purple coneflower, almost 30% in bladderwrack, and was found in three-quarters of the distilled waters studied.

Camphor

Properties:

Camphor gives a cool feeling to the skin and is an antiseptic, anaesthetic and is readily absorbed through the skin; may cause allergic reaction (Winter 1984, p. 59). allelopathic (Russell 1986), analgesic (Reynolds 1993, p. 1348), anaesthetic (Spring 1988, p. 65), antiacne (Nigg & Seigler 1992), antiemetic (Huang 1993), antifeedant (Lydon & Duke 1989), antineuralgic (Reynolds 1993, p. 1348), antipruritic (Reynolds 1993, p. 1348), antiseptic (Reynolds 1993, p. 1348), CNS-stimulant (Spring 1988), cancer-preventative (Stitt 1990), carminative (Reynolds 1993, p. 1348), convulsant (Huxtable 1992), counterirritant (Reynolds 1993, p. 1348), decongestant (Nigg & Seigler 1992), emetic (Reynolds 1993, p. 1348), expectorant (Reynolds 1993, p. 1348), fungicide (Keeler & Tu 1991), herbicide (Lydon & Duke 1989), irritant (Reynolds 1993, p. 1348), nematicide (Shoyakugaku Zasshi 45: 270), oculoirritant (Mitchell & Rook 1979), respirainhibitor (Reynolds 1993, p. 1348), rubefacient (Reynolds 1993, p. 1348), spasmolytic (Taddei et al 1988, p. 465), stimulant (Huxtable 1992), verrucolytic (Beckstrom-Sternberg & Duke 1996, p. 386).

Carvone

Properties:

allergenic (Mitchell & Rook 1979), antiseptic (Wagner & Wolf 1977), CNS-stimulant (Stitt 1990), cancer-preventative (Stitt 1990), carminative (Yamamoto et al 1994; Winter 1999, p. 113), insecticide (Jacobson 1990), insectifuge (Jacobson 1990), motor-depressant (Beckstrom-Sternberg & Duke 1996, p. 387), nematicide (Shoyakugaku Zasshi 44: 183), sedative (Beckstrom-Sternberg & Duke 1996, p. 387), stimulant (Winter 1999, p. 113), vermicide (Beckstrom-Sternberg & Duke 1996, p. 387). *(+)-carvone* is an ACE-inhibitor.

Carvone, in spite of being a ketone, is reported to have a very low toxicity (Budavari 1996, pp. 308, 1603) while Winter (1999, p. 113) reports that carvone has no known toxicity.

Thujone

Too high a dose of thujone can have a paralysing action (Duraffourd 1987). There are different configurations possible for the thujone molecule (Tyman 1990) and not all spatial arrangements may have the same effects.

Properties:

anthelmintic (Harborne & Baxter 1983), bactericide (Journal of Essential Oil Research 7: 271), cerebrodepressant, convulsant (Huxtable 1992), counterirritant (Harborne & Baxter 1983), epileptigenic (Beckstrom-Sternberg & Duke 1996, p. 418), hallucinogenic (Beckstrom-Sternberg & Duke 1996, p. 418), perfumery, respirainhibitor (Beckstrom-Sternberg & Duke 1996, p. 418), spasmolytic (Taddei et al 1988, p. 465), toxic (Beckstrom-Sternberg & Duke 1996, p. 418).

β-Thujone

Considered to be an insectifuge.

Oxides

Eucalyptol (1,8-cineole) is present in sage essential oil at between 5% and 14% whereas the water oil has 55%. It was present in all but three of the waters analysed: other oxides were found in the waters at low level (0.1–3%).

cis- and *trans*-carvone oxides in costmary
cis- and *trans*-linalyl oxides in orange flower water, rose
caryophyllene oxide in horsetail, lavender, wild marjoram
linaloyl oxide in helichrysum, lavender, geranium, clary, thyme linalool
cis- and *trans*-linalool oxide in lavender, lavandin, spike lavender, myrtle
nerol oxide is found in helichrysum, lavender, rose
cis- and *trans*-rose oxide in melissa, myrtle, geranium, rose.

1,8-Cineole

1,8-cineole – synonym: eucalyptol
$C_{10}H_{18}O$
Found in many essential oils in the Eucalypt and Melaleuca families, and spike lavender, basil, rosewood, etc.
Boiling point 177°[F]
Specific gravity 0.9267
Camphor-like odour, spicy, cooling taste.

Properties:
Cineole is widely used in pharmaceutical preparations. Internally it acts as a stimulating expectorant in cases of chronic bronchitis, etc. Locally, cineole is a mild anaesthetic and antiseptic in the treatment of inflammatory conditions (Guenther 1949, p. 710).

ACE-inhibitor (Beckstrom-Sternberg & Duke 1996, p. 377), allelopathic (Russell 1986), allergenic (Mitchell & Rook 1979), anaesthetic (Beckstrom-Sternberg & Duke 1996, p. 377), anthelmintic (Harborne & Baxter 1983), antiallergic (J. Food Hyg. Soc. Jap. 33(6): 569), antibronchitic (Beckstrom-Sternberg & Duke 1996, p. 377), anticatarrh (Reynolds 1993, p. 1354), antirhinitic (Beckstrom-Sternberg & Duke 1996, p. 377), antiseptic (Harborne & Baxter 1983), antitussive (Beckstrom-Sternberg & Duke 1996, p. 377), bactericide (Journal of Essential Oil Research), CNS-stimulant (Beckstrom-Sternberg & Duke 1996, p. 377), expectorant (Harborne & Baxter 1983), fungicide (Beckstrom-Sternberg & Duke 1996, p. 377), hepatotonic (Beckstrom-Sternberg & Duke 1996, p. 377), herbicide (Keeler & Tu 1991), hypotensor (Beckstrom-Sternberg & Duke 1996, p. 377), insectifuge (Jacobson 1990), nematicide (Nigg & Seigler 1992), perfume, rubefacient (Reynolds 1993, p. 1354), sedative (Ortiz de Urbina et al 1989, p. 165).

Phenols

Phenols were not found to any great extent in the waters tested. Carvacrol was present in *Balsamita suaveolens* (costmary) 0.1% and thymol in *Echinaceae purpurea* 0.2%, *Plantago major* 3.1%. The percentage of phenolic compounds, particularly carvacrol, in thyme essential oil is much less than that in the water oil.

Sulphides

An interesting fact is that in some of the hydrolats analysed there was a significant presence of dimethyl sulphide but the origin is unclear. Sulphides occur frequently in plants, probably in the form of glucosides which are decomposed by the process of distillation. It has been suggested (W. Morden, personal communication, 2003) that sulphides and dimethyl sulphide may possibly arise from any of the sulphur-containing amino acids, or the presence of iron pyrites (FeS_2) in the biomass. Dimethyl sulphide is found in rue, garlic, leek and the molecule $CH_3.CH_2.S.S.CH_2.CH_3$ is in garlic and onion (N. Revillion, personal communication, 2003).

Dimethyl sulphide

$(CH_3)_2S$ Used as a flavouring agent.

Hydrogen sulphide (H_2S) appears during the distillation of certain seeds: for example aniseed and caraway. Dimethyl sulphide occurs in American peppermint oil and is routinely removed by rectification to improve the odour of the oil. It is also found in geranium oils from Algeria and Réunion; sulphur is present in garlic and onion (Guenther 1949).

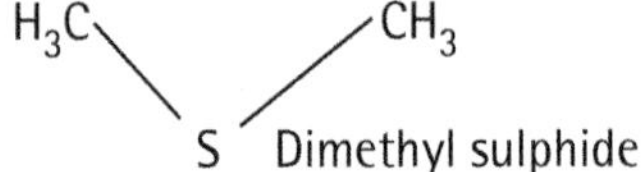

Dimethyl sulphide

Dimethyl sulphide was found in seventeen of the hydrolats tested, notably melissa 75%, nettle 71%, meadowsweet 70%, bladderwrack 60%, hawthorn 42%, horsetail 26%, St John's wort 25%, plantain 23%. Dimethyl sulphide can help break down ketones in the body because the sulphur atom latches on to the double-bonded oxygen of the ketone, opening the double bond; this helps to reduce the toxicity of ketones which would otherwise have to be metabolized by the body to deal with the toxicity (P. A. Whitton, personal communication, 2003).

Part 1: Table of molecules found in waters

Table 8.1 lists the water tested and summarizes the molecules found. Analyses of the water can be found in Appendix D.

Table 8.1 Summary of molecules found in the tested water

	Latin name	Common name	KETONES							
			Acetone	2-Butanone	Camphor	Hexanone isomers	Pino-camphone	Isopino-carvone	Carvone	Pino-carvone
1	*Achillea millefolium*	Yarrow			11.7		3.5–3.6			3.5
2	*Angelica archangelica*	Angelica	17.4	0.7	1.2	0.2				
3	*Balsamita suaveolens*	Costmary						0.1	75.0	0.6
4	*Calendula officinalis*	Marigold	0.7							
5	*Centaurea cyanus*	Cornflower	5.6		4.7					
6	*Chamaemelum nobile*	Roman chamomile	1.4	1.3	1.5		<6.5		<6.5	
7	*Citrus aurantium* (flos)	Orange flower								
8	*Crataegus oxyacantha*	Hawthorn	3.8							
9	*Equisetum arvense*	Horsetail	3.1		0.2	0.5			0.1	
10	*Daucus carota*	Carrot	1.5–2.2	0.5		0.4				
11	*Echinaceae purpurea*	Purple cone flower	17.4		0.4					0.7
12	*Filipendula ulmaria*	Meadowsweet	6.8	1.5	7.0					
13	*Fucus vesiculosus*	Bladderwrack	27.8							
14	*Helichrysum angustifolium*	Everlasting	0.7–5.8	0.5–4.1	0.2–0.4	30.2–35.7				
15	*Hypericum perforatum*	St John's wort	13.5	3.2						
16	*Hyssopus officinalis*	Hyssop					4.7–30.4	48.2–91.4		
17	*Juniperus communis* (fruct.)	Juniper berry	1.8	0.3		3.9			0.4	
18	*Lavandula angustifolia*	Lavender	2.2–10.1		1.0–2.4	2.7				
19	*Lavandula* x *intermedia* 'Grosso'	Lavandin grosso			0.8–11.0					
20	*Lavandula latifolia*	Spike lavender			32.3					
21	*Melaleuca alternifolia*	Tea tree								
22	*Malva sylvestris*	Mallow	10.2	5.1	0.3	0.9				
23	*Matricaria recutita*	German chamomile	1.0	0.9	<2.03	0.6	3.0			
24	*Melilotus officinalis*	Melilot	0.3		15.7					
25	*Melissa officinalis*	Lemon balm	1.8–19.8	2.1				0.6		
26	*Mentha* x *piperita*	Peppermint								
27		Wild marjoram	3.0				5.3	<24.6		
28	*Pelargonium graveolens*	Geranium	0.4–1.2							
29	*Pinus sylvestris*	Scots pine	9.6	1.9	6.6	0.3	3.0***			
30	*Plantago major*		0.5		1.6					
31	*Salvia officinalis*	Sage	0.1–1.5	0.3	24.5–28.7					
32	*Rosa damascena*	Damask rose	1.5–1.9		2.0					
33	*Rosmarinus off.* ct. verbenone	Rosemary verbenone			44.1		1.1			
34	*Salvia sclarea*	Clary	0.6							
35	*Thymus vulgaris* ct. linalool	Sweet thyme	1.6		3.1					
36	*Urtica dioica*	Nettle	0.5	0.8	7.5					
37	*Viola tricolor arvensis*	Heartsease			30.0					

*** two isomers

(Table 8.1 continued overpage)

(Table 8.1 - continued from previous page)

	KETONES		ALCOHOLS							
	3-octanone	Thujone	Endo-Borneol	Borneol	Cis-carveol	Transpino-carveol	Ethanol	Frenchyl Alcohol	Geraniol	Lavandulol
1	0.8–0.9	α- 2.2	2.8						0.7	
2			0.7							
3		α- 6.2 β- 0.6		0.4	2.2					
4									1.4	
5				4.5						
6	15.4		1.3			21	0.5			
7										
8										
9	1.0		0.5						1.3	
10										
11										
12							6.4			
13										
14				0.6			0.7–2.3	0.4		
15							5.0			
16	0.3	*cis* 0.4–0.5 *trans* 0.3–0.4							1.3	
17	0.3	*cis* 0.3 *trans* 1.5								
18	0–4.8			1.0–4.3					0.9–6.0	1.1–3.5
19	0.1–0.3			1.4–2.3					3.3–5.5	1.0–1.4
20	tr			2.3					1.8	<0.1
21										
22							1.6			
23	2.3								1.4	
24		*cis* 9.9 *trans* 2.8								
25	0.5–1.1		1.9						<12.4?	
26										
27	0.3–4.5								0.9	
28									1.0–38.4	
29	1.3		2.1					2.2		
30	4.9	*cis* 1.6 *trans* 0.3							1.6	
31	0.1	*cis* 8.4–8.6 *trans* 1.8–2.2	1.3–1.5				0.1			
32							up to 10.2**		14.1–27.9	
33	0.7		5.5					2.1		
34									0.6	
35				0.5					2.5	
36		*cis* 0.2	0.1				0.6			
37		*cis* 4.0 *trans* 0.3	3.9							
							** Max 4 Bulgarian			

ALCOHOLS					OXIDES			HYDROCARBONS		
Linalool	Nerol	α- and β-Terpineol	α-Terpineol	Terpinen-4-ol	Caryophyllene oxide	Eucalyptol (1,8-Cineole)	Nerol oxide	Cadinene	Caryophyllene	
1.1–8.8			0.7–2.8			50.0–64.2				1
53.1			1.8			6.5				2
0.1				0.3		3.5		delta tr		3
57.0			3.0			5.5				4
15.6–61.3			7.2–11.0			4.0–9.2				5
13.6			0.9			15.8				6
9.4			9.4							7
45.3			1.2			0.6				8
53.3	0.5		3.6			0.3			0.7	9
0.4–31.8			3.1–7.5			0.3–3.9				10
2.3			0.8			4.4				11
						3.3				12
6.1			1.5			1.0				13
11.2	0.7		6.5			4.5–14.4	2.1			14
						0.8				15
0.5–3.8						1.4–1.6			1.6	16
3.7			5.1			0.5				17
19.9–68.3	0.5–1.8	4.3–7.4	4.4–23.5	1.9–27.0	0.2–3.1	1.1–6.4	1.4		0.1–2.4	18
55.7–68.5	1.1–1.7	7.3–9.0		4.3–4.4		1.6–4.5			0.1	19
22.7	0.6	5.0		0.8		29.1			0.1	20
0–0.1			7.3–8.6	86		2.9–4.4				21
5.5			0.2			1.4				22
12.8						2.2				23
2.6			1.2			25.9				24
1.5–5.8					3.9			δ- 1.1	2.8–12.5	25
0.1–0.8	0.1		0.5		0.4	0.5–4.6			a 5.7 b 3.7	26
0.2–2.7					1.1	tr–3.8		d- 2.6	18.8	27
13.1–36.5	0.1–0.2		0–4.8			0–0.5				28
7.8–11.3			14.1–52.2			36.5				29
43.9	0.6		1.1			5.0				30
1.2			1.0–1.1			50.6–55.4				31
3.3–21.8	7.2–26.8		1.3–2.8							32
4.2			2.0			5.1				33
10.5–44.7	0.3		1.5–3.6			0.2			2.0	34
71.4	1.2		14.5			1.5				35
						3.7				36
23.5			3.2			19.4				37

(Table 8.1 continued overpage)

(Table 8.1. - continued from previous pages)

	HYDROCARBONS								COUMARIN	SULPHIDE	ALDEHYDES	
	Cymene isomers	Germacrene-D	Limonene	α-phellandrene	β-phellandrene	α-pinene	β-pinene	Sabinene	Coumarin	Dimethyl sulphide	Hexanal	2- propan
1			1.1								2.9	3.6
2	0.2–0.3			0.8	1.3					2.5		
3												
4												0.5
5												
6						0.3					1.5–4.7	
7												
8										42.5		
9										25.7		
10	<2.1		1.9–8.0			3.6–24.0	1.9–9.3	0–50.2		1.2	4.5	3.5
11	1.1									<5.5	15.6	
12										69.9		
13										60.1		
14	3.3		1.4							0.3		
15				7.8				<4.3		25.7	2.5	
16		7.5					0.5–3.1					1.5
17	0.1–0.4				1.6							
18	0–0.3		0.1–1.7		4.3		0.1–0.6		0.2–2.2	1.0	0–0.2	0.6
19			0.6–4.7				0.1		<0.1			
20							0.3		<0.1			
21												
22												
23												2.1
24										9.1		
25		4.2								75.4	1.1	0.7–
26												
27	3.05	14.8			0.4	0.4	0.3	27.1			0.1	9.8
28	4.6		0.1–3.4	0–4.6	0.2–2.8	0.5–1.6	0.6–2.6	0.4–6.2			0–1.3	0.2
29			0.3							0.7		
30										23.4		
31										0.3–1.2		0.4
32	<6.4		21.9*	3.5	*21.9							
33												
34		4.4			0.3							0.6
35												
36										71.5		
37										1.7		

*Limonene + β-phellandrene

ALDEHYDES		ACETATES			
3-Methyl-butanal	2-Methyl-butanal	Bornyl acetate	Lavandulyl acetate	Linalyl acetate	
4.9	2.9				1
		0.8			2
					3
0.8			0.4–3.1		4
					5
5.1	3.0				6
					7
					8
		0.3			9
19.9	9.9	*endo-* 0.8–12.6		0.2	10
10.4	7.59?				11
					12
					13
0.7–1.2	1.3–5.5	0.2			14
8.3	1.8?				15
0.5–0.8	0.3–0.4			0.5	16
					17
1.2?	0.5		0.5–6.5	0.1–41.8	18
				0.1	19
				0.1	20
					21
					22
			43.9		23
		1.2			24
4.1–19.8	12.9			12.4	25
					26
14.2	7.4				27
0.3	0.2				28
		0.9			29
					30
		0.3			31
					32
		endo- 12.43			33
1.1	1.0		0.4–0.5	76.1	34
0.4					35
					36
					37

Part 2: Chemistry of aromatic molecules

A smattering of chemistry

Water plays a central part in hydrolats (distilled plant waters) and the nature and structure of water is discussed in Chapter 3. Here we attempt to understand the chemical structure of the hydrophilic compounds found in the hydrolats, and to help us with this a little basic chemistry is set out below.

Organic and inorganic chemistry

When hydrolats are under consideration we are involved in both organic and inorganic chemistry. *Organic* chemistry, also called the chemistry of the carbon compound, concerns the three basic building blocks of life: namely, carbon (chemical symbol C), hydrogen (H), which occurs in heavenly bodies and the sun, and oxygen (O), which is one-fifth of the world's atmosphere and accounts for nine-tenths of our own human bodies. All three occur in abundance in nature. The plant essential oils and the plant molecules found in the hydrolats used in aromatherapy are composed chiefly of these three basic building blocks in differing combinations. Others are nitrogen (N), which is four-fifths of the world's atmosphere, sulphur (S) and phosphorus (P). All of these – C, H, O, N, S, P – are present in DNA and all living things.

The dead (never living) part of the world (e.g. water, salt) is covered by that part of chemistry known as *inorganic* chemistry, which is a much smaller branch of chemistry; there are about 100 000 inorganic compounds known, compared to over 1 million organic compounds.

Atoms

The origin of the word atom (from the Greek *tom* (*temnein*) = to cut, *a* = not) indicates that the atom, when first discovered, was thought of as indivisible: it is now known that each atom consists of a number of smaller particles, such as electrons, protons and neutrons, and that it can be split up.

An atom has size, shape and weight and consists of a *nucleus* at the centre with *electrons* in orbit around it. The nucleus, which can be regarded here as a minute particle that cannot be divided, is very small and the electrons in orbit are even tinier, and so most of the volume occupied by the atom is actually empty space, as the diameter of an atom is about 10 000 times that of the nucleus – to give an idea, if the nucleus were the size of a pea, then the atom would be about 200 feet (65 metres) in diameter. This means that all material, even our own body, is 99.9% empty space.

In the nucleus there are positively charged bodies called *protons*, and neutral bodies called *neutrons*.

For example, within the nucleus of the helium atom (Fig. 8.1) there are two protons – which have a positive electric charge, and two neutrons – which are neutral, having no electric charge. The electrons and protons, with their negative and positive charges respectively, are equal in number in an atom, therefore the whole atom is electrically neutral. As far as weight (mass) is concerned, that of a proton or neutron is 1840 times greater than that of an electron, so the weight of the electrons can be ignored.

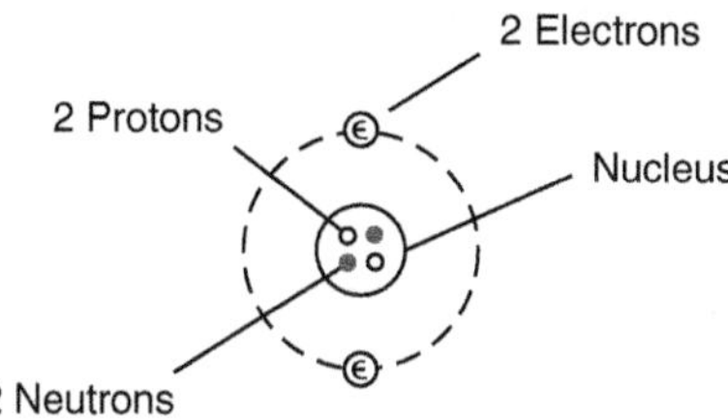

Figure 8.1 Helium atom; two protons, two neutrons, two electrons.

Remember when looking at a diagram such as Figure 8.1 that it is merely a poor two-dimensional representation of a three-dimensional energetic, vibrant entity.

The electrons in an atom occupy a series of concentric zones (called energy shells or orbitals) around the nucleus; the electrons in the shells nearest to the nucleus have less energy than those further away. The shell nearest the nucleus can accommodate two electrons, the next shell eight electrons, and we can consider the third energy shell also as accommodating eight electrons. If the outer shell does not contain all the electrons of which it is capable, then the scene is set for chemical reactions to take place, because the law of molecular stability is that all atoms seek to have their outer orbitals filled. Once filled to capacity, stability is achieved and no further reaction can take place.

For the atom to achieve stability and be in a state of equilibrium, each shell should have the requisite number of electrons. In the case of hydrogen (Fig. 8.2), for the first shell two electrons are needed to give a state of equilibrium; as the hydrogen atom has only one, it is necessary for this hydrogen atom to join with

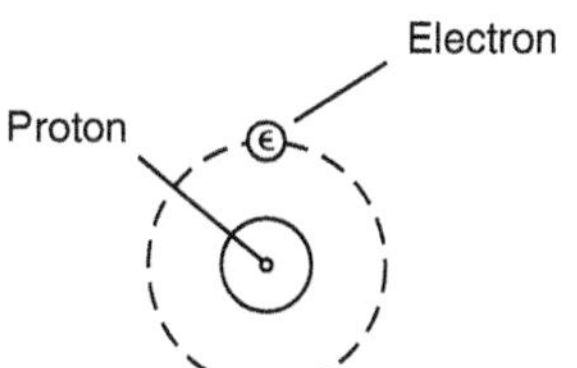

Figure 8.2 Hydrogen atom.

another atom to gain access to another electron: thus if it joins with another hydrogen atom a hydrogen molecule is formed (Fig. 8.3).

Bonds between atoms: molecules

A molecule is two or more atoms joined together and acting as a single entity. How does this molecule hold itself together?

Atom plus atom = molecule

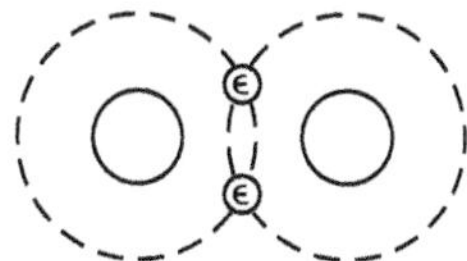

Figure 8.3 Hydrogen molecule, single bond (H–H).

The atoms bond together in a variety of ways to maintain this togetherness:

- by sharing of electrons (*covalent* bond) as in the hydrogen molecule above
- by mutual attraction due to the loss or gain of electrons (*electrovalent* or *ionic* bond)
- by means of the *hydrogen* bond, discussed in Chapter 3, on water.

Single/double bonds

If an atom shares an electron with another atom then it is said to be a *single* bond, as in the case of the hydrogen molecule (see Fig. 8.3) where there are two hydrogen atoms sharing a pair of electrons (H–H).

It is possible for two atoms to share *two* pairs of electrons between them and this is known as a *double* bond: double bonds provide a certain rigidity to the molecule because they are not as flexible as single bonds.

A double bond makes for a rigid molecule which cannot deform, has no opportunity for rotation and has a definite shape. This rigidity is a feature which is easily attacked by light and oxygen causing rancidity. Carbon dioxide and oxygen are examples of molecules with double bonds.

O=C=O	carbon dioxide, two double bonds
O=O	oxygen molecule, one double bond

Bonds show stability of a substance, and this includes essential oils and hydrolats. When two atoms share a pair of electrons and have a single bond, it is a dynamic relationship with three possible ways of changing shape:

1. Constantly moving away from and towards each other, but there are limits with a minimum and a maximum distance deviation
2. Atoms can move slightly up or down as well as sideways
3. Rotation round the bond can occur causing distortion.

Thus most molecules have a flexible shape and any therapeutic qualities which are related to molecular shape are variable. This perhaps helps to explain how most volatile molecules found in essential oils and hydrolats can have a positive therapeutic effect on many diverse problems.

Electrovalent or ionic bond

This type of bond means that there is a transference of electrons from one atom to another: a donation of electron(s) can take place between atoms which means that although the atoms are then stable each atom now has an electrical charge. If we look at the example of salt, made up of chlorine and sodium atoms, we see that the sodium gives one electron and chlorine receives this gift of one electron with its negative charge, with the result that the sodium atom now has a positive charge and the chlorine atom has a negative charge. Consequently they are attracted to each other, and this bond between them is called an electrovalent bond (also known as an ionic bond). However, *ionic compounds do not occur in essential oil compounds* (Clarke 2002, p. 20).

Covalent bond

This type of bond means that to form the molecule there is a sharing of electrons between atoms of different elements, for example hydrogen and carbon. The simplest example is the hydrogen molecule. In this case each atom has only one electron and the simple solution to their problem of stability is to share electrons with each other. This is the covalent bond, a very strong type of bond; the compounds found in essential oils and the carrier oils are all covalently bonded (Clarke 2002, p. 22). The hydrogen, carbon dioxide and oxygen molecules shown above are all examples of covalent bonding, as also is the methane molecule (see Fig. 8.5).

The carbon atom (Fig. 8.4) has six electrons. It satisfies the stability requirement of having two electrons in its first shell, but to be stable it also needs eight electrons in its second shell, and only has four. Four more are needed: one solution is to combine with four hydrogen atoms for mutual sharing of the electrons (Fig. 8.5).

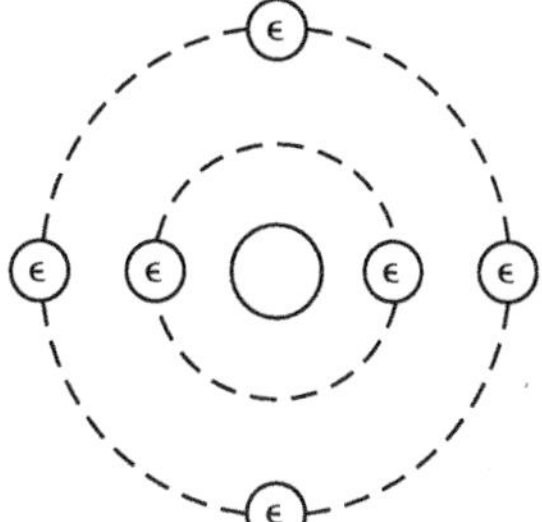

Figure 8.4 Carbon atom.

Now we have the situation where each hydrogen atom has two electrons in its orbit shell, and the carbon atom has eight in its outer orbit shell, so all are satisfied due to this system of sharing electrons, producing a stable system.

To describe a molecule in the simplest way we need only count the number of each kind of atom in the molecule. In the example given, one carbon atom and four

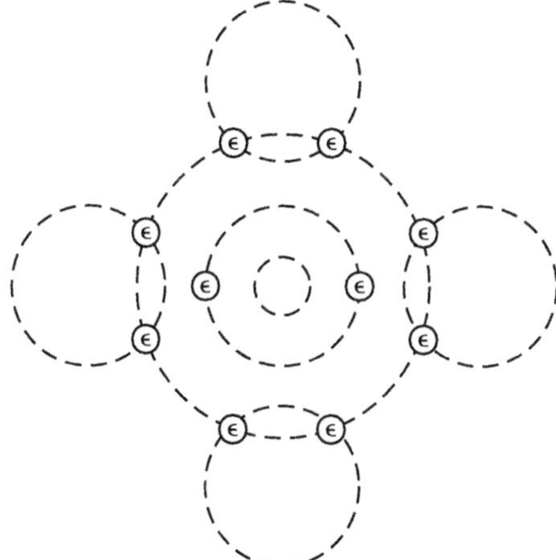

Figure 8.5 Methane molecule (CH_4).

hydrogen atoms together form the molecule, i.e. one C (for carbon) plus four Hs (for the hydrogen atoms), or – in the rather neat special shorthand adopted by chemists – CH_4. The molecule CH_4 is a gas.

Graphic representation

Molecules can also be written in a graphic way which is simple to understand and gives some idea of the possible shape of the molecule and this is the style adopted in this book. Figure 8.6 is a graphic representation of the same molecule as the one in Figure 8.5. This is only a crude representation for it has to be borne in mind that this is an attempt to represent a three-dimensional molecule on a two-dimensional page; it cannot be done with complete success.

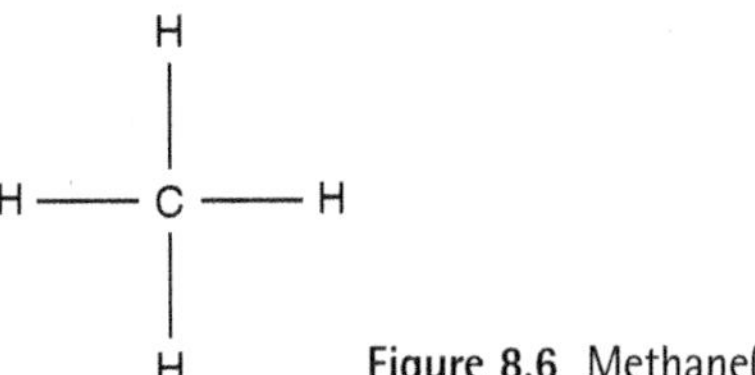

Figure 8.6 Methane(Ch_4).

Carbon atoms have the unique capacity to join with other carbon atoms in straight and branched chains, to give rise to C_2H_6, C_3H_8, C_4H_{10}, etc. (C_nH_{2n+2}) (Fig. 8.7).

Sometimes the carbon chain will attach itself to itself and thus form a cyclic arrangement, which is often found in the volatile molecules (Fig. 8.8).

To simplify the diagram even further, the hydrogen atoms also are often omitted and their presence taken as read. Even the carbon atoms are not always shown, only the bonds between them, so cyclohexane is usually shown simplified as in Figure 8.9.

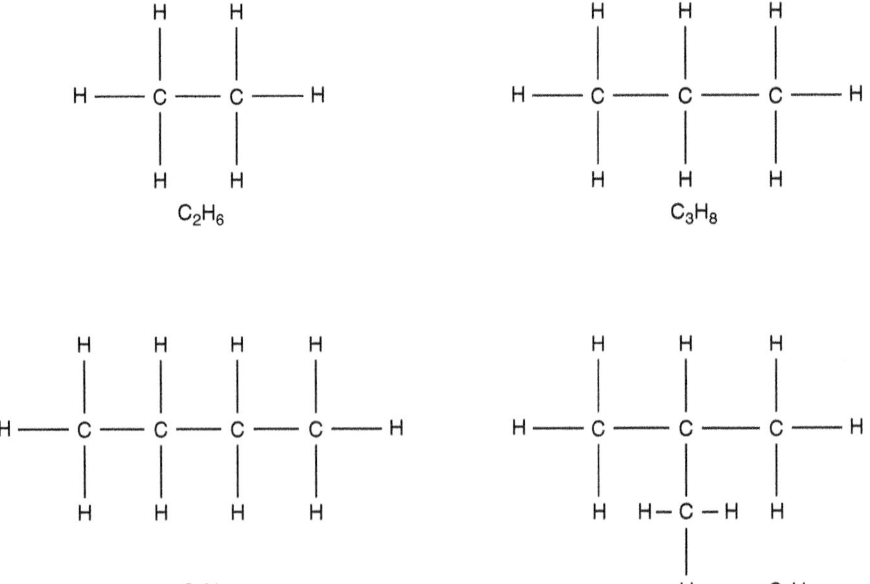

Figure 8.7 Carbon atoms, straight and branched chains.

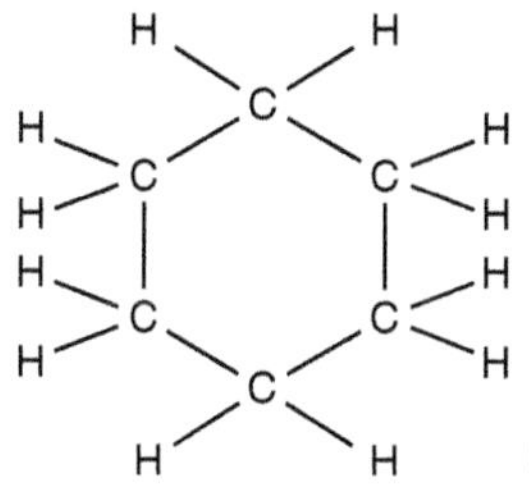

Figure 8.8 Cyclohexane.

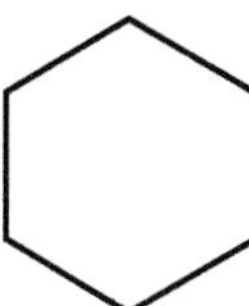

Figure 8.9 How cyclohexane is represented in formulae.

The isoprene unit

Isoprene molecules are found within the plant and are part of the process which forms the terpenes; each isoprene unit is made up of a branched chain of five carbon atoms (with the necessary hydrogen atoms) and is not capable of independent existence. It is a fundamental unit and is to be found in many organic compounds, including rubber and the molecules in essential oils. Isoprene units have double bonds and these are important because they provide sites where activity can occur, offering an opportunity for more atoms to attach to form larger structures (Fig. 8.10).

Two isoprene units joined together make a 10-carbon molecule known as a *monoterpene* (Fig. 8.11).

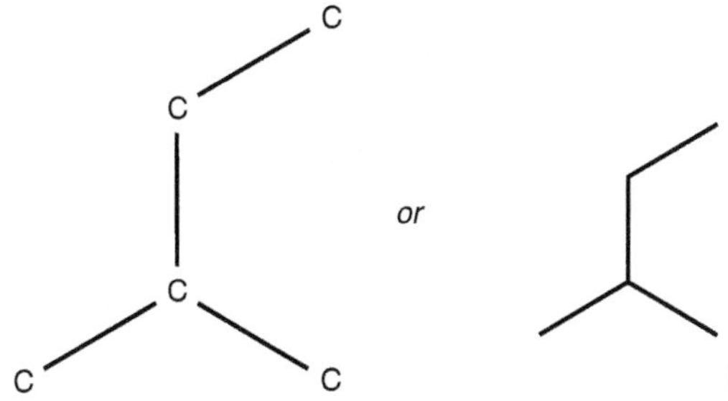

Figure 8.10 Isoprene.

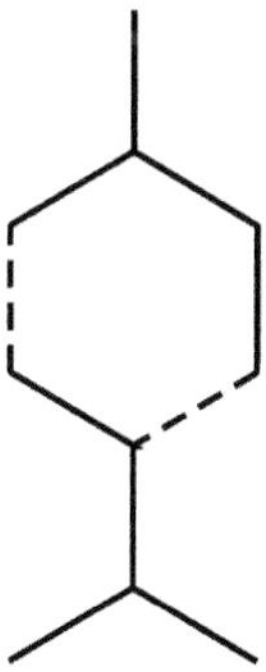

Figure 8.11 Monoterpene.

Three isoprene units join together to make a 15-carbon molecule called a *sesquiterpene* (Fig. 8.12).

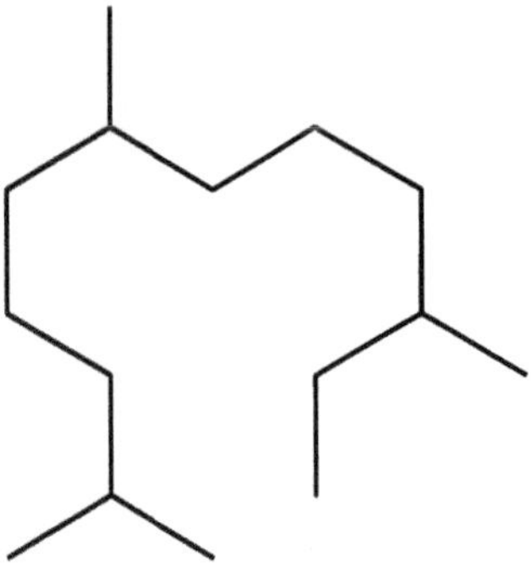

Figure 8.12 Sesquiterpene.

Hydrocarbons sometimes found in distilled waters are shown in Figure 8.13.

Four isoprene units can join together (and this happens only rarely in essential oils) to make a *diterpene* (20 carbon atoms in one molecule). Molecules larger than this do not occur in essential oils nor in distilled plant waters because their molecular weight is too great for the distillation process.

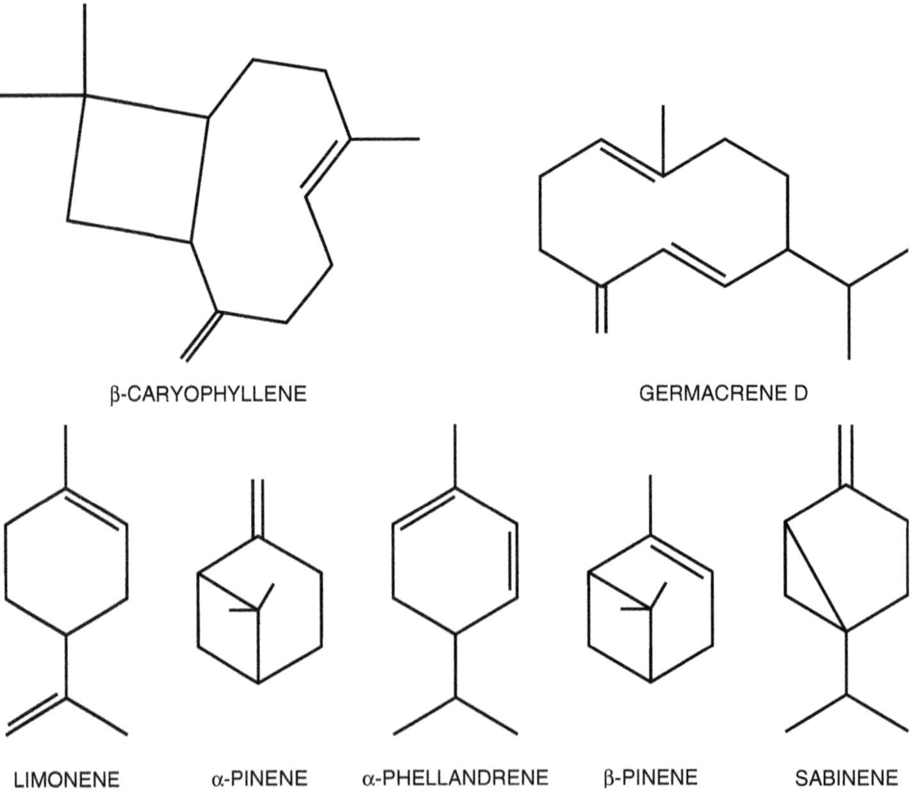

Figure 8.13 Hydrocarbons found in distilled waters.

The aromatic ring

Apart from the chain formation, another arrangement is possible. The carbon atoms of molecules found in essential oils may be joined not only in a straight chain, but also in a ring (cf. cyclohexane C_6H_{12}). This ring, being composed only of carbon and hydrogen atoms and three double bonds, is a hydrocarbon C_6H_6 (benzene). The ring system is often called an 'aromatic compound' because it is found so often in odorous compounds.

The benzene ring is flat and rigid and is the simplest member and starting point of a huge family of complex ring compounds of infinite variety. This ring molecule has three names, all of them in use, and is known not only as the *benzene ring* (because the basic ring of six carbon atoms is benzene) but also as the *phenyl ring* and the *aromatic ring*. The formula for benzene is C_6H_6, different from cyclohexane (Fig. 8.9). Benzene (phenyl ring, aromatic ring) may be shown in diagrammatic form in two ways (Fig. 8.14).

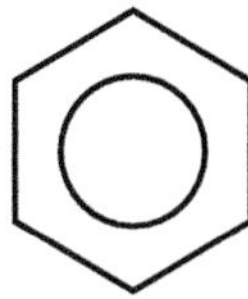

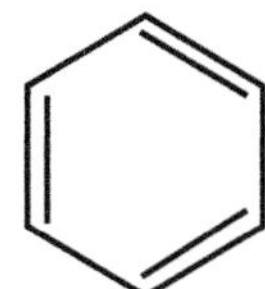

Figure 8.14 Benzene, phenyl ring

Molecules which are made up only of the atoms of carbon and hydrogen are known as hydrocarbons.

Oxygen

So far only molecules consisting only of hydrogen and carbon have been dealt with. We now look at compounds containing not only hydrogen and carbon, but also oxygen. Oxygen has a combining power of 2 and it is not usually found alone, often being part of a little group. In chemistry terminology such a group would be called a *radical*, and a commonly found group is made up of oxygen and hydrogen. This group is denoted as -OH, and is called the 'hydroxyl radical' or 'hydroxyl group'. A radical is a group of elements which stick together and act as a single entity during a chemical reaction

Oxygen molecule:	O=O
Hydroxyl group:	-O–H
usually written as:	-OH

Alcohols and phenols

The hydroxyl group –OH

If we take another look at our original molecule CH_4 (methane), we find that one of the hydrogen atoms can be replaced by the hydroxyl group giving CH_3OH, which is an *alcohol*. There are many alcohols and some of the alcohols found in hydrolats are shown in Figure 8.15.

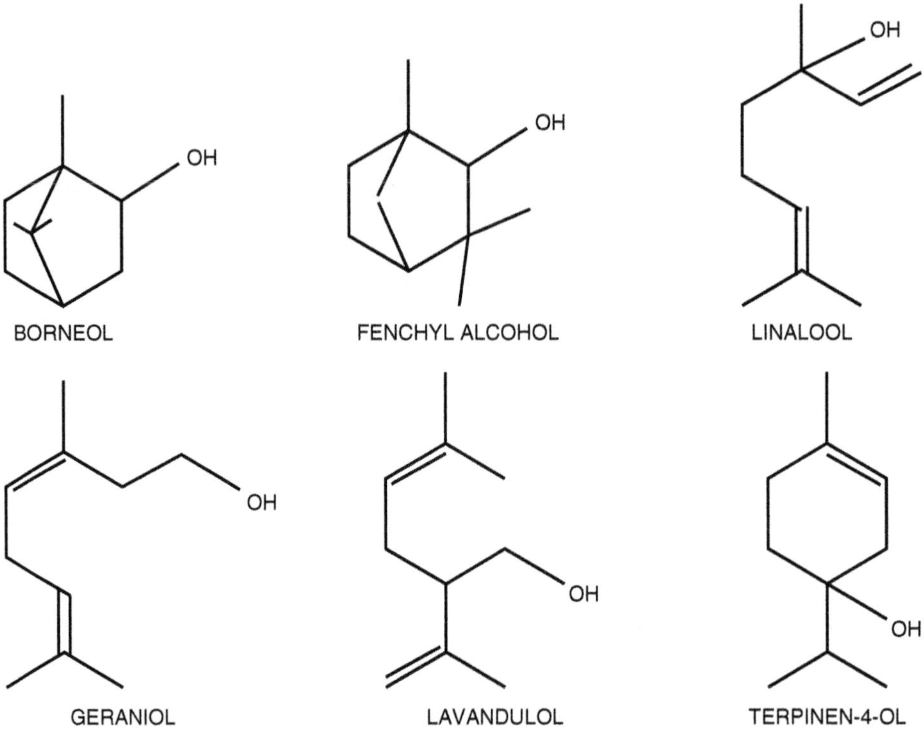

Figure 8.15 Alcohols found in distilled waters.

If, however, the hydroxyl group –OH is attached to a benzene ring, then what we have is a special kind of alcohol called a *phenol*. Examples of phenols which may be found occasionally in hydrolats are eugenol (clove bud), thymol, carvacrol (thyme) (Fig. 8.16), anethole (dill), etc.: all phenols have antiseptic properties in common with the basic phenol (carbolic acid).

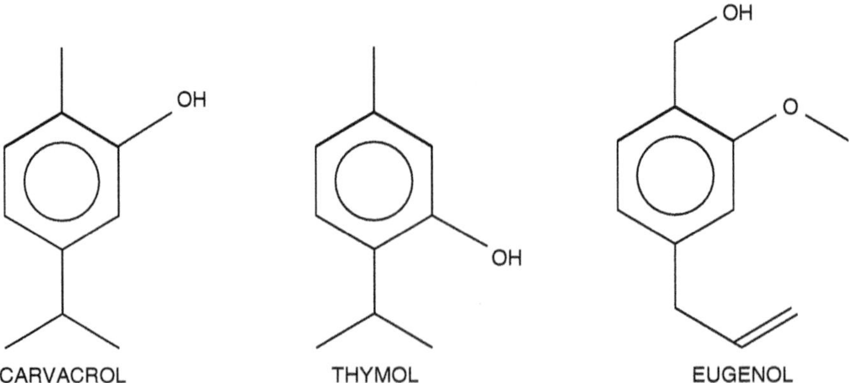

Figure 8.16 Phenols found in distilled waters.

Aldehydes and ketones

The ketones and aldehydes are closely related and both have the carbonyl group –C=O in their structure, and so have properties in common.

Aldehydes

In the case of aldehydes, the carbonyl group is attached to the end carbon of a carbon chain (Fig. 8.17). Aldehydes are present in many essential oils such as cinnamic aldehyde (cinnamon bark), citral (lemon). As can be seen, the name of an aldehyde ends in -*al* (short for aldehyde) or else the word aldehyde appears in full, so there is no trouble identifying aldehydes from their name.

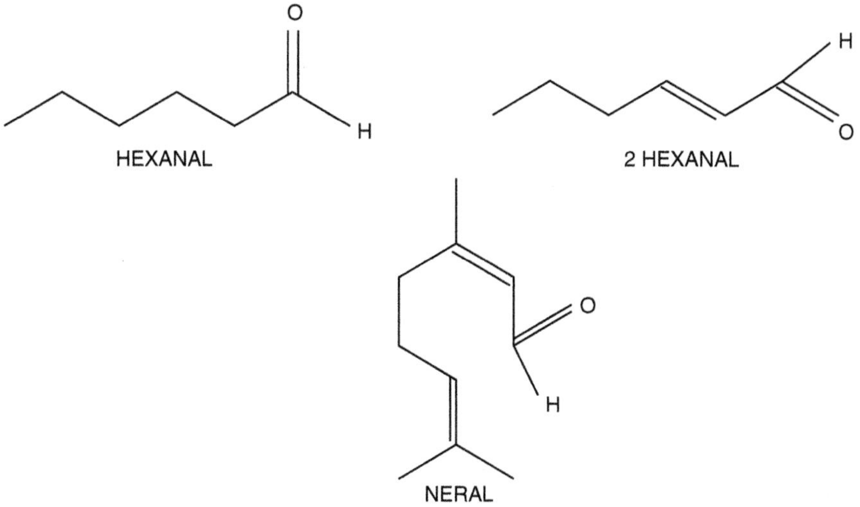

O H HEXANAL

H O 2 HEXANAL

O H NERAL

Figure 8.17 Aldehydes found in distilled waters.

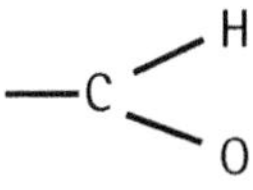

—C(H)(O) carbonyl group forming an aldehyde, usually written -CHO

It is moderately easy for an alcohol to turn into an aldehyde and it is very easy for the aldehydes to go into acids thus losing some of their therapeutic qualities. Alcohols oxidize to aldehydes: aldehydes oxidize to acids very easily (this is why citrus essential oils go off very easily): acids are very stable.

Ketones

Ketones have a structure in which the carbonyl group is attached to a carbon which is itself attached to two other carbons, either in a chain or a phenyl ring (Fig. 8.18).

Acetone, shown in Figure 8.18, is the simplest ketone. The word ketone is derived from the basic member of the family *acetone*. They are easy to identify from the name as all of them end in -*one*.

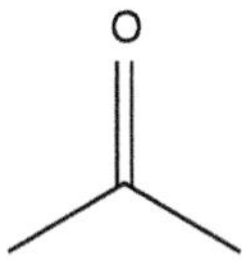

O

Figure 8.18 Acetone.

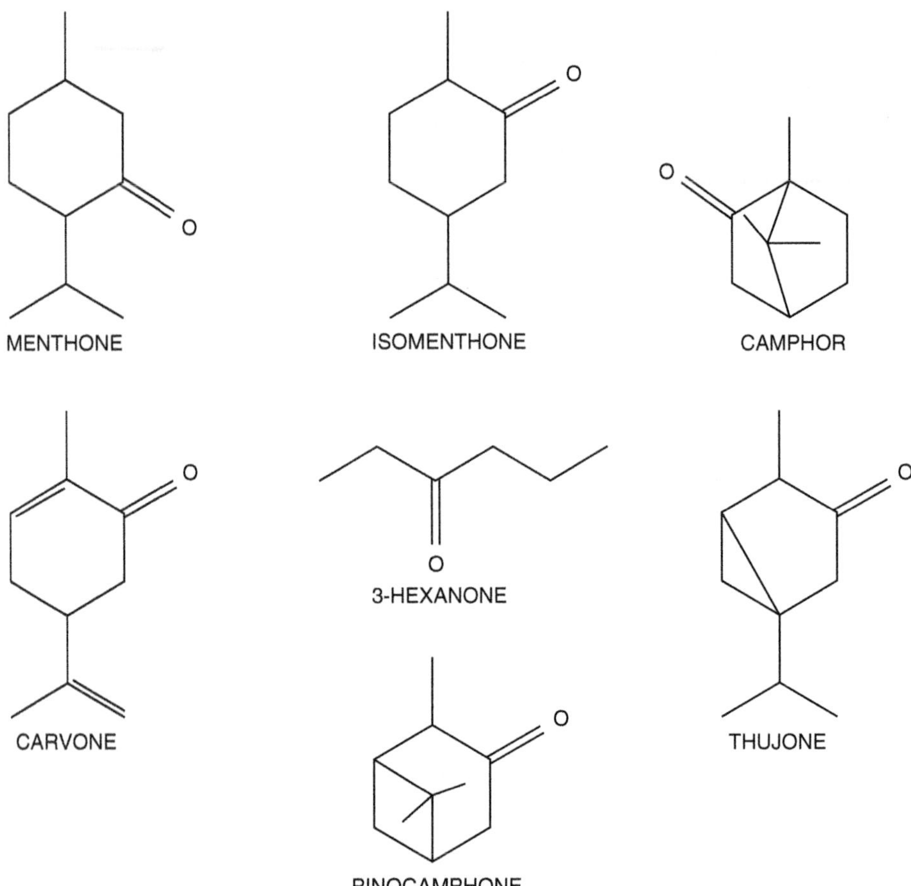

Figure 8.19 Ketones found in distilled waters.

Ketones have to be used with care as some are considered neurotoxic. Fortunately they are not present in the majority of essential oils in any significant amount. Some of the more notorious ketones are pulegone (pennyroyal), thujone (thuja) and pinocamphone (hyssop), and although these may be found in hydrolats, together with camphor and other ketones, the very low quantities present are such that they should present no hazard. Some ketones found in distilled waters are shown in Figure 8.19.

Acids

The carboxyl group -COOH

When the -COOH group is attached to a ring or a chain we have what is known as an organic acid. Free acids may be found in the distilled waters but are quite rare in

Figure 8.20 Acetic acid.

essential oils, occurring naturally only in tiny quantities. They are normally found in essential oils only in a combined state in the esters, hardly ever in the free state, and then only in short chain acids of less than 10 carbon atoms. The organic acids found in distilled waters have no known risks attached to them. The carboxylic acids are easily soluble in water because, firstly, the C=O and -OH groups are attached to the same carbon atom, reinforcing the hydrogen bonding and, secondly, the non-polar, hydrophilic carbon chain tends to be short (two to five carbon atoms) (Fig. 8.20).

Esters

Esters are made up of an organic acid and an alcohol, and are named after the two molecules which go to form them. Esters as a class are very aromatic and are much used in flavourings for food and drink.

Acetic acid + linalool = linalyl acetate + water
(Organic acid + alcohol = ester + water)

Examples of esters found in the hydrolats are linalyl acetate, geranyl acetate, and lavandulyl acetate (Fig. 8.21).

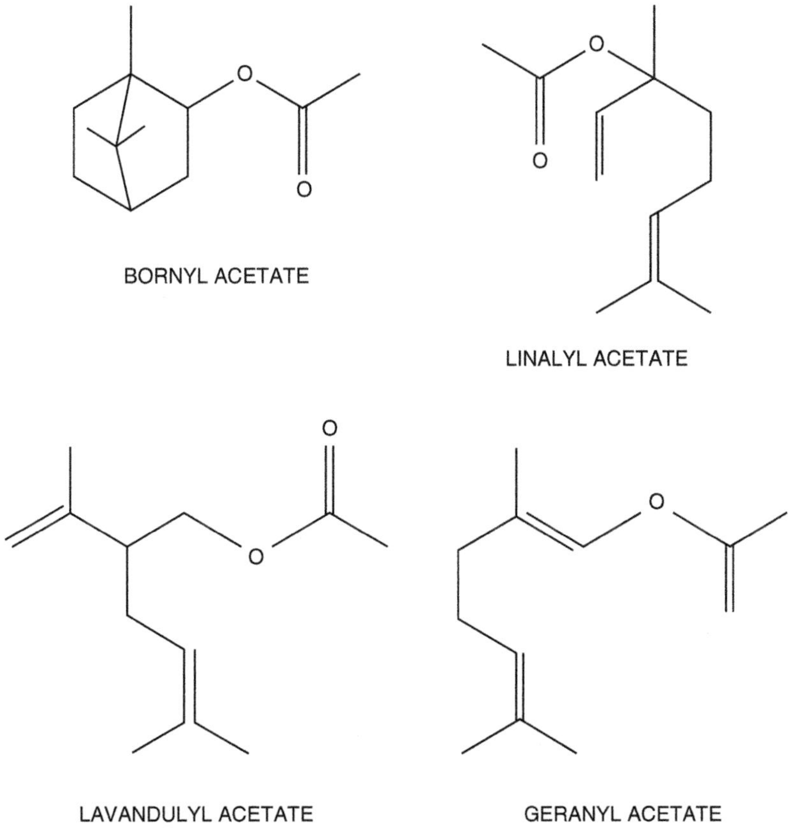

O
O
BORNYL ACETATE
O
O
LINALYL ACETATE
O
O
LAVANDULYL ACETATE
O
GERANYL ACETATE

Figure 8.21 Esters.

Oxides

These are derived from alcohols but instead of adding a new group to the oxygen, a closed ring is formed like an internal ether. The most common oxide found in essential oils and in hydrolats is eucalyptol, otherwise known as 1,8-cineole, which may also be described as a bicyclic ether. The oxides encountered in aromatherapy have an oxygen atom within the ring structure (Fig. 8.22).

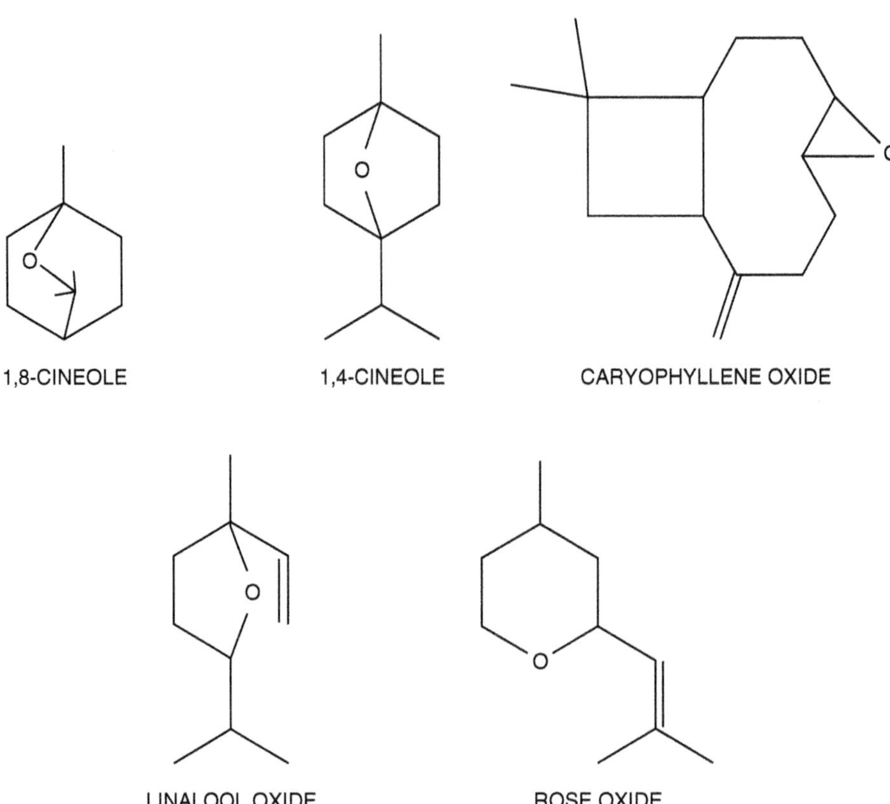

Figure 8.22 Oxides.

Isomers

Molecules which have precisely the same number and kind of atoms, but in a different spatial arrangement, are known as isomers. For example, many monoterpene hydrocarbons are made up of 10 carbon atoms and 16 hydrogen atoms, but there are many different structures made from these atoms with differing properties – these are called isomers.

Structural isomers: to help explain this concept, these many different molecules – made from the same quantity and quality of atoms – are, in a tenuous way, somewhat analogous to an anagram; for example the words *time, item, mite, emit* are all made up of the same letters but are different in structure and meaning.

Optical isomers: some molecules have the capacity to rotate light; carvone, a ketone, is such a one and exists in two forms, (+)–carvone being present in spearmint and (–)–carvone being in caraway (Fig. 8.23). These two molecules have the respective

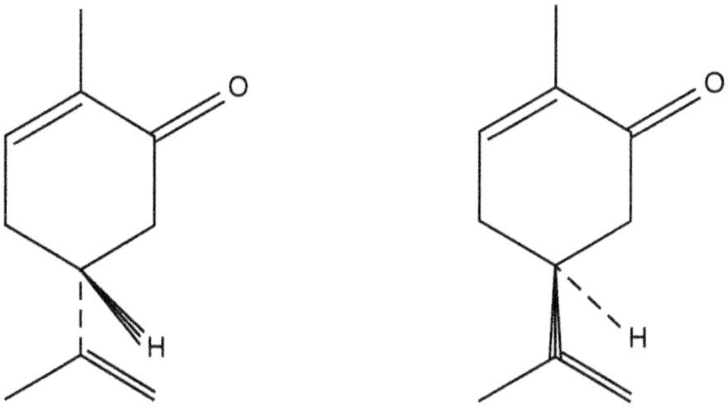

Figure 8.23 (-) and (+) carvone.

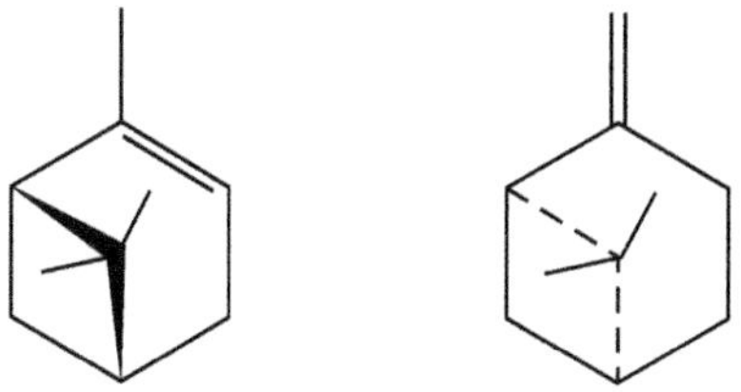

Figure 8.24 Alpha- and beta-pinene.

aromas of the plants, showing that quite a small change in the spatial arrangements of atoms within the molecules can have a significant effect. These are known as *optical isomers*, sometimes called molecules in the mirror, rather like a pair of hands which are a mirror image of each other.

Geometric isomers: the terpene pinene occurs in two slightly different forms (distinguished nominally by the Greek letters α and β), with only a change in the position of the double bond (Fig. 8.24). The aldehydes geranial and neral are very similar in structure and are said to be *geometric isomers.*

The prefixes *cis-* and *trans-* are used to describe the positioning of groups on either side of a double bond. Neral is a *cis*-isomer and geranial the *trans*-isomer, and because they often occur together and it is difficult to discriminate between the two during analysis; the mixture of these two isomers is called citral (Fig. 8.25).

The terpene cymene has three isomers, *para-*, *meta-* and *ortho-* respectively, denoting the positions of side groups attached to the benzene ring (Fig. 8.26).

Positive/negative molecules

All chemical products which are made up of only one kind of atom are electrically neutral, but aromatic molecules have a negative or positive energy depending on whether there is a receiving or a giving of electrons (as with molecules of all metabolic chains).

When an oxygen atom is present as part of a hydroxyl group (-OH) there is a similarity with the water molecule (with its hydrogen bonding) but it is more positive. The less a molecule is oxygenated (e.g. hydrocarbons, saturated terpenes, alcohols, phenols, oxides, ether-oxides), the more positive it is. The terpenes, which consist only of hydrocarbons, have a negative carbon nucleus with a positive hydrogen envelope.

When oxygen is double bonded to a carbon atom (e.g. aldehydes, ketones, esters) then the aromatic molecule seems to be negative. This can be seen only when the aromatic molecules are dispersed as in an emulsion, dispersion or aerosol. The more

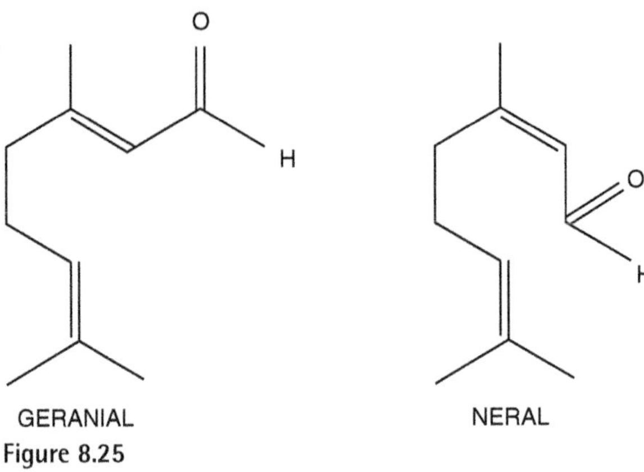

Figure 8.25

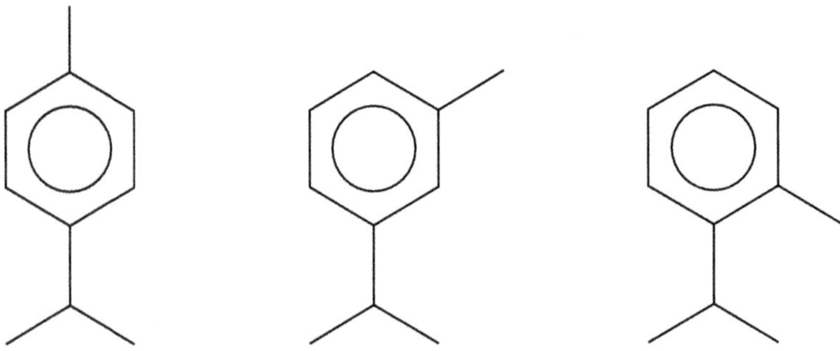

Figure 8.26 *Para-*, *ortho-* and *meta-*cymene.

a molecule is oxygenated by the addition of oxygen (ketones, aldehydes, esters, polyunsaturated terpenes) the more negative it is.

Jean Mars, a French engineer, developed a machine with an ultra-fine generator, which could determine whether a molecule had a negative or a positive charge. The information gained from this machine using single components of essential oil molecules was used by Franchomme & Pénoël (1990, pp. 96–104) who were able to discover which components were weakly/strongly negative and which were weakly/strongly positive. For example, linalool was found to be strongly positive, the citrals geranial and neral being moderately negative. After much work, it was found that the components, the alcohols, terpenes, esters, etc., each fell into natural

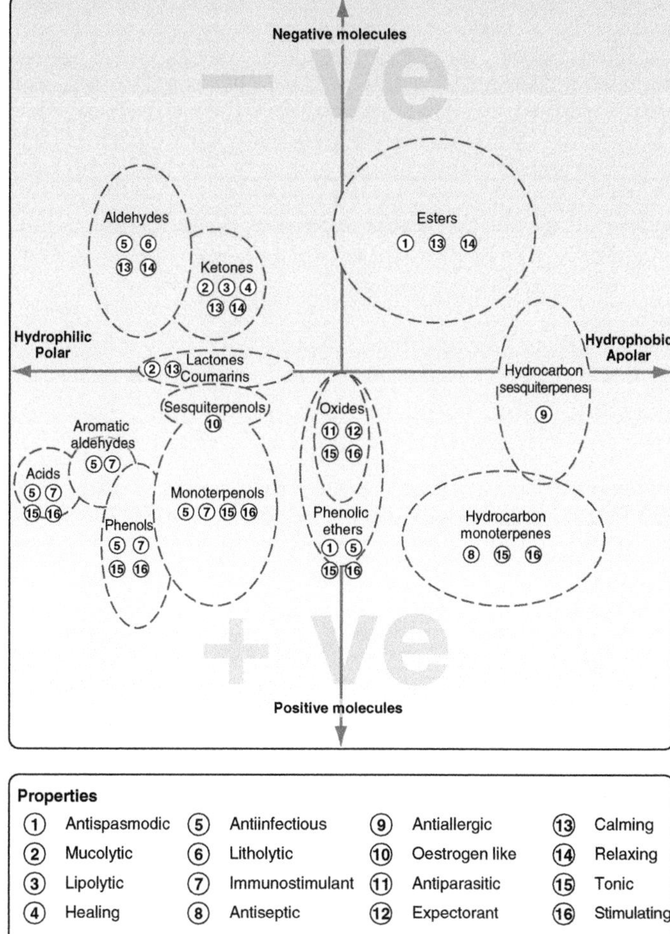

Figure 8.27 Positive and negative molecules.

'groupings' and so it was possible to plot the results on a grid. From these results, it was believed that, speaking generally, negative molecules such as aldehydes, ketones and esters were relaxing and positive ones such as phenols, alcohols and terpenes were stimulating. Still further work identified which groupings were antibacterial, antiseptic, antispasmodic, mucolytic and so on. To verify their findings, the two men carried out many studies and the work is summarized in Figure 8.27 (ascribed to Roger Jollois), published in Franchomme & Pénoël (1990).

9

Alphabetical listing of hydrolats with description, properties and indications

- Introduction 93
- Arrangement of the text 94
- Alphabetical list of hydrolats 95

Introduction

Some writers suggest that decoctions or/and tisanes possess some of the same properties as hydrolats obtained from the same part of the plant and the authors tend, from personal experience, to agree with them. Some of the waters listed below are known to be produced perhaps only occasionally or in small quantities; they are included for the sake of completeness, even though little or nothing has been written about their therapeutic properties and uses.

The authors have had many hydrolats analysed; some of these have the same botanical name but are from more than one source, and the results are not always the same. In such cases, the average has been taken. This is important to note, because it shows that, as with essential oils, analyses can vary between batches and between suppliers. Terpenes are not expected to be found in hydrolats, but are occasionally present in very small amounts (rarely more than 1–2%). The analysed waters showing a higher percentage of terpenes (8–20%) may be 'false' waters which include essential oil in their make-up. None of these 'suspect' analyses have been used in this chapter, although they appear in Appendix D for interest and comparison. It is possible also that occasionally additional properties found by therapists may be due to their having used a fragrant (prepared) water which has essential oils incorporated, when properties due to hydrocarbons may have come into play.

Information for the properties listed has been taken from the authors' own experience, from old books on herbal medicine, from the work of Mars, Franchomme and Pénoël (see p. 91), and from various modern writers. 'Guesswork' on the authors' part has been avoided, but the information gathered from some other sources must be assessed by the reader (for further referenced properties, see Appendices A and B).

It is only a theory that functional groupings of molecules found in essential oils and hydrolats have similar effects on the body – these are 'family' characteristics and, as in all families, there are some 'black sheep'. For instance, ketones as a group can be described as sedative and while this is largely true, the ketone camphor is stimulating. Esters as a group are described as safe to use, but one exception is methyl salicylate which is readily absorbed through the skin and is toxic if ingested (Winter 1999, p. 298). Alcohols as a group are stimulating and uplifting, yet the linalool found in lavender essential oil is known to be a factor in the sedative property of lavender oil (Buchbauer et al 1993, p. 661). When describing the effects of a particular compound, it must be borne in mind that the action of the whole oil or hydrolat cannot necessarily be forecast from the characteristics of a single molecule, even though that molecule is a large part of the whole, for that would be to ignore the influence of synergistic and quenching (antagonistic) effects, where the effects of one compound may be enhanced or diminished by another. This interraction is complex and is not predictable, therefore the overall effects of a whole essential oil or hydrolat cannot necessarily be forecast from knowing the composition or the effects of the individual components.

Henri Viaud (1983) spent many years of his life distilling both essential oils and hydrolats and researching their effects; he was in the middle of writing a book when the authors visited him at his still and workshop in Provence. Sadly he died before the book was completed, but hopefully his good work will be continued by his wife; his findings to that date are to be trusted.

Jeanne Rose was one of the first English-speaking authors to pass on her knowledge of hydrolats, one book (1992, p. 172) containing information on how to make your own hydrolats and other waters, the second (1999) having a useful table presenting the properties she attributes to them.

Suzanne Catty (2001), in her useful and informative book on hydrosols (hydrolats), gives many health attributes for so many of the hydrolats that one may wonder how this can be possible. Having said that, the authors have found from experience with essential oils that they can be unexpectedly effective for many problems for which they are not normally recommended – and the same could also apply to hydrolats. Although Catty's book has a long bibliography, references in the text to the findings of others are rarely given, and perhaps some of the waters used may have been prepared using essential oils, when properties associated with the essential oils may have shown themselves. Nevertheless we are grateful for her suggestions and her extensive research.

Arrangement of the text

In the text, under each hydrolat:

- the properties found by the practitioners quoted are shown in italics
- where the authors have received an analysis giving the composition of a hydrolat, the properties which may (repeat, *may*) be attributed according to the studies by Franchomme & Pénoël are summarized in italics below the analysis
- those properties suggested by the practitioners which agree with the findings of Franchomme & Pénoël are highlighted in bold
- properties from infusions, etc. are shown in parentheses
- where a plant contains a volatile oil, this is noted.

It is to hoped that practitioners will use these waters as indicated and report any results so that all therapists may benefit from shared experience.

Alphabetical list of hydrolats

Abies balsamea [BALSAM FIR, BALM OF GILEAD] Pinaceae

(contains a volatile oil)

analgesic, calming, circulatory, diuretic, immunostimulant, mucolytic, tonic

A general tonic, mild diuretic, it supports the immune system, reduces seasonal affective disorder (SAD), is mucolytic and is used as a base for cough syrups. It is gently stimulating to the circulation, though calming to the mind, and is used in compresses for rheumatic, arthritic and joint pains (Catty 2001, p. 73).

Acacia decurrens [MIMOSA]

detoxifying (hepatic cleanser and gall bladder drainer) (Viaud 1983)

Achillea millefolium [YARROW] Asteraceae

(contains a volatile oil)

Achillea is named after the Greek warrior Achilles because, during the siege of Troy, achillea was used to heal the soldiers' wounds.

The main components of the hydrolats analysed suggest the following properties may apply:

50–64% eucalyptol	expectorant, mucolytic
10–19% alcohols	antiinfectious, antiviral, bactericidal, decongestant, stimulating
17–19% aldehydes	antiinfectious, antiinflammatory, antiviral, calming, circulatory (hypotensor), febrifuge, tonic
7–13% ketones	analgesic, anticoagulant, antiinflammatory, calming, cicatrizant, digestive, expectorant, lipolytic, mucolytic, sedative, stimulant

Summary of the above properties:

analgesic, anticoagulant, antiinfectious, **antiinflammatory,** *antiviral,* **bactericidal, calming,** *cicatrizant,* **circulatory** *(hypotensor), decongestant,* **digestive,** *expectorant, febrifuge, lipolytic, mucolytic, sedative, stimulating,* **tonic**

The highlighted properties appear in the text below, and the following have also been suggested:

antiirritant, antiseptic, antispasmodic, astringent, diuretic

According to Viaud (1983) and Price & Price (1999), yarrow hydrolat is useful for easing circulation problems in women.

Apart from suggesting it has the mental properties of being good for spiritual healing, Rose (1999, p. 171) gives yarrow as being energizing, antiinflammatory and antiseptic and effective on cellulite.

Catty (2001, p. 74) gives many other uses for this water, citing it as being antispasmodic, mildly antibacterial, antiseptic, digestive, diuretic and giving relief in premenstrual syndrome (PMS). She says also it is helpful for varicose veins and cellulite.

Skin
Historically, an infusion of yarrow was used to wash the skin to soothe cases of dermatitis and eczema (Clair 1961, p. 260).

Rose (1999, p. 171) uses yarrow hydrolat for acne and damaged skin, naturesgift.com/hydrosols saying it is both antiinflammatory and antirritant, while innerself.com/magazine/herbs/essential_oils (2001) adds that it is also astringent.

Agaricus campestis [MUSHROOM] Agaricaceae
antiallergic, detoxifying, hepatic drainer (Viaud 1983)

Aloysia triphylla (Aloysia citriodora, Lippia citriodora) [LEMON VERBENA] Verbenaceae (contains a volatile oil)
antiinflammatory, balancing, calming, digestive, general tonic
Rose (1999, p. 173) has found lemon verbena hydrolat balancing and stimulating and an aid to a good night's sleep (delicious in a tea).

Apart from the property of calming stage fright 'nerves', Catty (2001, p. 107) has found it to be a general tonic to the system, a powerful relaxant, being calming for both stress and PMS. She considers it a strong antiinflammatory, with an affinity for the mucus membranes of the mouth and nose. According to innerself.com/magazine/herbs/essential_oils (2001), lemon verbena hydrolat can be taken internally to help an upset stomach.
Skin
Rose (1999, p. 173) finds lemon verbena hydrolat balancing and revitalizing to normal skin types, while Catty (2001, p. 107) suggests its use as a toner for normal to combination skin. innerself.com/magazine/herbs/essential_oils (2001), recommends it for an acne-prone skin and skin hydration.
Culinary use
Catty (2001, p. 107) has found it to be delicious in beverages, with seafoods and in desserts.

Anagallis arvensis [SCARLET PIMPERNEL, POOR MAN'S WEATHERGLASS] Primulaceae
skin cleanser and smoother
Culpeper, on the use of scarlet pimpernel, informs us that 'the distilled water or juice is much celebrated by French dames to cleanse the skin from any roughness, deformity or discolourings thereof' (cited in Grieve 1992, p. 633).

Stuart (1987, p. 151) writes that, cosmetically, 'pimpernel water' is used for freckles. He tells us that the scarlet pimpernel is an interesting herb which merits modern research. The name is derived from the Greek 'to delight', supposedly given by Dioscorides, and the leaves were once used in salads.

Anemone hepatica [AMERICAN LIVERWORT, KIDNEYWORT] Ranunculaceae
Skin
A distilled water was once used for freckles and sunburn, but even though it has been in use from ancient days its very mild character has resulted in it being little used today (Grieve 1992, p. 494). The tisane is used for liver congestion, kidney, gall bladder and digestive disorders (Stuart 1987, p. 152).

Anethum graveolens [DILL WEED] Apiaceae
(contains a volatile oil)
The earliest recorded use of dill in medicine is in ancient Egyptian medical papyri. Their word for dill was *imse*, from which is derived the Coptic (a medieval Egyptian language) *emise* or *amise*. According to one authority, this word is wrongly translated in the Authorized Version of the Bible (Matthew 23: 23) as anise (Clair 1961, p. 154).
carminative

Dill water has long been in popular use as a carminative and the essential oil of dill has been much used for the same purpose in mixtures, or given in doses of 5 drops on sugar. Dill weed has been (and still is) most commonly used in the preparation of dill water (Grieve 1992, p. 256). Every parent knows that it is safe to use dill water as a cheap and safe domestic remedy for wind in babies; it can be a useful vehicle for children's medicines generally. In 1525 the popular Banckes's *Herbal* (Larkey & Pyles 1941) said that it 'destroyed the yexing' – meaning to say that it got rid of hiccups.

Angelica archangelica [ANGELICA] Apiaceae
(contains a volatile oil)
The main components of the hydrolat analysed suggest the following properties may apply:

18–20% ketones analgesic, anticoagulant, antiinflammatory, antiviral, calming, cicatrizant, digestive, expectorant, mucolytic, sedative, stimulant

53–54% alcohols antiinfectious, antiviral, bactericidal, decongestant, stimulating

Summary of the above properties:
analgesic, anticoagulant, antiinfectious, antiinflammatory, antiviral, bactericidal, **calming,** *cicatrizant,* **digestive,** *expectorant, mucolytic,* **sedative, stimulating**

The highlighted properties appear in the text below, and the following property has also been suggested, using an infusion:
(*emmenagogic*)

Catty (1998a, p.76) suggests that angelica hydrolat increases the appetite, tones the digestion and, being a strong sedative, is calming in anxious and very stressful conditions.

An infusion can be made from bruised angelica root (500 ml of boiling water to 30 g of root) and given to relieve flatulence or as a stimulating bronchial tonic; it may also be used as an emmenagogue (Grieve 1992, p. 38). The hydrolat may have digestive and bronchial actions in common with the infusion, as these effects are suggested by the above theoretical properties.

Apium graveolens [WILD CELERY, SMALLAGE] Apiaceae
(contains a volatile oil)
anticancerous, carminative, diuretic (Viaud 1983)

Arbutus uva ursi **(*Arctostaphylos uva-ursi*)** [BEARBERRY, MOUNTAIN BOX] Ericaceae
antiseptic, renal cleanser (Viaud 1983)

Arctium lappa [GREATER BURDOCK, BEGGAR'S BUTTONS] Asteraceae

(contains a volatile oil)
The following property is from an infusion:
(*antirritant*)

John Wesley (1792), who was a great believer in, and advocate for, plant remedies, recommended an infusion made from dried burdock as a remedy for 'King's evil' (scrofula) (Clair 1961, p. 129). If infusions have similar properties to hydrolats, burdock hydrolat could possibly be antirritant.

Arnica montana [ARNICA] Asteraceae

(contains a volatile oil)
Arnakis meaning 'lamb's skin' was the Greek name for the plant, because of the softness of the leaves. No anecdotal or other evidence is available for this hydrolat.

Artemisias (see below)

NB: there are many artemisias – the user should be sure to check the full Latin name before using the hydrolat for a specific purpose.

Artemisia abrotanum [SOUTHERNWOOD, LAD'S LOVE] Asteraceae

(contains a volatile oil)
aphrodisiac, revitalizing
In former times, Culpeper wrote that 'the distilled water of the herb is said to helpe . . . diseases of the spleen. The Germans commend it for a singular wound herb [but] Wormwood has thrown it into disrepute' (cited in Grieve 1992, p. 755). In modern times, Viaud (1983) gives this water as being revitalizing and aphrodisiac.

Artemisia absinthium [WORMWOOD] Asteraceae

(contains a volatile oil)
(*digestive*)
Wormwood has long been an important ingredient in aperitifs and herbal wines, which suggests that the hydrolat also may possess digestive qualities. In *Delightes for Ladies* by Sir Hugh Plat (1609), there is a recipe for making 'wormwood wine verie speedily and in great quantitie' (Clair 1961, p. 256) and Estienne wrote that 'for the stomacke oppressed with flegmaticke humours there is a wine made of wormwood and called by the same name'.

Artemisia arborescens [TREE WORMWOOD] Asteraceae

(contains a volatile oil)
antiinflammatory, antispasmodic, calming (mild), stomachic, revitalizing
The distilled water of *Artemisia arborescens* (tree wormwood) is said to be stomachic, revitalizing and a muscle regenerator. It eases joint pain, is antiinflammatory and antispasmodic (Rose 1999, p. 170). Rose also suggests that it is mildly calming and strongly energizing.
Skin
Rose (1999, p. 170) recommends it for damaged skin; innerself.com\magazine\herbs\essential_oils 2001 suggests its use for sensitive skin.

Artemisia dracunculus [TARRAGON] Asteraceae

(contains a volatile oil)

analgesic, anticancerous, antiinflammatory, antispasmodic, carminative

Viaud (1983) gives tarragon as anticancerous.

According to Catty (1998b), it is very powerful in low concentrations, easing muscle and joint pain. It is antiinflammatory, antispasmodic and carminative (Catty 2001, pp. 76–77).

Culinary use

Tarragon vinegar is made simply by steeping 8 oz leaves in 4 pt of wine vinegar; it has culinary uses only, e.g. for mixing mustard (Clair 1961, p. 247).

The distilled water can be used to give added aroma to vegetable juices and salad dressings (Grosjean 1993a, p. 118).

Artemisia vulgaris [MUGWORT, FELON HERB] Asteraceae

(contains a volatile oil)

The leaves are used by the Chinese in moxibustion.

antiparasitic, circulatory, energizing, expectorant (mild), general tonic, sedative (mild)

Mugwort distillate stimulates circulation, strengthens capillaries and peripheral circulation and is a general tonic; it is antiparasitic, a mild expectorant, mildly sedative and highly energizing (Catty 2001, p. 77).

Balsamita suaveolens [COSTMARY, ALECOST, BALSAM HERB] Asteraceae

(contains a volatile oil)

This plant is known by several common and Latin names such as herbe Sainte-Marie, *Balsamita mas*, maudlin, *Achillea ageratum*, and *Balsamita foemina*. It is more widely called costmary (from the Latin *costus*, an oriental plant whose roots were used as a spice and as a preservative, and from Mary, in reference to the biblical Mary) or alecost because it was used to flavour and clarify beer. Also known as bibleleaf because its broad, long leaves have often been used as aromatic bookmarks in the Bible (Palma 1964). The species is native to Asia Minor, Asia and Australia but has now become naturalized in many parts of southern Europe, where it is well known and used in folk medicine mainly for antimicrobial properties due to its essential oil (Kubo & Kubo 1995).

Different liquid preparations and tablets based on the essential oil and aromatic water of *B. suaveolens* are produced in Florence, using plant material cultivated in Tuscany. For these preparations original recipes of a Dominican monk, Angiolo Marchissi, have been used since 1614. They are traditionally used for their sedative properties, although no pharmacological investigations have supported this application so far. The essential oil is used to prepare some products (0.03% w/w), whereas the aromatic water is employed for the formulation of others (31.23 and 94.75% w/w). More than 150 000 tablets and more than 560 litres of liquid preparations are marketed every year (Gallori et al 2001).

The main components of the hydrolat analysed suggest the following properties may apply:

77–83% ketones analgesic, anticoagulant, **antiinflammatory**, calming, cicatrizant, **digestive**, expectorant, lipolytic, mucolytic, sedative, stimulant

The highlighted properties appear in the text below, and the following have also been suggested for the juice and an infusion:
(*diuretic, emmenagogic*)

Grieve (1992, p. 226) quotes Green's *Universal Herbal* (1532) which stated 'a strong infusion of the leaves to be good in disorders of the stomach and head' and much celebrated for its efficacy as an emmenagogue.

Salmon (1710) recommends the juice of the herb as a diuretic and 'good in cases of Quotidien Ague' (inflammation and swelling due to a cold). Perhaps the antiinflammatory property may also be present in the hydrolat.

Betonica officinalis [BETONY] see **Stachys officinalis**

The hydrolat has been produced but no information is available.

Betula alba and ***Betula pendula*** [WHITE BIRCH and SILVER BIRCH] Betulaceae

(*antiinflammatory, antiseptic, diuretic, litholytic*)
Stuart (1982, p. 23) tells us that the leaves of silver birch are diuretic and mildly antiseptic, being used in urinary tract infections. As it is likely that hydrolats contain some of the constituents which are extracted simply with boiling water, as when making a tea, it follows that the effects of the hydrolat may be similar. Grieve (1998, p. 104) says that the leaves of white birch have been used in tea for gout, rheumatism, and the tea is also a reliable solvent of kidney stones. This suggests that both varieties of birch are useful for the urinary system generally.

Borago officinalis [BORAGE] Boraginaceae

(contains a volatile oil)
(*antiinfectious, antiinflammatory, diuretic, energizing, euphoric*)
These properties apply to the wine and the tisane made from borage, but it could be possible that at least some of the properties apply also to the hydrolat. Borage tisane is a mild diuretic, once used for kidney inflammations, and now for rheumatism and respiratory infections (Stuart 1987, p. 163). Evelyn writes that sprigs of borage in wine 'are of known Vertue to revive the Hypochondriac and chear the hard Student' (Clair 1961, p. 123). According to Dioscorides, borage was the famous *nepenthe* of Homer which Polydamna, wife of Thonis, sent to Helen for a token 'of such rare virtue that when taken steeped in wine, if wife and children, father and mother, brother and sister, and all thy dearest friends should die before thy face, thou could'st not grieve or shed a tear for them'. From this I suppose we may take it that borage wine is uplifting to the spirits; it was called *Euphrosinum* by Pliny because of its euphoric effect.

Buxus sempervirens [BOX] Buxaceae

(contains a volatile oil)
anticancerous (Viaud 1983)

Calendula officinalis [MARIGOLD, POT MARIGOLD] Asteraceae

The main components of the hydrolat analysed suggest the following properties may apply:

57–64% alcohols antiinfectious, antiviral, bactericidal, decongestant, stimulating

15% esters	antifungal, antiinflammatory, antispasmodic, balancing (to nervous system), calming, cicatrizant, uplifting

Summary of the above properties:
antifungal, **antiinflammatory,** *antispasmodic, antiviral,* **bactericidal,** *balancing (to nervous system), calming,* **decongestant,** *stimulating*

The highlighted properties appear in the text below, and the following have also been suggested:
analgesic, diaphoretic, emmenagogic, hypotensive, ophthalmic, skin cleanser, sudorific

The distilled water of *Calendula officinalis* (calendula) is listed by Viaud (1983) and Price & Price (1999) as a skin drainer, useful for pyodermatitis, eczema; it is active against *staphylococcus*, is an emmenagogue and helpful in cases of hypertension.

'The floures and leaves of Marigolds being distilled, and the water dropped into red and watery eies, ceaseth the inflammation, and taketh away the paine' (Gerard 1964, p. 169). Grieve (1992, p. 518) tells us that a lotion made from the flowers is useful for sprains and wounds. She goes on to say that an infusion of the freshly gathered flowers is employed on fevers, as it gently promotes perspiration and throws out any eruption. Grieve also tells us that a decoction of the flowers (see glossary) is much in use in country districts to bring out smallpox and measles, in the same manner as saffron.

Carum carvi [CARAWAY] Apiaceae

(contains a volatile oil)

digestive

Distilled caraway water is considered a useful remedy in the flatulent colic of infants, and is an excellent vehicle for children's medicine. When sweetened, the flavour is agreeable (Grieve 1992, p. 158).

Cedrus atlantica [ATLAS CEDAR] Abietaceae

(contains a volatile oil)

antibacterial, regenerative

Grosjean (1993a, p. 105) recommends its use on damaged hair to restore strength and condition; it may also help with regrowth. She also advocates it in compresses for chickenpox and measles.

naturesgift.com/hydrosols says it is strongly antibacterial, and has been recommended for treating cystitis or bladder and kidney infections.

Skin

Grosjean (1993a, p. 105) suggests it may be beneficial on scars, and naturesgift.com/hydrosols uses it on oily skin and dandruff, and recommends it as an aftershave.

Centaurea cyanus [CORNFLOWER, BLUEBOTTLE, BATCHELOR'S BUTTON] Asteraceae

The main components of the hydrolats analysed suggest the following properties may apply:

4–9% eucalyptol	expectorant, mucolytic
35–72% alcohols	antiinfectious, antiviral, bactericidal, decongestant, stimulating

22–26% aldehydes	antiinfectious, antiinflammatory, antiviral, calming, circulatory (hypotensor), febrifuge, tonic

Summary of the above properties:
antiinfectious, antiinflammatory, *antiviral, bactericidal,* **calming,** *circulatory (hypotensor), decongestant,* **febrifuge, stimulating, tonic**

The highlighted properties appear in the text below, and the following have also been suggested:
antiirritant, astringent, diuretic (mild), ophthalmic, soothing

Cornflower water is given not only the properties of being astringent and ophthalmic but also as being useful for skin problems of intestinal origin (Viaud 1983, Price & Price 1999); it is also used in compresses and eyebaths to soothe conjunctivitis, styes and blepharitis.

The water distilled from cornflower petals was formerly in repute as a remedy for weak eyes. The famous French eyewash 'eau de casse lunettes' used to be made from them (Grieve 1992, p. 224). A decoction (see glossary) is used as an eyewash to counteract eye irritation and tiredness (Stuart 1987, p. 169); it is wonderfully soothing to the delicate tissue around the eye (6scent). The seeds or leaves (or the distilled water of the herb) used to be taken in wine as it was thought to be very good against the plague and all infectious diseases, and also was very good in pestilent fevers.

Cornflower floral water has a stimulating effect on the skin and a soothing effect for irritated eyelids thanks to its astringent and antiinflammatory properties (Sanoflore 2000). Cornflower water is a general system tonic and mild diuretic and can be used as a douche for urinary or reproductive infections (Catty 2001, naturesgift.com/hydrosols). It makes a calming and relaxing tea and is good for 'hot flashes' (hot flushes) (Rose 1999, p. 170).

Skin

The hydrolat tones crepey skin and is the aesthetician's choice for dry, devitalized or mature skin or bruising (Rose 1999, p. 170).

Chamaemelum nobile [ROMAN CHAMOMILE] Asteraceae

(contains a volatile oil)

The main components of the hydrolats analysed suggest the following properties may apply:

5–33% esters	antifungal, antiinflammatory, antispasmodic, balancing (to nervous system), calming, cicatrizant, uplifting
11–23% alcohols	antiinfectious, antiviral, bactericidal, decongestant, stimulating

Summary of the above properties:
antifungal, **antiinfectious, antiinflammatory, antispasmodic,** *antiviral, bactericidal, balancing (to nervous system),* **calming, cicatrizant,** *decongestant, stimulating, uplifting*

The highlighted properties appear in the text below, and the following have also been suggested:
analgesic, antiallergic, antiirritant, astringent (mild), digestive, purifying

Viaud (1983) gives it as healing and ophthalmic. It can be used in compresses for all eye tiredness also for inflammation due to conjunctivitis, repeating the treatment many times during the day if necessary. Franchomme & Pénoël (1996, p. 86) write that distilled waters are often useful in the treatment of pain, saying (p. 287) that Roman chamomile water is active in combating some post zoster pain and also painful eye problems such as infectious conjunctivitis.

Both Viaud and Grosjean (1993a, p. 97) attribute to Roman chamomile hydrolat a calming property, useful for helping with sleeping difficulties if taken as a drink before retiring; it is also a cardiac calmative. naturesgift.com/hydrosols suggests a compress of Roman chamomile hydrolat to ease a migraine.

Skin

Claeys (1992) gives chamomile water as purifying and cicatrizant; he also says that it is suitable for all types of skin (including mucous surfaces), although he does not identify the specific chamomile. The floral water of Roman chamomile has a calming and purifying effect. It helps to give the right balance to dry, irritated and fragile skins and calms tired eyes (Sanoflore 2000, Price & Price 1999).

The authors have found Roman chamomile water to be antiinflammatory and antiinfectious, making it useful for calming inflamed and irritated skin conditions (Rose 1999, p. 170) such as rosacea, burns, sunburn and razor rash (Catty 2001, p. 82; Battaglia 1995, p. 425).

Goëb (1998) specifies that the water is used in aesthetics for face care for delicate skins with allergic tendency, as does Bego (1995), and that chamomile is an excellent cutaneous antiinflammatory and antiallergic. As it is mildly astringent (Catty 2001, p. 82) it makes an effective skin tonic, but she advises against long-term use on very dry skin.

Chamomile water is excellent to calm the itching of eczema and psoriasis (6scent). naturesgift.com/hydrosols claims it also soothes flaky, itchy skin, rashes and acne, including the mucous membranes (mouth, gums, respiratory tract and anal and genital areas), which may safely be treated with this relaxing antiinflammatory water.

Baby care

Chamomile water is considered to be very suitable – equal with lavender water – for baby care in general, to calm when teething, calm diarrhoea and promote sleep (Grosjean 1993a, pp. 97–98).

Hair

Chamomile water is traditionally used as rinse on hair, to lighten it (Grosjean 1993a, p. 98; Sanoflore 2000).

Chelidonium majus [GREATER CELANDINE] Papaveraceae

calming to the eyes (Montesinos 2001)

Chenopodium album [FAT HEN, WHITE GOOSEFOOT] Chenopodiaceae

antiinfectious

Viaud (1983) tells us that distilled water of fat hen can be used to help in cases of intestinal problems with taenia (tapeworm) infection.

Chrysanthemum parthenium [FEVERFEW] Asteraceae

The water can be obtained but no information is available.

Cinnamomum verum [CINNAMON] Lauraceae

(antiinfectious, digestive, stimulating)

An infusion of the bark is used at a dilution of 8–15 g in 1 litre of water, or 10–50 g in syrups and draughts. Used for general debility, for people suffering from melancholia or digestive problems; it is also useful to older people during the winter months against chills and influenza (Valnet 1980, p. 110).

Cistus ladaniferus [ROCK ROSE] Cistaceae
(contains a volatile oil)
antiviral, antiwrinkle, astringent, cicatrizant, immunostimulant, styptic
This hydrolat has shown a capacity to bring about certain mental states where the patient is 'disconnected' (out of touch with themselves), which can be put to good use with those who have a dependence on certain drugs, e.g. alcohol, cigarettes, etc., by helping them to break the habit (Franchomme & Pénoël, 1990, p. 300); the hydrolat also aims at viral conditions (Franchomme & Pénoël 1990, p. 286).

Catty (2001, p. 84) gives several attributes for the hydrolat of rock rose; it is highly astringent, cicatrizant, an immune system booster, styptic, useful for cleaning wounds; it is an effective douche for endometriosis and healing to mind, body and spirit.
Skin
She tells us that it is an excellent and powerful antiwrinkle treatment, its micro-cluster behaviour plumping up cells and smoothing fine lines; it is a good aftershave too.

***Citrus aurantium* (flos)** [ORANGE FLOWER] **General information**
Often when orange flower water is mentioned, no distinction is made as to whether it is the sweet or bitter variety for which the properties are given. Orange flower water of either variety is always given as calming. Distilled orange flower water is also known as neroli water. Winter (1999, p. 322) gives orange flower water as being the watery solution of the sweet smelling principles of the flowers of *Citrus sinensis*. Orange flower water is used to flavour medicines (Stuart 1987).

***Citrus aurantium* var. *amara* (flos)** [BITTER ORANGE FLOWER] Rutaceae
(contains a volatile oil)
The main components of the hydrolat analysed suggest the following properties may apply:

20–21% alcohols antiinfectious, antiviral, bactericidal, decongestant, **stimulant**

The highlighted property appears in the text below, and the following have also been suggested:
antiinflammatory, antiseptic, antispasmodic, astringent, calming, cooling, digestive, sedative

The authors have found that, like the essential oil, orange flower water is calming and uplifting (Price & Price 1999, p. 115) and so can be put to good use for people suffering from SAD and to relieve stressed or emotionally upset people. It is calming in the bath for over-excited children, being sedative without causing sleepiness. Rose (1999, p. 171) tells us that while it is gentle for babies, it is also aphrodisiac and uplifting.

A few drops in a glass of water is soothing and emotionally settling, and similarly a drop added to a cup of black coffee can help calm the effects of the caffeine (naturesgift.com/hydrosols). Rose (1999, p. 171) advises a teaspoonful to a cup of coffee, which sounds much more likely for a hydrolat, a drop being more the quantity necessary for an essential oil. Catty (2001, p. 86) gives the hydrolat as antiseptic and suggests various digestive attributes, such as stimulating bile, relieving heartburn – due to its antispasmodic action.

Skin

Together with lavender and rose hydrolats, orange blossom hydrolat contains skin-soothing substances that are not found in the corresponding essential oils; these waters are also free of irritating terpenes and other hydrocarbons. Their effects are antiseptic, antiinflammatory, cooling and astringent (Keller 1991).

Universally regarded as astringent and toning to the skin, orange flower water strengthens the skin and is particularly beneficial for the skin of nervous and stressed people with drawn features (Bego 1995, Goëb 1998).

Orange flower water appears to be much used for all types of skin:

- calms and rebalances dry skins (Sanoflore 2000)
- calming and hydrates dry, wrinkled skin (sabia.com 1997–1999)
- helps slow down the production of oil on the face and has an astringent effect that helps refine pores (6scent, Bego 1995)
- tones the skin – especially suitable for oily skin (Goëb 1998; Catty 2001, p. 86)
- delicate, sensitive skin (Catty 2001, p. 86)
- hydrating to dry skin (Rose 1999, p. 171)
- mature skin (innerself.com\magazine\herbs\essential_oils 2001)
- clears acne, irritated skin (Catty 1998b)

Culinary use

As well as its cosmetic use, it is widely known and used in the world of confectionery for its aromatic qualities (Sanoflore 2000) and it is delicious added to desserts, drinks, fruit salads, curries, etc. Rose (1992, p. 118) considers it perfect in 'all sorts of chocolate foods and drink'.

Grieve (1992, p. 602) says that it gives a gentle aroma to pastries; 'orange flower water is being increasingly used in France by biscuit makers to give crispness to their products, and some of the English biscuit makers have also adopted it for this purpose'.

Citrus aurantium var. ***amara*** **(fol.)** [PETITGRAIN] Rutaceae

(contains a volatile oil)

soporific

Petitgrain hydrolat can be used by both adults and infants for insomnia – 1–2 teaspoons at night (Franchomme & Pénoël 1990, p. 286).

Citrus aurantium var. ***sinensis*** **(flos)** [SWEET ORANGE FLOWER] Rutaceae

(contains a volatile oil)

antibacterial, antidepressive, antispasmodic, calming, carminative, digestive, nerve tonic

Sweet orange flower water is given by Viaud (1983) as being a cardiac calmative and an anticollibacillus agent; he claims that it is also useful for people suffering from seasonal nervous depression.

In Lebanese folk medicine it is used as a calming nervine (Nasr 2000, p. 26) in cases of acute anxiety and distress. Used as a facial splash for fainting due to emotional shock or psychological strain and traditionally employed as an antispasmodic and carminative taken neat to relieve intestinal colic, bloating due to trapped wind. Nasr claims that the therapeutic effects are immediate, implying an action through the inhaled volatile principles. He also tells us that in the Middle East, a mixture of warm boiled orange flower water and sugar, called white coffee, is sometimes given to children before bedtime to relax and aid digestion.

The flowers and leaves of the orange tree are used in infusions to act as sedative stomachics (Stuart 1987).

Citrus limon [LEMON] Rutaceae
(contains a volatile oil)
No information is available.

Cnicus benedictus (***Carbenia benedicta***) [HOLY THISTLE, BLESSED THISTLE] Asteraceae
antiinflammatory, calming (diaphoretic emmenagogic, stimulant)
An infusion of the herb is used medicinally as a stimulant and emmenagogue and the warm infusion is a diaphoretic in cases of bad colds. Parkinson says 'the distilled water hereof is much used to be drunk against agues of all sorts, either pestilential or humoral' and the water used to be popular as evidenced by the mention in Shakespeare: 'Get you some of this distilled *Carduus Benedictus*, and lay it to your heart: it is the only thing for a qualm' (*Much Ado About Nothing*, III, iv). [Ague is a swelling and inflammation due to a cold.]

Convallaria magalis [LILY OF THE VALLEY] Liliaceae
antiinflammatory (eyes), mental stimulant
Grieve (1992, p. 482) states that special virtues were once thought to be possessed by water distilled from the flowers, which was known as *Aqua aurea* (Golden water); it was deemed worthy to be preserved in vessels of gold and silver. Dodoens (1554) points out how this water 'doth strengthen the Memorie and comforteth the Harte'.

A wine may be prepared from the flowers mixed with raisins, as is done in some parts of Germany. Coles (1657) gives directions for the preparation of a wine: 'Take the flowers and steep them in New Wine for the space of a month; which being finished, take them out again and distil the wine three times over in a Limbeck. The wine is more precious than gold, for if anyone troubled with apoplexy drink thereof with six grains of Pepper and a little Lavender water they shall not need to fear it that moneth' (Grieve 1998, p. 482).

Gerard (1964, p. 104) said 'the floures of the Valley Lillie distilled with wine, and drunke the quantity of a spoonefull, restoreth speech unto those that have the dumb palsi and that are falne into the Apoplexie, and are good against the gout, and comforteth the heart. The water aforesaid doth strengthen the memory that is weakened and diminished; it helpeth also the inflammations of the eies, being dropped thereinto.'

Coriandrum sativum [CORIANDER] Apiaceae
(contains a volatile oil)
carminative
Coriander water was formerly much esteemed as a carminative for windy colic (Grieve 1992, p. 222).

Cotinus coggygria [SMOKE TREE] Anacardiceae

(contains a volatile oil)
antirheumatic

Cotyledon umbilicus [KIDNEYWORT] Crassulaceae

analgesic, antiinflammatory, cicatrizant, cooling, decongestant, digestive, litholytic
'The juice or distilled water if drunk is good to cool inflammations and unnatural heats, a hot stomach, a hot liver, or the bowels; the herb, juice, or distilled water applied outwardly, heals pimples, St. Anthony's fire and other outward heats' (Culpeper n.d., p. 206). He also recommends the juice or distilled water for ulcerated kidneys, gravel and stone, and an ointment made with it for painful piles and the pains of gout and sciatica.

The dried leaves and flowers are used to make a tisane for liver congestion, kidney, gall bladder and digestive disorders (Stuart 1987, p. 152).

Crataegus monogyna, C. oxyacantha [HAWTHORN, WHITETHORN] Rosaceae

The main components of the hydrolat analysed suggest the following properties may apply:

48–50% alcohols	antiinfectious, antiviral, bactericidal, decongestant, stimulating
42% dimethyl sulphide	(see p. 70)

Summary of the above properties:
antiinfectious, antiviral, bactericidal, decongestant, stimulating
The following properties have also been suggested:
antidepressive, calming (to the heart), muscle regenerator (Viaud 1983)
Fischer-Rizzi (1990) suggests taking this hydrolat to regulate high blood pressure.

Crocus sativus [SAFFRON] Iridaceae

The scent of this plant was valued as much as the dye; saffron water was sprinkled on the benches of the theatre, the floors of banqueting-halls were strewn with crocus leaves, and cushions were stuffed with it (Grieve 1992, p. 700).

Cuminum cyminum [CUMIN] Apiaceae

Found to have antibacterial activity against *Bacillus brevis, Enterobacter aerogenes* and one strain of *Escherischia coli* (Sağdiç & Özcan 2003).

Cupressus sempervirens [CYPRESS] Cupressaceae

(contains a volatile oil)
circulatory, diuretic
Viaud (1983) and Price & Price (1999) say that cypress hydrolat is a circulatory stimulant, useful for haemorrhoids, broken and varicose veins. It is also a diuretic (therefore good for counteracting water retention). Catty (2001, p. 89) advises avoiding this water in the first 3 months of pregnancy and in cases of kidney and urinary tract disease, although no reference or reason is given.
Hair
Useful for fragile hair and for diseases of the scalp (Grosjean 1993a, p. 116).

***Daucus carota* (sem.)** [CARROT SEED] Apiaceae

(contains a volatile oil)

The main components of the hydrolats analysed suggest the following properties may apply:

28–49% alcohols	antiinfectious, antiviral, bactericidal, decongestant, stimulating
12–36% esters	antifungal, antiinflammatory, antispasmodic, balancing (to nervous system), calming, cicatrizant, uplifting

Summary of the above properties:
antifungal, antiinfectious, **antiinflammatory,** *antispasmodic, antiviral, balancing (to nervous system), bactericidal,* **calming, cicatrizant,** *decongestant,* **stimulating, uplifting**

The highlighted properties appear in the text below, and the following property has also been suggested:
antiirritant, detoxifying, diuretic (mild)

Wild carrot seed hydrolat is considered by Catty (2001, p. 90) to cleanse and support the liver, gall bladder and kidneys, as it is mildly diuretic. As it is also restorative and tonic, it can be used as part of a detoxification plan in colonics, when it is healing and calming to irritations in the smooth muscle tissue.

Skin

Carrot seed hydrolat is antiinflammatory, soothing irritated, itchy, dry skin, says Rose (1999, p. 172). It can also be used in acne treatments and impetigo, as well as for calming eczema and psoriasis. It can be added to face scrubs and masks and for men in an aftershave (Catty 2001, p. 90). The hydrolat is also a useful toner or cleanser for mature skin (naturesgift.com/hydrosols).

Culinary use

Catty (2001, p. 90) finds it delicious in soups and juices (sweet and savoury) and in salad dressings and sauces.

Dictamnus albus [BURNING BUSH] Rutaceae

(contains a volatile oil)

The *distilled water* is used as a cosmetic. An *infusion* of the leaves is regarded as a substitute for tea (Grieve 1992, p. 147).

Echinacea purpurea [PURPLE CONEFLOWER] Asteraceae

The main components of the hydrolat analysed suggest the following properties may apply:

50–53% aldehydes	antiinfectious, antiinflammatory, antiviral, calming, circulatory (hypotensor), febrifuge, tonic
17–18% ketones	analgesic, anticoagulant, antiinflammatory, calming, cicatrizant, digestive, expectorant, lipolytic, mucolytic, sedative, stimulant

Summary of the above properties:
analgesic, anticoagulant, antiinfectious, antiinflammatory, antiviral, calming, cicatrizant, circulatory (hypotensor), digestive, expectorant, febrifuge, lipolytic, mucolytic, sedative, **stimulant, tonic**

The authors have found this hydrolat to be an effective immune booster.

Elettaria cardamomum [CARDAMOM] Zingiberaceae

antiinfectious, antispasmodic, calming, sedative (mild)
Cardamom hydrolat quickly calms spasms in the digestive tract and appears to be relaxing (Catty 2001, p. 91).
Culinary
The same writer tells us it is 'delightful in both savoury and sweet dishes'.

Equisetum arvense [FIELD HORSETAIL] Equisetaceae

The main components of the hydrolat analysed suggest the following properties may apply:

62–64% alcohols antiinfectious, antiviral, bactericidal, decongestant, stimulating

Erigeron canadensis [FLEABANE] Asteraceae

analgesic, antibacterial, antiinflammatory, circulatory, digestive, diuretic, styptic
Viaud (1983) says that fleabane stimulates the circulation and helps joints (possibly due to its analgesic and antiinflammatory properties). He also recommends it for uterine and nasal haemorrhages. Catty (2001, p. 92) says it is antibacterial, digestive and diuretic in renal infections. It is currently being researched in veterinary medicine as a treatment for high blood pressure.

Eucalyptus dives [BROAD LEAVED PEPPERMINT] Myrtaceae

nasal mucolytic (Franchomme & Pénoël 1990 p. 302)

Eucalyptus globulus [TASMANIAN BLUE GUM] Myrtaceae

(contains a volatile oil)
antidiabetic, antiinfectious, antioxidant, stimulating
Viaud (1983) gives this hydrolat as antidiabetic and also helpful for the kidneys and pancreas. He also suggests its use on the bronchi. Rose (1999, p. 172) says the water is respiratory, and for colds, respiratory infections and sore throats. Catty (2001, p. 93) suggests combining it with Inula for infections and liver support. She gives it as a strong antioxidant, free radical scavenger and stimulating to mind and body.

Grosjean (1993a, p. 120) suggests putting 2 tablespoonfuls of the distilled water in 1½ litres of water to drink during the day in cases of diabetes, alternating daily with juniper water. She also recommends it for respiratory problems in babies and children. As the taste is strong and not altogether pleasant, it can be sweetened with honey (Catty 2001, p. 93) and diluted well for children.
Skin
Eucalyptus hydrolat is helpful in cases of acne (Price & Price 1999; Rose 1999, p. 172) and it helps repel biting insects (6scent).

Eucalyptus polybractea [BLUE LEAVED MALLEE] Myrtaceae

bronchitis (Catty 1998)

Eupatorium cannabinum [HEMP AGRIMONY] Asteraceae

chronic cystitis, mineral deficiency, pulmonary (Viaud 1983)

Euphrasia officinalis [EYEBRIGHT] Scrophulariaceae

Although rather neglected nowadays, many modern herbalists still retain faith in this herb and recommend its use in diseases of the sight, weakness of the eyes, ophthalmia, etc., combining it often with golden seal in a lotion stated to be excellent for general disorders of the eyes.

(analgesic), ophthalmic

An infusion of 1 oz (28 g) of the herb to a pint (500 ml) of boiling water should be used and the eyes bathed three or four times a day. Ordinarily a cold application will suffice, but when there is a lot of pain, it is considered desirable to use a warm infusion rather more frequently for inflamed eyes until the pain has gone. (Grieve 1998, p. 292).

Culpeper (n.d.) considered eyebright to be an excellent hydrolat to clear the sight; 'the juice or distilled water of eyebright taken inwardly in white wine or broth, or dropped into the eyes, for divers days together helps all infirmities of the eyes that cause dimness of sight' (p. 134).

'Eyebright stamped and laid upon the eyes, or the juice thereof mixed with white wine, and dropped into the eyes, or the distilled water, taketh away the darknesse and dimnesse of the eyes, and cleareth the sight' (Gerard 1964, p. 151).

***Filipendula ulmaria* (*Spirea ulmaria*)** [MEADOWSWEET] Rosaceae

The main components of the hydrolat analysed suggest the following properties may apply:

69% dimethyl sulphide (see p. 70)	
14–15% ketones	analgesic, anticoagulant, antiinflammatory, calming, cicatrizant, digestive, expectorant, lipolytic, mucolytic, sedative, stimulant
10–11% eucalyptol	expectorant, mucolytic
8–9% alcohols	antiinfectious, antiviral, bactericidal, decongestant, stimulating

Summary of the above properties:

analgesic, *anticoagulant, antiinfectious,* **antiinflammatory**, *antiviral, bactericidal, calming, cicatrizant, decongestant, digestive, expectorant, lipolytic, mucolytic, sedative,* **stimulant**

The highlighted properties appear in the text below, and the following have also been suggested:

antiirritant, ophthalmic, (sudorific), uplifting

Grieve (1992, p. 525) tells us that an infusion of the fresh tops produces perspiration, and a decoction of the root, in white wine, was formerly considered a specific in fevers.

Gerard (cited in Grieve 1992, p. 524) says that 'It is reported that the floures boiled in wine and drunke do take away the fite of the quartaine ague and make the heart merrie.' Grieve herself says: 'An infusion of 1 oz of the dried herb to a pint of water is the usual mode of administration, in wineglassful doses. Sweetened with honey, it forms a very pleasant diet-drink, or beverage both for invalids and ordinary use.' In his own book Gerard (1964, p. 245) adds: 'The distilled water of the floures dropped into the eies taketh away the burning and itching thereof and cleareth the sight.' Culpeper (n.d., p. 230) says the water is also 'good for inflammation of the eyes.'

Foeniculum vulgare* var. *dulce (sem.) [FENNEL] Apiaceae

(contains a volatile oil)

analgesic, anticatarrhal, antiseptic, antispasmodic, carminative, digestive, lactogenic, stimulating

'Aqua Foeniculi (fennel water) is prepared by distilling, till one gallon comes over, one pound of bruised sweet fennel-fruit and two gallons of distilled water . . . It is stimulant, aromatic, and carminative, and is used to relieve flatulence and diminish griping' (Newcastle Chronicle 1896).

Viaud (1983) credits the hydrolat with being antiseptic and a useful galactogen.

Grieve (1992, p. 296) says that fennel water has properties similar to those of anise and dill water: mixed with sodium bicarbonate and syrup, these waters make the domestic 'gripe water', used to correct the flatulence of infants. Volatile oil of fennel has these properties in concentration. The authors have in the past, used a few drops of fennel essential oil in a litre of water as a preventative against digestive infections and against stomach pains. However, they now use the hydrolat as a prophylactic (1 teaspoonful – 5 ml – daily, in 1 or 2 teaspoons of water), which is easier, and equally effective.

Catty (2001, p. 94) says fennel hydrolat is antiseptic and antispasmodic for digestive, respiratory and muscular conditions. She also credits it with helping lung congestion and catarrh and says it may promote lactation in nursing mothers. She tells us not to give the hydrolat to children under 6 years and to avoid long-term use, although she does not say why.

Fennel tea, formerly also employed as a carminative, is made by pouring half a pint of boiling water on a teaspoonful of bruised fennel seeds. It has a distinctive aroma and flavour.

Fragaria vesca [STRAWBERRY] Rosaceae

(cooling), uplifting

'The leaves boyled and applied in manner of a pultis taketh away the burning heate in wounds. The distilled water drunke with white Wine is good against the passion of the heart, reviving the spirits, and making the heart merry' (Gerard 1964, p. 237).

Fucus vesiculosus [BLADDERWRACK] Fucaceae

Bladderwrack is one of several seaweeds which have long been used in medicine and for culinary purposes. Iodine, essential for an underactive thyroid, was first discovered by distilling bladderwrack in the early nineteenth century and for 50 years most supplies were obtained in this way (Stuart 1982, p. 193).

The main components of the hydrolat analysed suggest the following properties may apply:

60% dimethyl sulphide (see p. 70)

27–28% ketones	analgesic, anticoagulant, antiinflammatory, calming, cicatrizant, digestive, expectorant, lipolytic, mucolytic, sedative, stimulant
9–10% alcohols	antiinfectious, antiviral, bactericidal, decongestant, stimulating

Summary of the above properties:

analgesic, *anticoagulant, antiinfectious,* **antiinflammatory,** *antiviral, bactericidal, calming, cicatrizant,* **decongestant,** *digestive, expectorant, lipolytic, mucolytic, sedative, stimulant*

The highlighted properties appear in the text below, and the following have been suggested for a decoction:

(antiobesic, antirheumatic, thyroid stimulant)

Stuart also tells us that this plant is of specific use in obesity which is linked with underactive thyroid glands. He goes on to say that a decoction (see glossary) of the whole fresh plant can be applied externally for rheumatism and rheumatoid arthritis.

Fumaria officinalis [FUMITORY] Fumariaceae

Physicians and writers from Dioscorides to Chaucer, and from the 14th century to Cullen and to modern times, value this herb's purifying power. The thickened juice, syrups, powders, tinctures and the distilled water were used. The distilled water has the same virtues as the juice, but is much weaker and may be used as a vehicle for any of the other preparations (Grieve 1998, p. 330).
antiseptic, cicatrizant, cooling, purifying

Culpeper (n.d., p. 157) wrote that the distilled water of the herb was an excellent preventative against the plague and Gerard put forward that it helped 'those troubled with scabs'.

Clair (1961, p. 171) wrote that the herb was at one time commonly used for making a cosmetic water to purify the skin and, two decades later, Kresanek (1982, p. 90) reiterated that the water is popularly used as a skin cleansing agent.

An old rhyme has it that the flowers were:

– Cropped by maids in weeding hours,
To boil in water, milk, or whey,
For washes on a holiday;
To make their beauty fair and sleek,
And scare the tan from summer's cheek.

Another old rhyme indicates that the water of fumitory has hepatic properties:

– Get water of fumitory, liver to cool,
And others the like, or else go like a fool.
Thomas Tusser

Galega officinalis [GOAT'S RUE] Papilionaceae

antidiabetic, detoxifying, lactogenic
Viaud (1983) says that goat's rue is helpful for breast abscesses, the pancreas and the respiratory mucous membranes because of its antitoxic and antidiabetic action. A tea of goat's rue has supportive antidiabetic action and it is employed as a galactogogue in both humans and animals (Stuart 1987, p. 194).

Gentiana lutea [YELLOW GENTIAN] Gentianaceae

Fresh gentian root is largely used in Germany and Switzerland for the production of an alcoholic beverage. The roots are cut, macerated with water, fermented and distilled; the distillate contains alcohol and a trace of volatile oil, which imparts to it a characteristic odour and taste (Grieve 1998, p. 349).
uplifting, energizing (Viaud 1983)

Glechoma hederacea [FIELD BALM, GROUND IVY] Lamiaceae

People used to make gill (ground ivy) tea which was mixed with honey or sugar to take away the bitterness, as a remedy for coughs and colds (Clair 1961, p. 177).

Hamamelis virginiana [WITCH HAZEL, WINTERBLOOM] Hamamelidaceae

This extract is made from the autumn collection of leaves and twigs and has an ethanol content of 70–80% and a tannin content of 2–9%. However, when the product is bought at a store it contains 15% ethanol (Winter 1999, p. 458). The plant is distilled solely for the hydrolat although it contains a very small percentage of volatile oil.

Distilled witch hazel extract was official in the USP (United States Pharmacopoeia) from 1905 to 1926 and in the NF (National Formulary) from 1888 to 1905 and from 1926 to the present day.

In a study on witch hazel, Korting et al (1993) compared the antiinflammatory properties of witch hazel with hydrocortisone cream and concluded that although not as efficient as hydrocortisone, witch hazel was effective and offered the advantage of not having the serious adverse side effects of hydrocortisone, such as skin atrophy and suppression of the hypothalamic–pituitary–adrenal system.

Mills (1985, p. 219) notes that the distilled witch hazel widely sold commercially is not as astringent as other preparations as no tannins are present. Tyler (1993) agrees that no tannin is present in the distilled plant water and adds that red wine, which contains some tannin, has a therapeutic value as an astringent exceeding that of witch hazel.

analgesic, antibacterial, antifungal, antiinflammatory, antiirritant, antioxidant, antiseptic, astringent, cicatrisant, cooling, ophthalmic, sedative, styptic, tonic

Aqueous extracts of the shrub plant, hamamelis water, have been applied as cooling agents to sprains and bruises, and also as a haemostat on small wounds. The hydrolat can be used as a haemostat and sedative in veterinary medicine also. Ody (1997) advises using the distilled water for cooling minor burns, sunburn and insect bites.

Well diluted, Lower (1999) tells us that the extract has also been included in eye lotions, while Mabey (1988) says that conjunctivitis can be treated with compresses of the distilled water. Diluted with warm water, Grieve (1998, p. 851) recommends the extract be used for inflammation of the eyelids, using ½ to 3 drachms of liquor hamamelidis (a distillate of the fresh leaves). It can also be used in a compress for bags under the eyes.

For nose bleeds an effective treatment is to plug the nostril with cotton wool saturated in the distilled water (Bartram 1995). Bartram also mentions it as being useful for treating skin that has been thinned by long steroid therapy; the astringent action could help toughen the skin.

Its astringent action is further extolled by Grieve (1998, p. 851) when she tells us that witch hazel is excellent in cases of both internal and external bleeding, for example from the lungs or from the nose, as well as other internal organs. This could be due to its action on the muscular fibre of the veins.

Varicose veins can be eased by using compresses of the distilled water, helping to relieve heat, pain and itching (Mabey 1988) while toning the vein walls, and it is also useful for phlebitis (Bartram 1995). In the treatment of varicose veins, Grieve (1998, p. 851) advises it be applied on a lint bandage, which must be constantly kept moist (cling film?). In fact, she goes on to say that a pad of witch hazel applied to a burst varicose vein will stop the bleeding and often save life by its instant application. Catty (2001, p. 96) recommends witch hazel hydrolat in a sitz bath for haemorrhoids.

naturesgift.com/hydrosols says it is antibacterial, soothing and antiinflammatory and for fungal infections in 'delicate' places when no other remedy seems to help.

In Grieve (1998, p. 851) we find that a tea made with the leaves or bark may be taken freely with advantage, being good for bleeding of the stomach and in complaints of the bowels, and an injection of this tea is excellent for inwardly bleeding piles, the relief being marvellous and the cure speedy.

One further use for witch hazel hydrolat is in cases of bites from insects and mosquitoes, when a pad of cotton wool, moistened with the hydrolat and applied to the spot, will soon cause the pain and swelling to subside (Grieve 1998, p. 851).

Skin

Witch hazel is considered an effective astringent by the FDA (Food and Drug Administration of the US Health Department). Commission E (a German authority) considers aqueous extracts of witch hazel leaves to be an astringent for inflammation of the skin and mucous membranes. Sanoflore (2000) also states that witch-hazel floral water is an astringent which stimulates micro-circulation and calms congestive eruptions of the face.

It is very widely used as a cosmetic ingredient and as a skin freshener; it is a local anaesthetic and also an astringent (Winter 1999, p. 458). Wren (1975) tells us that a simple, pleasant skin toner can be made by mixing equal parts of rose water and witch hazel.

Being antioxidant, antiinflammatory and cicatrizant, witch hazel hydrolat heals cracked or blistered skin and is useful as an anti-age treatment; it is also antiseptic and makes a good astringent toner for a teenage skin (Catty 2001, p. 96).

Harpagophytum procumbens [DEVIL'S CLAW] Pedaliaceae

anticancerous, renal cleanser (Viaud 1983)

Hedera helix [IVY] Araliaceae

An infusion of the leaves in wine was once considered to be an effective preventative and treatment for drunkenness and a decoction of the leaves in vinegar may be used as a mouth rinse in cases of toothache (Stuart 1987, p. 200).

Helichrysum italicum, Helichrysum angustifolium [EVERLASTING] Asteraceae

(contains a volatile oil)

The main components of the hydrolats analysed suggest the following properties may apply:

38–41% ketones	analgesic, anticoagulant, antiinflammatory, calming, cicatrizant, digestive, expectorant, lipolytic, mucolytic, sedative, stimulant
19–20% alcohols	antiinfectious, antiviral, bactericidal, decongestant, stimulating
14–16% eucalyptol	expectorant, mucolytic

Summary of the above properties:

analgesic, **anticoagulant,** *antiinfectious,* **antiinflammatory,** *antiviral, calming,* **cicatrizant, digestive,** *expectorant, lipolytic, mucolytic,* **sedative, stimulant**

The highlighted properties appear in the text below, and the following have also been suggested:

antidiabetic, antiirritant, detoxifying, lung cleanser, soothing

Viaud (1983) recommends the hydrolat of helichrysum for diabetes, nervous depression and aerophagy, saying it is also a pulmonary depurative. Rose (1999, p. 172) says it is detoxifying and soothing to the heart. For liver and gall bladder problems, she recommends taking it in mineral water or wherever a honey scent is desired.

The authors have found it to be sedative (Price & Price 1999) and also effective in a compress for bruises and abscesses. Catty (2001, p. 96) says it is a powerful antiinflammatory and mild analgesic. It is an effective mouthwash for gingivitis and receding gums, having good results also as a gargle for a sore throat. She advocates it too for an upset stomach.

Skin

Rose (1999, p. 172) tells us that everlasting heals and soothes irritation, being good for inflamed conditions. She says it is also helpful in reducing scarring when used on fresh wounds.

naturesgift.com/hydrosols says the hydrolat is a useful toner for rosacea, couperose (thread veins) and inflamed skin.

Hieracium pilosella [MOUSE EAR, HAWKWEED] Asteraceae

(contains a volatile oil)

(antipyretic), (antibiotic), diuretic

Viaud (1983) recommends this hydrolat as a diuretic, saying also that it breaks urinary stones.

It is an effective gargle (presumably as an infusion or decoction) and possesses antibiotic action; various claims have been made for its beneficial effect on eye conditions (Stuart 1987, p. 202).

Hydrocotyle asiatica [INDIAN PENNYWORT] Apiaceae

No information on the distilled water is available, but the plant is used as diuretic, tonic and purgative.

Hypericum perforatum [ST JOHN'S WORT] Hypericaceae

(contains a volatile oil)

The main components of the hydrolat analysed suggest the following properties may apply:

25% dimethyl sulphide (see p. 70)	
15–17% alcohols	antiinfectious, antiviral, bactericidal, decongestant, stimulating
28–36% aldehydes	antiinfectious, antiinflammatory, antiviral, calming, circulatory (hypotensor), febrifuge, tonic
17–20% ketones	analgesic, anticoagulant, antiinflammatory, calming, cicatrizant, digestive, expectorant, lipolytic, mucolytic, sedative, stimulant

Summary of the above properties:

analgesic, anticoagulant, antiinfectious, antiinflammatory, antiviral, bactericidal, calming, cicatrizant, circulatory (hypotensor), decongestant, digestive, expectorant, febrifuge, lipolytic, mucolytic, sedative, stimulating, tonic

A host of virtues has been ascribed to this plant, including the following:

anticancerous (Viaud 1983)

Hyssopus officinalis [HYSSOP] Lamiaceae

(contains a volatile oil)

The main components of the hydrolats analysed suggest the following properties may apply:

89–90% ketones analgesic, anticoagulant, antiinflammatory, calming, cicatrizant, digestive, expectorant, lipolytic, mucolytic, sedative, stimulant

Summary of the above properties:

analgesic, anticoagulant, antiinflammatory, calming, cicatrizant, **digestive, expectorant,** *lipolytic,* **mucolytic,** *sedative, stimulant*

The highlighted properties appear in the text below, and the following has also been suggested:

antiepileptic

Viaud (1983) considers a low dose of hyssop hydrolat clears the lungs and that a high dose is antiepileptic. The authors find this particularly interesting, as they have used hyssop essential oil in a low concentration several times on young adults with epilepsy with positive results.

The authors have used the fresh flower tops in an infusion for coughs and bronchial ailments with some success, and hyssop tea, brewed from the green tops of the herb, has long been an accepted country remedy all over Europe for colds and anaemia (Clair 1961, p. 184).

Grosjean reminds us that although the essential oil of hyssop is not suitable for babies and certain adults, the distilled water can be used instead – a teaspoonful in water three to five times per day (Grosjean 1993a, pp. 133–134).

In former days, the remedy *Diatron piperion* was much used for medicinal purposes, and was said (in *The Widdowes Treasure*, 1595) to aid digestion, expel wind, keep ill vapours from the brain and restore lost memory. The ingredients of this remedy were white pepper, black pepper, long pepper, thyme, ginger and aniseed pounded and boiled in a solution of sugar in *hyssop water* (Clair 1961, p. 69). This remedy had great virtues, according to *The Widdowes Treasure*, which gives a recipe for making the best *Diatrion piperion* and adds:

This decoction is good to eat
alwaies before and after meate.
For it will make digestion good,
and turne your meat to pure blood.
Besides all this it doth excell
all windines to expell;
And all groce humors colde and rawe
that are in belly, stomacke or mawe,
It will dissolve without paine,
and keep ill vapors from the braine.
Besides all this it will restore
your memory though lost before.
Use it therefore when you please,
for therein resteth mightie ease.

Inula graveolens, I. helenium [ELECAMPANE] Asteraceae

(contains a volatile oil)

liver stimulant (Catty 2001, p. 99), *mucolytic, respiratory*

The mucolytic effects of this hydrolat make it useful for leucorrhoea, chest congestion and phlegm and it is particularly effective on bronchitis – in short, a respiratory tonic. Use it in a douche for thrush or vaginitis (Catty 2001, p. 99). The Chinese use it for conditions of the lungs and liver; it has a long record of use for coughs – tuberculosis, whooping cough, croup (Bartram 1995, p. 164) and it is almost exclusively employed in respiratory disorders (Stuart 1987, p. 206).

Skin

Catty tells us that it also balances an oily skin and calms acne and can be used in a sauna, steam or humidifier.

Iris pseudacorus [IRIS] Iridaceae

ophthalmic

Culpeper says that the distilled water of the whole herb is a sovereign remedy for weak eyes, either applied on a wet bandage, or dropped into the eye (Grieve 1992, p. 439).

Juglans regia [WALNUT] Juglandaceae

antidiabetic (Viaud 1983)

[The dried leaves are weakly hypoglycaemic, astringent, antiinflammatory (Stuart 1987, p. 209).]

Junipers (see below)

NB: As many of the sources do not give the Latin name, or discriminate between the hydrolat obtained from the branches (wood, needles and berries) and that obtained only from the berries, the authors have listed both under the one heading.

Juniperus communis [JUNIPER BRANCH AND JUNIPER BERRY] Cupressaceae

(contains a volatile oil)

The main components of the juniper hydrolat analysed (not specified whether branches or berries) suggest the following properties may apply:

74–78% alcohols	antiinfectious, antiviral, bactericidal, decongestant, stimulating
8–9% ketones	slightly – analgesic, anticoagulant, antiinflammatory, calming, cicatrizant, digestive, expectorant, lipolytic, mucolytic, sedative, stimulant

Summary of the above properties:

analgesic, *anticoagulant, antiinfectious*, **antiinflammatory**, *antiviral, bactericidal, calming, cicatrizant, decongestant, digestive, expectorant, lipolytic, mucolytic, sedative*, **stimulant**

The highlighted properties appear in the text below, and the following have also been suggested:

antidiabetic, astringent, circulatory, detoxifying, diuretic

Viaud (1983) considers juniper (unspecified) hydrolat to be diuretic, a kidney deflocculant (cleanser) and helpful to rheumatoid arthritis and the skin.

Grosjean (1993a, p. 123) recommends juniper (unspecified) hydrolat for all sufferers of rheumatism and persons with acid constitution. She suggests putting 2 tablespoonfuls of the distilled water in 1½ litres of water to drink during the day in cases of diabetes; alternating daily with eucalyptus. In her book in English (1993b, p. 36), she recommends it as an effective slimming drink.

Rose (1999, p. 172) considers juniper berry hydrolat to be detoxifying, diuretic and simulating to both the mind and the circulation. Catty (2001, p. 101) uses juniper berry hydrolat for water retention and related issues, including cellulite. She especially recommends it to ease rheumatic and arthritic conditions.

Skin

Juniper branch hydrolat is a refreshing astringent toner for oily and acneic skin (Price & Price 1999).

Culinary use

The berry hydrolat is considered to be delicious in marinades, sauces and gravies (Catty 2001, p. 101) and Rose (1999, p. 173) uses it in marinades.

Lactuca hortensis, Lactuca sativa [LETTUCE] Asteraceae

hepatic depurative, vermifuge (Viaud 1983)

Lactuca virosa [WILD LETTUCE] Asteraceae

hepatic depurative (Viaud 1983)

Lamium album [DEAD NETTLE] Lamiaceae

refreshing, uplifting

'The floures are baked with sugar as Roses are, which is called Sugar roset: as also the distilled water of them, which is used to make the heart merry, to make a good colour in the face, and to refresh the vital spirits' (Gerard 1964, p. 158).

***Laurus nobilis* (fol.)** [BAY LAUREL, BAY LEAF] Lauraceae

(contains a volatile oil)

analgesic, antibacterial, antiinfectious, antiseptic, antispasmodic, circulatory stimulant, digestive, immunostimulant, toning, uplifting

Viaud (1983) recommends bay hydrolat as an intestinal antiseptic, digestive (aiding flatulence) and an antispasmodic.

Franchomme & Pénoël (1990) write that the hydrolat is antiinfectious and analgesic, excellent in a compress for varicose ulcers.

Catty (2001, pp. 103–104) has found it stimulates the lymph and circulation and is a broad-acting antiseptic and bactericide; it tones the intestines and may relieve gas; it is an excellent tonic and immune booster and is suitable as a mouthwash and gargle for infections and dental hygiene.

In San Francisco, Catty (1998a) reported that in over two dozen cases of long-term palpable swollen lymph nodes in breast tissue, *Laurus nobilis* (bay leaf) hydrolat effected a complete disappearance of the swelling and tenderness within 5 days by dilute internal use. She went on to say that given before and after vaccinations, bay leaf hydrolat acts prophylactically to prevent many of the associated side effects and helps the body deal with the vaccination process.

Skin

Rose (1999, p. 170) suggests its use as a man's aftershave, both for the toning effect and the scent.

Culinary use
Bay hydrolat has a strong 'food' type aroma and taste and is good in all savoury cooking, with fish or meat, and can be sprinkled on steaming vegetables (Rose 1999, p. 172). Catty (2001, p. 104) finds it indispensable in the kitchen, saying it can be added to any savoury dish – pastas, sauces, soups, fish or meat and salad dressings.

Lavandula angustifolia (L. officinalis, L. vera) [LAVENDER] Lamiaceae
(contains a volatile oil)
In the past, the distinction between true lavenders, lavandins and spike lavender was not always observed and all species and their varieties were referred to as 'lavender'. Lavender water has a long history of use. The aroma of lavender hydrolat is not the same as the essential oil, probably because of the lack of linalyl acetate, and the author suggests adding a small amount of geranium or peppermint hydrolats. When the authors first marketed lavender water, many years ago, some clients returned it because it did not have the expected aroma.

The main components of the hydrolats tested suggest the following properties may apply:

56–69% alcohols	antiinfectious, antiviral, bactericidal, decongestant, stimulating
18–19% ketones	analgesic, anticoagulant, antiinflammatory, calming, cicatrizant, digestive, expectorant, lipolytic, mucolytic, sedative, stimulant

Summary of the above properties:
analgesic, *anticoagulant, antiinfectious,* **antiinflammatory,** *antiviral,* **bactericidal, calming, cicatrizant,** *decongestant, digestive, expectorant, lipolytic, mucolytic, sedative, stimulant*

The highlighted properties appear in the text below, and the following have also been suggested:
antiirritant, balancing, soothing

Viaud (1983) and Fischer-Rizzi (1990) both give true lavender hydrolat as an intestinal antibiotic.

Grieve (1992, p. 472) recommends it as a gargle and for hoarseness and lack of voice.

It is useful in lotions and friction rubs for rheumatism (Price & Price 1999) and for cleansing wounds.

The authors have found lavender hydrolat to be relaxing and revitalizing, and to reduce headaches and ease stress and mental fatigue; however, unless used in a compress, a more acceptable aroma can easily be achieved by adding a little of a pleasant smelling hydrolat with similar properties. In any case, as with essential oils, a synergy of two or three hydrolats will have an enhanced effect.

Rose (1999, p. 170), among the other attributes she gives for lavender water, says it is a must for long aeroplane flights, being helpful against jet lag.

naturesgift.com/hydrosols and Grosjean (1993a, p. 138) suggest it calms and relaxes babies after the bath as a lotion. It should be equally effective adding a tablespoonful to the bath.

Skin
Being antiseptic, lavender hydrolat is helpful to all skin problems including acne, pimples and eczema and is soothing to burns and insect bites (Price & Price 1999).

Lavender water is gentle, balancing for all skin types, cooling in summer's heat, soothing sunburn, razor rash and healing irritation. It gently and safely cleanses and tones oily, dry and mature skin (Rose 1999, p. 170; Catty 2001, pp. 104–105; naturesgift.com/hydrosols).

Lavender hydrolat is chiefly used to cleanse and soften facial skin and the hair (Grosjean 1993a, p. 138). Sanoflore (2000) adds that lavender floral water not only purifies and balances greasy skins, but is also used to strengthen the hair.

Claeys (1992) says lavender water is cicatrizant, bactericidal and suitable for greasy skin, although he does not specify which lavender.

Culinary use
Rose (1999, p. 170) recommends its use in mineral water and all dessert foods, though the essential oil is preferable in the experience of Maria Kettenring who in 1995 prepared a delicious lavender ice cream for our students (for recipe see Kettenring 1994, p. 140).

Keville & Green (1995) have made lavender lemonade, using 2 cups of lemonade to 1–2 tablespoons of lavender hydrolat. For a special touch, they suggest adding ice cubes with fresh lavender flowers frozen into them.

Lavandula × intermedia (LAVANDIN) Lamiaceae
(contains a volatile oil)
The main components of the hydrolat analysed suggest the following properties may apply:

70–87% alcohols	antiinfectious, **antiviral**, bactericidal, decongestant, **stimulating**

The highlighted properties appear in the text below, and the following have also been suggested:
antiseptic, relaxing

Price & Price (1999) have found lavandin hydrolat to be helpful to acneic skin and herpes; Rose (1999, p. 171) says it is toning, relaxing and revitalizing.

Lavandula latifolia [SPIKE LAVENDER] Lamiaceae
(contains a volatile oil)
The main components of the hydrolat tested suggest the following properties may apply (they also suggest that this could be a very useful hydrolat for the therapist:

29% eucalyptol	expectorant, mucolytic
30–32% alcohols	antiinfectious, antiviral, bactericidal, decongestant, stimulating
32% ketones	analgesic, anticoagulant, antiinflammatory, calming, cicatrizant, digestive, expectorant, lipolytic, mucolytic, sedative, stimulant

Summary of the above properties:
analgesic, *anticoagulant, antiinfectious, antiinflammatory, antiviral, bactericidal, calming, cicatrizant, decongestant, digestive, expectorant, lipolytic, mucolytic,* **sedative, stimulant**

The highlighted properties appear in the text below, and the following have also been suggested:

antiepileptic, strengthening

In Culpeper (n.d., pp. 210–211) we learn that two spoonfuls of spike lavender hydrolat help people who have lost their voice. He goes on to say that it also helps 'the tremblings and passions of the heart, and faintings and swoonings, applied to the temples or nostrils, to be smelt unto'.

Gerard (1964, p. 132) echoes the effects on the heart, but with a synergy of spices:

> *The floures of (spike) Lavander picked from the knaps, I meane the blew part and not the husk, mixed with Cinnamon, Nutmegs, & Cloves, made into pouder, and given to drinke in the distilled water thereof, doth helpe the panting and passion of the heart, prevaileth against giddiness, turning, or swimming of the braine, and members subject to the palsie.*

Regarding the use of spike lavender on its own, he recommends inhaling, or bathing the temples and forehead with, distilled water of spike lavender to refresh those that have a light migraine, faint a lot or suffer from falling sickness (epilepsy). He also says it will aid those with catalepsy (a neurosis characterized by a temporary loss of the senses and the power to move the muscles; trance-like).

Coles (in Adam and Eve) describes the many virtues of the distilled water of spike lavender; he warns, as did Culpeper, that 'it is not safe to use it when the body is full of humours, mixed with blood, because of the hot and subtill spirits wherewith it is possessed' (Clair 1961, p. 186).

Ledum groenlandicum [GREENLAND MOSS] Ericaceae

antiinfectious, detoxifying, immunostimulant, sedative

According to Catty (2001, p. 106), this rare and expensive hydrolat is the most powerfully therapeutic of all hydrolats and should be used at half the strength recommended for other hydrolats. Because of its strength, she recommends avoiding it if pregnant or where there is a tendency to epilepsy and not using it on children under 6 years old.

A liver detoxifier, it improves liver function and is generally good for the health. It is excellent for postoperative use or infections and seems to strengthen the immune system. It is strongly sedative, with an unusual fragrance and flavour.

Levisticum officinale [LOVAGE] Apiaceae

(contains a volatile oil)

detoxifying, ophthalmic

Viaud (1983) recommends this hydrolat as a skin purifier.

In the opinion of Culpeper (n.d., p. 219), gargling with the distilled water relieves quinsy (inflammation of the throat due to abscesses on the tonsils) and helps pleurisy if drunk three or four times. He goes on to say that the hydrolat, 'if dropped into the eyes', takes away the redness and dimness of the eyes; it also removes spots and freckles from the face.

Linaria vulgaris [TOADFLAX] Scrophulariaceae

antiinflammatory, (astringent), cleansing, (diuretic), ophthalmic, (tonic)

The juice of the herb, or the distilled water, has been considered a good remedy for inflammation of the eyes, and for cleansing ulcerous sores (Grieve 1992, p. 816).

The tea and compress of this plant is given as astringent, detergent, diuretic, hepatic, antiscrofula, blood tonic (Bartram 1995, p. 425).

Lippia citriodora [LEMON VERBENA] (see ***Aloysia triphylla***)

Malva sylvestris [MALLOW] Malvaceae

The main components of the hydrolat tested suggest the following properties may apply:

68% dimethyl sulphide	(see p. 70)
6–7% alcohols	antiinfectious, antiviral, bactericidal, decongestant, stimulating
15–16% ketones	analgesic, anticoagulant, antiinflammatory, calming, cicatrizant, digestive, expectorant, lipolytic, mucolytic, sedative, stimulant

Summary of the above properties:
analgesic, anticoagulant, antiinfectious, antiinflammatory, antiviral, bactericidal, calming, cicatrizant, decongestant, digestive, expectorant, lipolytic, mucolytic, sedative, stimulant

Matricaria recutita, Chamomilla recutita [GERMAN CHAMOMILE] Asteraceae

(contains a volatile oil)

The hydrolat from this plant is quite rare.

The main components of the hydrolat analysed suggest the following properties may apply:

14–16% alcohols	antiinfectious, antiviral, bactericidal, decongestant, stimulating
57–59% esters	antifungal, antiinflammatory, antispasmodic, balancing (to nervous system), calming, cicatrizant, uplifting

Summary of the above properties:
antifungal, antiinfectious, antiinflammatory, antispasmodic, *antiviral, bactericidal, balancing (to nervous system),* **calming, cicatrizant,** *decongestant, stimulating, uplifting*

The highlighted properties appear in the text below, and the following have also been suggested:
antiirritant, digestive, sedative, soothing, styptic

Fischer-Rizzi (1990) recommends this hydrolat for stomach and intestinal disorders, and Rose (1999, p. 170) tells us that German chamomile hydrolat is emotionally calming.

According to Catty (2001, p. 108), German chamomile hydrolat is blessed with many attributes: being antifungal it is useful for *Candida albicans*, thrush, etc. She recommends it as a douche or taken internally for urinary tract infections and says it is antispasmodic to the intestinal tract, being useful in colonics. Topically, it is useful on varicose veins and haemorrhoids, etc.

Skin

Catty says further that German chamomile hydrolat is antiinflammatory in both compresses and lotions, calms sensitive skin, rashes and itching and is recommended for eczema and psoriasis. It is an excellent skin cleanser, useful in masks, although it has a powerful aroma. naturesgift.com/hydrosols.htm gives it as cooling, soothing, and healing for baby's bottom. It can be used in a spray for sunburn and as a toner for skin with acne; its powerful antiinflammatory action makes it suitable for rosacea, couperose, and other inflamed skin conditions.

Melaleuca alternifolia [TEA TREE] Myrtaceae

(contains a volatile oil)

This gentle, safe hydrolat is usually distilled locally from the dried leaves which are transported in preference to the distilled water, because of costs and difficulty in providing the proper storage conditions.

The main components of the hydrolats analysed (Australian and French) suggest the following properties may apply:

93–94% alcohols	antiinfectious, antiviral, bactericidal, decongestant, stimulating

antiinfectious, *antiviral,* **bactericidal,** *decongestant, stimulating*

The highlighted properties appear in the text below, and the following have also been suggested:

antifungal, antiirritant, antiseptic, expectorant, mucolytic

Catty (2001, p. 109) recommends tea tree hydrolat for wounds, skin irritations, infections, fungal conditions such as thrush, *Candida albicans* and fungal infections under the nails. It is useful as a gargle or mouthwash for a sore throat or cough and is mildly mucolytic and expectorant.

Skin

naturesgift.com/hydrosols continues its praises, saying it is also a superb toner for acne, makes a good base for a deodorant or foot spray – and will treat hot spots on dogs or cats!

Melilotus officinalis [COMMON MELILOT] Leguminosae

The water distilled from melilot flowers was said to improve the flavour of other ingredients (in a preparation) (Grieve 1992, p. 527).

The main components of the hydrolat analysed suggest the following properties may apply:

25% eucalyptol	expectorant, mucolytic
8–9% alcohols	antiinfectious, antiviral, bactericidal, decongestant, stimulating
34% ketones	analgesic, anticoagulant, antiinflammatory, calming, cicatrizant, digestive, expectorant, lipolytic, mucolytic, sedative, stimulant

Summary of the above properties:

analgesic, anticoagulant, *antiinfectious,* **antiinflammatory,** *antiviral, bactericidal, calming, cicatrizant, decongestant, digestive, expectorant, lipolytic, mucolytic, sedative,* **stimulant**

The highlighted properties appear in the text below, and the following have also been suggested:

antispasmodic, circulatory, (ophthalmic)

Culpeper (n.d., pp. 231–232) tells us that boiled in wine, melilot is good for inflammation of the eye or other parts of the body, and steeped in vinegar or rose water, it alleviates a headache. He goes on to say:

> *that if the head is washed often with the distilled water of the herb and flowers, it has a beneficial effect on those who faint frequently and will comfort the head and brain, preserving them from pain ... it will also strengthen the memory and comfort the apoplexy.*

This water has traditionally been used for hundreds of years to help with problems of circulation, and in the 20th century Henri Viaud confirmed this traditional use when he listed melilot as being antispasmodic, anticoagulant, useful against embolism, phlebitis and blocked circulation (Viaud 1983).

Melissa officinalis [LEMON BALM, BALM] Lamiaceae

(contains a volatile oil)

Grieve (1998, p. 77) tells us that John Hussey of Sydenham, who lived to the age of 116, breakfasted for 50 years on balm tea sweetened with honey, and herb teas were the usual breakfast of Llewelyn, Prince of Glamorgan, who died in his 108th year. Carmelite water, of which balm was the chief ingredient, was drunk daily by the Emperor Charles V.

The essential oil of melissa is difficult to distill well as it is composed of many molecules which are hydrophilic, thus the water, when correctly obtained and of good quality, has properties which are quite close to those of the essential oil. Micro-molecules of essential oil are in fact left in this aqueous solution, which has a lemony scent.

In her book *The Herb Garden* (referred to by Grieve 1998, p. 77), Mrs Bardswell gives a recipe for a refreshing tea for a fever:

> *Put two sprigs of Balm, and a little woodsorrel, into a stone jug, having first washed and dried them; peel thin a small lemon, and clear from the white; slice it and put a bit of peel in; then pour in 3 pints of boiling water, sweeten and cover it close.*

The main components of the hydrolats analysed suggest the following properties may apply:

69–73% aldehydes	antiinfectious, antiinflammatory, antiviral, calming, circulatory (hypotensor), febrifuge, tonic
10% ketones	analgesic, anticoagulant, antiinflammatory, calming, cicatrizant, digestive, expectorant, lipolytic, mucolytic, sedative, stimulant

Summary of the above properties:

analgesic, *anticoagulant,* **antiinfectious, antiinflammatory, antiviral, calming,** *cicatrizant, circulatory (hypotensor),* **digestive,** *expectorant, febrifuge, lipolytic, mucolytic,* **sedative, stimulant, tonic**

The highlighted properties appear in the text below, and the following have also been suggested:

antiirritant, antioxidant, antispasmodic, immunostimulant

The antiinflammatory properties of melissa hydrolat are helpful in blepharitis and conjunctivitis (Viaud 1983, Price & Price 1999). The authors have always regarded melissa essential oil as the principal choice for women's problems and the hydrolat certainly lives up to this, as well as being more affordable. Like its expensive partner, it is effective against irregular periods and alleviates period pains; its calming properties relieve headaches and help control PMS (it is uplifting and antidepressive also). Its digestive qualities even include soothing morning sickness and its lemony taste makes it pleasant to take internally.

naturesgift.com/hydrosols recommends it to settle upset stomachs, nausea and indigestion, and suggest adding a teaspoon of the hydrolat to water every day during the flu and virus season. innerself.com/magazine/herbs/essential_oils (2001) advocates it for throat infections.

Catty (2001, pp. 110–111), tells us that it reduces the intestinal spasms and cramps associated with colitis and Crohn's disease, although she suggests being prudent with its use for this, as with some people it has a laxative effect. It is a moderate antioxidant and also antiviral; it helps treat water retention and is immunostimulant.

In southern Europe this plant is known as 'heart's delight' and the aromatic water makes an excellent general tonic, being both uplifting, relaxing and sedative (Price & Price 1999) and therefore recommended for times of emotional crisis. It makes an effective relaxing drink and can be added to the bath, also for relaxation. Rose (1999, p. 173) recommends it for herpes, insomnia, hot flushes and mental stress, and Kresanek (1982, p. 130) tells us that the distillate is very effective and popular (in drops, up to one teaspoonful 3–4 times per day) for migraines and other pains.

Melissa tea is reputed to encourage longevity – and is used to this day, with lemon juice and sugar, as a remedy for feverish colds (Claire 1961, p. 114). Although not a water, the restorative cordial called Carmelite water (based on melissa) was also supposed to confer longevity; it was at the same time deemed highly useful against nervous headache and 'neuralgic affections' (Grieve 1998, p. 76). It was made by macerating the fresh flowers and tops of lemon balm in fortified white wine, together with lemon peel, cinnamon, cloves, nutmeg and coriander.

Skin

Melissa hydrolat is soothing to insect bites, and Grosjean (1993b p. 145) and Price & Price (1999) recommend it as an effective toner for an irritated skin, naturesgift.com/hydrosols saying that it is also a great toner/astringent for an oily skin. Catty (2001, p. 110) recommends it as a cleanser for all skin types and says it is good for babies for cradle cap and nappy rash. innerself.com/magazine/herbs/essential_oils (2001) recommends it for ageing skin and throat infections.

Culinary use

The hydrolat of melissa has a lemony scent and taste and is excellent in all beverages and recipes both sweet and savoury. Catty (2001, p. 110) says it is delicious for steaming vegetables and fish, and Rose (1999, p. 173) says it acts as a viricide in water, for cooking lamb or adding to punches.

Mentha × piperita [PEPPERMINT] Lamiaceae

(contains a volatile oil)

In the time of Grieve (1998, p. 542) the preparation most in general use was peppermint water, peppermint water and spirit of peppermint being official preparations in the British pharmacopoeia (Grieve 1992, p. 542).

The main components of the hydrolats analysed suggest the following properties may apply:

23–64% ketones	analgesic, anticoagulant, antiinflammatory, calming, cicatrizant, digestive, expectorant, lipolytic, mucolytic, sedative, stimulant
31–48% alcohols	antiinfectious, antiviral, bactericidal, decongestant, stimulating

Summary of the above properties:
analgesic, anticoagulant, antiinfectious, **antiinflammatory,** *antiviral, bactericidal, calming, cicatrizant,* **digestive,** *expectorant, lipolytic, mucolytic, sedative,* **stimulant**

The highlighted properties appear in the text below, and the following have also been suggested:
antiirritant, antiseptic, cooling, febrifuge

Viaud (1983) gives this hydrolat as being eupeptic (digestive) and antiseptic.

Price & Price (1999) have found it to be cooling, antiinflammatory and refreshing to the emotions. It can be used in the bath for an invigorating effect. Claeys (1992) agrees with its refreshing property but does not say which variety of mint he is talking about or whether its action is on a mental or physical plane.

For a digestive or a cooling drink, add about 75 ml of distilled peppermint water to a litre of water (Grosjean 1993a, p. 42).

Both Rose (1999, p. 174) and Catty (2001, pp. 112–113) have found the hydrolat to be cooling (therefore helpful to hot flushes), antiirritant, antiinflammatory, uplifting and mentally stimulating. She adds that the French recommend it for toning the bust line.

naturesgift.com/hydrosols says peppermint hydrolat is a wonderful 'spritzer' in the car, both to keep the driver alert, and also to allay any possible car sickness among the passengers. The site goes on to say that the hydrolat is a great mouthwash/breath freshener and is mildly antiseptic. As it is soothing, it will ease the itchiness of rashes, making a great soothing aftershave. As it settles the stomach and is energizing, it is helpful in combating a hangover.

Grieve (1998, p. 543) suggests peppermint tea for palpitations of the heart and says that boiled in milk and drunk hot, the peppermint herb is good for abdominal pains.

She goes on to tell us about a concoction to alleviate internal pains:

> 'Aqua Mirabilis' *is a term applied on the Continent to an aromatic water which is taken for internal pains. It is a water distilled from herbs, sometimes used in the following form:*
> *cinnamon oil, fennel oil, lavender oil, peppermint oil, rosemary oil, sage oil, of each 1 part; spirit 350 parts; distilled water, 644 parts.*

Grieve gives two further suggestions for slight colds or early indications of disease, saying that free use of peppermint tea will, in most cases, effect a cure. She recommends an infusion of 1 pint of boiling water poured over 1 oz of the dried herb, taken in wineglassful doses and adding sugar and milk if desired. Her second recipe is for an infusion made with peppermint and elderberry flowers, which she says will banish a cold or mild attack of influenza within 36 hours, and there is no danger of an overdose or any harmful action on the heart.

6scent says that peppermint hydrolat can bring a fever down and is safe to use on children, although Catty (2001, p. 113) suggests that it should not be used on children under 3 years of age.

Skin

Rose (1992, p. 124) suggests peppermint hydrolat as a skin cleanser, while Grosjean (1993a, p. 148) recommends it as a deodorizing foot spray and as an aid for 'heavy legs', hot feet and feet tired after walking, to refresh and soothe. During the summer months it can be kept in the fridge for a cooling facial spray

Culinary use

Catty, at the Nice conference in 2000 (poster display), said the hydrolat was delicious hot or cold and can be used in sweets, fruit and preserves. In her book (2001, p. 113) she suggests the hydrolat is good in ice cubes and is sweet enough to use as a replacement for sugar.

Mentha pulegium [PENNYROYAL] Lamiaceae

(contains a volatile oil)

antiinfectious, antiseptic, antispasmodic, calming, sedative

Pennyroyal water distilled from the leaves was formerly given as an antidote to spasmodic, nervous and hysterical affections. It was also used against colds and 'affections of the joints' (Grieve 1992, p. 626). The infusion of 1 oz of herb to a pint of boiling water is taken warm in teacupful doses, frequently repeated.

Mentha spicata (SPEARMINT) Lamiaceae

(contains a volatile oil)

analgesic, (antiinflammatory), digestive

The distilled water of spearmint was said by Mrs Grieve (1992, p. 536) to relieve hiccups and flatulence as well as the giddiness of indigestion.

She goes on to say that for infantile trouble generally, a pint of boiling water poured onto 1 oz of the dried herb, then strained and sweetened, is an excellent remedy. It is also a pleasant beverage in fevers, inflammatory diseases, etc. taken in doses of a wineglassful or less. The same infusion is considered as specific in allaying nausea and vomiting and will relieve the pain of colic.

Mentha sylvestris (HORSEMINT) Lamiaceae

anticancer, antispasmodic, bactericidal, euphoric (Viaud 1983)

Culpeper (n.d., p. 236) says that: 'The decoction or distilled water helps a stinking breath, proceeding from corruption of the teeth; and snuffed up the nose, purges the head. It helps the scurf or dandruff of the head used with vinegar.'

Myrtus communis [MYRTLE] Myrtaceae

(contains a volatile oil)

This hydrolat has not been analysed for this book, but the authors have been told it contains the following components:

terpineol
linalool

myrtol
1,8-cineole

Alcohols and oxides, according to the studies by Franchomme & Pénoël, may have the following properties, which are therefore listed below:
antiinfectious, antiviral, **bactericidal, decongestant, expectorant, mucolytic, stimulating**

The highlighted properties appear in the text below, and the following have also been suggested:
antiallergic, antiirritant, antiseptic, ophthalmic, soothing

Viaud (1983) says this hydrolat is soothing and antiseptic.

Franchomme & Pénoël (1996, p. 86) tell us that it is suitable for calming pain due to an inflammatory state of the eyes. It is reputed to be very gentle and can be sprayed into the eyes to calm allergic reactions. Schnaubelt (1999) tells us that it is effective in most cases of occasional conjunctivitis, while innerself.com\magazine\herbs\essential_oils 2001 recommend the hydrolat as eye drops for infected or irritated eyes.

Catty (2001, p. 115) includes in her attributes for this hydrolat the fact that it is mucolytic and a strong expectorant – calming sore throats and coughs, useful in bronchitis and asthma (particularly where this is triggered by allergens or pollutants).

Skin
Rose (1999, p. 173) recommends myrtle hydrolat for all over skin care, saying it is both refreshing and reviving.

Culinary use
Rose also says it has some use in the cooking of meats and fish.

Ocimum basilicum [SWEET BASIL] Lamiaceae

(contains a volatile oil)
calming, carminative, digestive, stimulating
Both Viaud (1983) and Price & Price (1999) credit this hydrolat with carminative and digestive properties.

Rose (1999, p. 172) gives the hydrolat as being stimulating for hair loss and calming to nausea, Catty (2001, pp. 116–117) adding that it is also calming to the nervous system.

When it was first introduced into the UK basil was used mainly for the preparation of sweet waters, scent bags and nosegays. John Swan, in his *Speculum Mundi*, says 'we in England seldome or never eat it; yet we greatly esteem it because it smelleth sweet, and (as some think) it comforteth the brain' (Clair 1961, p. 116).

Culinary use
Rose (1999, p. 172) extols its culinary value, telling us that the water has a slightly liquorice taste and that it gives a boost to pastas and any vegetable dish. Grosjean (1993, p. 87) suggests its use in salad dressings and soups.

Olea europaea [OLIVE] Oleaceae

Olive hydrolat is obtained from the distillation of the leaves.
cardiac protector, hypotensive (Viaud 1983)

The tea and decoction of olive leaves are given as hypoglycaemic, hypotensive, diuretic, mild antispasmodic, febrifuge, vulnerary, vasodilator, cholagogue (Bartram 1995, p. 318).

Origanum majorana [SWEET MARJORAM] Lamiaceae

(contains a volatile oil)

Sweet marjoram essential oil, one which the authors find as indispensable as lavender on account of its many and varied properties, is not always given the credit it deserves. The hydrolat, it would seem, from the impressive components which follow, could be used much more than it appears to be.

The main components of the sweet marjoram hydrolats analysed suggest the following properties may apply:

32–35% aldehydes	antiinfectious, antiinflammatory, antiviral, calming, circulatory (hypotensor), febrifuge, tonic
30–34% ketones	analgesic, anticoagulant, antiinflammatory, calming, cicatrizant, digestive, expectorant, lipolytic, mucolytic, sedative, stimulant
13–18% alcohols	antiinfectious, antiviral, bactericidal, decongestant, stimulating

Summary of the above properties:

analgesic, *anticoagulant, antiinfectious,* **antiinflammatory,** *antiviral, bactericidal,* **calming,** *cicatrizant, circulatory (hypotensor), decongestant,* **digestive,** *expectorant, febrifuge, lipolytic, mucolytic, sedative, stimulant, tonic*

The highlighted properties appear in the text below, and the following have also been suggested:

antispasmodic, detoxifying, soothing

The authors have found this hydrolat to be helpful added to a tea and applied in a compress for muscular aches and the inflamed swelling of a twisted ankle.

Viaud (1983) tells us that the hydrolat of sweet marjoram clears the liver and gall bladder, Fischer-Rizzi (1990) suggesting its use also for stomach and intestinal cramps.

It is soothing to the stomach (innerself.com/magazine/herbs/essential_oils 2001) and is generally regarded as good for the digestive system. Taken in water daily it is good for anxious and nervous persons (Grosjean 1993a, p. 143).

Origanum onites [FRENCH MARJORAM] Lamiaceae

(contains a volatile oil)

circulatory stimulant, digestive

This herb is best known as being a substitute for thyme and the hydrolat is popular today for various therapeutic purposes in Turkey (where it is known as kekik water). It has inhibitory effects on the gastrointestinal system and has been found to be stimulating to the cardiovascular system (Aydin et al 1996).

Origanum vulgare, Oheracleoticum [OREGANO, WILD MARJORAM] Lamiaceae

(contains a volatile oil)

antibacterial, antifungal, antiseptic, antiviral, calming, tonic

Viaud (1983) suggests this hydrolat is calmative to the central nervous system.

Catty (2001, p. 118) echoes Rose (1999, p. 173) when she suggests that oregano hydrolat is strongly antiseptic, antibacterial, antiviral and antifungal and can be used in a douche or sitz bath both for reproductive and urinary tract care. Rose says it makes a good daily tonic drink, and Catty says it supports a weakened immune system too delicate to handle essential oils and that it is delicious in cooking.

Grosjean (1993b, p. 156) recommends it for colds and flu.

naturesgift.com/hydrosols, echoing the thoughts of the authors, says that this 'gentle hydrosol' is a much safer and more effective way to experience the germ killing effects of oregano essential oil, as it is much gentler and lighter in aroma. The site recommends its use as a mouthwash and a gargle for sore throats.

Found to have antibacterial activity against *Bacillus amyloliquefaciens, B. brevis, B. cereus, B. subtilis* var. *niger, Enterobacter aerogenes, Escherischia coli, Klebsiella pneumoniae, Proteus vulgaris, Salmonella enteritidis, S. gallinarum, S. typhimurium, Staphylococcus aureus, Yersinia enterocolitica* (Sağdiç & Özcan 2003).

Skin

The same website uses it to moisten a clay mask for its antibacterial effect on acne.

Ormenis mixta [MOROCCAN CHAMOMILE] Asteraceae

relaxing (Paris 2000)

Passiflora incarnata [PASSIONFLOWER] Passifloraceae

Bartram (1995, p. 330) suggests using the tea against sleeplessness.

Pelargonium graveolens [GERANIUM] Geraniaceae

(contains a volatile oil)

The main components of the hydrolats analysed suggest the following properties may apply:

30–45% alcohols	antiinfectious, antiviral, bactericidal, decongestant, stimulating
39–42% ketones	analgesic, anticoagulant, antiinflammatory, calming, cicatrizant, digestive, expectorant, lipolytic, mucolytic, sedative, stimulant

Summary of the above properties:

analgesic, anticoagulant, antiinfectious, **antiinflammatory,** *antiviral, bactericidal, calming,* **cicatrizant,** *decongestant,* **digestive,** *expectorant, lipolytic, mucolytic, sedative,* **stimulant**

The highlighted properties appear in the text below, and the following have also been suggested:

antidepressive, (antispasmodic), balancing, cooling

Boukef (1986), Peyron (1962) and Loeper & Lesure (1948) offer the following information on the hydrolat and infusion of geranium:

- it is valued for its tonic and stimulating properties for use in cosmetic waters
- the aromatic water has analeptic cardiac qualities and is used on the head in case of sunstroke
- the leaves can be used in an infusion, together with tea, as a stomachic and antispasmodic.

Rose (1999, p. 174) finds it cooling for hot flushes and generally good for women's hormonal imbalances. She also says it is a cell regenerator, antidepressant and stimulating to the adrenal cortex.

The authors have found geranium hydrolat to be useful in balancing the sebum production in either an oily or dry skin and scalp.

Catty (2001, p. 119) finds it mildly antiinflammatory for sunburn, rashes and insect bites and says that with continued use it promotes healing on rough elbows, calluses and children's scabby knees. She says geranium hydrolat is effective on broken capillaries and rosacea (combined with German chamomile for best results).

Culinary use

Geranium aromatic water has numerous uses in Tunisia, especially within the family. Here it is used to flavour pastries, sweets, creams, fruit salads, drinks, toppings and sometimes as a sweetener. Rose (1999, p. 174) says it is good in jellies and fruit desserts.

Petroselinum crispum, P. sativum [PARSLEY] Apiaceae

(contains a volatile oil)

Grieve (1992, p. 614) gives a recipe for the preparation and dosage using the root, hydrolat and essential oil of parsley. Fluid extract root, $\frac{1}{2}$ to 1 drachm; fluid extract seeds, $\frac{1}{2}$ to 1 drachm; apiol (oil), 5–15 drops in a capsule.

anticancerous, carminative, digestive, litholytic

Viaud (1983) has found parsley water to be anticancerous, a red cell regenerator and litholytic (to the kidneys).

'The distilled water of parsley is a familiar medicine with nurses to give children when troubled with wind in the stomach or belly [as dill water still is] and it is also of service to grownup persons' (Culpeper n.d., p. 258).

Peumus boldus [BOLDO LEAF] Monimiaceae

(contains a volatile oil)

liver decongestant (Viaud 1983)

Bartram (1995, p. 64) gives boldo as a cholagogue, liver tonic, choleretic and liver protector, among other properties.

Phytolacca americana, P. decandra [POKE ROOT] Phytolaccaceae

Viaud (1983) tells us that poke root hydrolat corrects the accumulation of local fat in the tissues (e.g. thighs, hips). He does not say whether it is used externally or internally, but Grieve (1998, p. 648) tells us that an overdose, taken internally, causes unpleasant side effects (e.g. vomiting). The plant itself is given as toxic and dangerous (Stuart 1987, p. 238).

Picea mariana [BLACK SPRUCE] Pinaceae

(contains a volatile oil)

analgesic, antiinflammatory, antiirritant, calming, stimulating, tonic

Rose (1999, p. 172) recommends the hydrolat of black spruce for stress and relieving pain and itching. Internally, she recommends it as a tonic.

Catty (2001, p. 120) suggests the use of this hydrolat for pain and inflammation in a compress or bath (together with Scots pine). She has found it to be a stimulating and restorative body tonic.

Pimento officinalis [PIMENTO] Myrtaceae
(contains a volatile oil)
digestive, purgative, sedative
Grieve (1998, p. 20–21) tells us that pimento water (*Aqua pimentae*) is used as a vehicle for stomachic and purgative medicines and is made by taking five parts of bruised pimento to 200 parts of water and distilling down to 100, the dose being 1–2 fluid ounces. She recommends this distilled water for flatulent indigestion and for hysterical paroxysms.

Pimpinella anisum [ANISEED] Apiaceae
The tea is carminative, expectorant, antispasmodic (Bartram 1995, p. 23; Stuart 1987, p. 239).

Found to have antibacterial activity against one strain of *Escherischia coli*, and one strain of *Staphylococcus aureus* (Sağadiç & Özcan 2003).

Pimpinella magna [SAXIFRAGE, GREATER BURNET] Apiaceae
antispasmodic
The distilled water, boiled with castoreum, is good for cramps and convulsions (Culpeper n.d., p. 320).

Pinus sylvestris [SCOTS PINE] Pinaceae
(contains a volatile oil)
A dark deposit may form at the bottom of the bottle when pine water is stored; this can be removed by filtration.

The main components of the hydrolat analysed suggest the following properties may apply:

36% eucalyptol	expectorant, mucolytic
29–31% alcohols	antiinfectious, antiviral, bactericidal, decongestant, stimulating
13–16% ketones	analgesic, anticoagulant, antiinflammatory, calming, cicatrizant, digestive, expectorant, lipolytic, mucolytic, sedative, stimulant

Summary of the above properties:
analgesic, anticoagulant, antiinfectious, **antiinflammatory,** *antiviral,* **bactericidal, calming,** *cicatrizant,* **decongestant,** *digestive, expectorant, lipolytic,* **mucolytic,** *sedative,* **stimulant**

The highlighted properties appear in the text below, and the following have also been suggested:
antifungal, antiseptic, diuretic

Viaud (1983) considers this hydrolat to be balsamic and diuretic.

Grosjean (1993a, p. 46) finds pine hydrolat very suitable for babies and children, recommending it as a soothing, hygienic drink and as a friction rub on the back and chest when they are suffering from chills.

Among the many attributes given to this hydrolat by Catty (2001, p. 121) are that it is antiseptic, antibacterial, antifungal, a good decongestant for the respiratory and lymphatic systems, a general system tonic, mucolytic, an effective antiinflammatory compress when used with black spruce, stimulating to the adrenals, and mentally calming used in the bath, steam, sauna or humidifier.

Piper nigrum [PEPPER] Piperaceae
(contains a volatile oil)
No information is available

Pistacia lentiscus [PISTACHIO] Anacardiaceae
reticulo-endothelial decongestant (Viaud 1983)

Plantago major [PLANTAIN] Plantaginaceae
The main components of the hydrolat analysed suggest the following properties may apply:

eucalyptol	expectorant, mucolytic
46–48% alcohols	antiinfectious, antiviral, bactericidal, decongestant, stimulating
7–9% ketones	analgesic, anticoagulant, antiinflammatory, calming, cicatrizant, digestive, expectorant, lipolytic, mucolytic, sedative, stimulant

Summary of the above properties:
analgesic, anticoagulant, **antiinfectious,** *antiinflammatory, antiviral,* **bactericidal,** *calming, cicatrizant, decongestant, digestive, expectorant, lipolytic, mucolytic, sedative, stimulant*

'The distilled water with a little alum and honey dissolved in it is of good use for washing, cleansing and healing a sore ulcerated mouth or throat' (Salmon's *Herbal* (1710), cited in Grieve 1992, p. 642).

Polygonatum multiflorum [SOLOMON'S SEAL] Liliaceae (Convallariaceae)
Skin
Parkinson says 'The Italian dames, however, doe much used the distilled water of the whole plant of Solomon's seal – for their complexions, etc.' (Grieve 1992, p. 750).

In Galen's time the distilled water of the herb was used by ladies for removing freckles and pimples, and the expressed juice of the rhizome is said to be good for the complexion. In parts of Europe it is blended into a pomade for use on boils and abscesses (Clair 1961, p. 240).

'The distilled water of the whole plant takes away morphew, freckles &c., from any part of the body' (Culpeper n.d., p. 339).

Portulaca sativa [GOLDEN PURSLANE] Portulacaceae
(One) authority declared that the distilled water took away pains in the teeth (Grieve 1992, p. 660).

Potentilla anserina [SILVERWEED] Rosaceae
(antiseptic, styptic)
Grieve (1998, pp. 740, 741) gives us the following information about silverweed hydrolat:

> *A strong infusion of silverweed, if used as a lotion, will check the bleeding of piles, the ordinary infusion (1 oz. to a pint of boiling water) being meanwhile taken as a medicine. The same infusion, sweetened with honey, constitutes an excellent gargle for sore throat.*
>
> *On the continent, a tablespoonful of the herb, boiled in a cup of milk, has been recommended as an effective remedy in tetanus or lockjaw; the tea should be drunk as hot as possible.*

Skin
Grieve continues by saying that a distilled water of the herb was in earlier days much in vogue as a cosmetic for removing freckles, spots and pimples, and for restoring the complexion when sunburnt.

Primula veris [COWSLIP] Primulaceae

Alexander, in Grieve (1998, p. 231), tells us that cowslip water was considered to be good for the memory.

Grieve herself tells us that the old writers considered the water of the flowers to be 'very proper medicine for weakly people'.

Prunus laurocerasus [CHERRY LAUREL] Rosaceae

Grieve (1998, p. 465) informs us that cherry laurel water (*Aqua laurocerasi*) has been used in Paris fraudulently to imitate the cordial called Kirsch and according to the British pharmacopoeia, it is prepared as follows:

'One pound of fresh leaves of cherry-laurel, 2½ pints of water. Chop the leaves, crush them in a mortar, and macerate them in the water for 24 hours; then distill one pint of liquid; shake the product, filter through paper, and preserve it in a stoppered bottle'. In America, oil of bitter almonds is often substituted, owing to the variability of the above.
digestive, expectorant

Used for asthma, coughs, indigestion and dyspepsia; 1 drop of sulphuric acid added to a pint of cherry laurel water will keep it unchanged for a year.

Robinia pseudoacacia [FALSE ACACIA] Papilionaceae

antidiabetic, circulatory
Viaud (1983) recommends acacia hydrolat for capillary problems of the skin and the arterial circulatory system; it is also antidiabetic.

Rosa canina [WILD ROSE] Rosaceae

(contains a volatile oil)
cicatrizant, *cooling, opthalmic, refreshing*, **rejuvenating**, *uplifting*
Culpeper considered *Rosa canina* to be superior to *Rosa damascena*:

> *the distilled water of roses, vinegar of roses, ointment and oil of roses and the rose leaves dried are of very great use and effect. . . . Red rose [i.e. Rosa canina] water is well known, and better than damask rose water, it is cooling, cordial, refreshing, quickening the weak and faint spirits, used either in meats or broths to smell at the nose, or to smell the sweet vapours out of a perfume pot, or cast into a hot fire-shovel. It is of much use against the redness and inflammation of the eyes to bathe therewith and the temples of the head . . . and to stay and dry up the rheums and watering of them. (Culpeper n.d., pp. 300–301)*

He then refers to *Rosa rubra* (p. 302) saying: 'The distilled water, made of the full blown flower is cooling, of good use in recent inflammations of the eyes, if it be dissolved in a small quantity of rock saltpetre' (Culpeper n.d., p. 302) and on the same page he refers to the flowers of *Rosa alba* when he recommends that the distilled water from them is used in 'collyriums' (colorye is an archaic word for eye ointment) for sore inflamed eyes.

Grosjean (1993) finds wild rose hydrolat to be very beneficial to the skin. She mentions its efficacy on a dry skin (p. 57) and tells us that it is also cicatrizant

(p. 87), being helpful to scars (p. 95) – and finally, that it makes an excellent rejuvenating tonic (p. 114).

Rosa centifolia [CABBAGE ROSE] Rosaceae
(contains a volatile oil)
This rose is often referred to as *rose de mai* and is considered to have similar properties to *Rosa damascena* below.

Rosa damascena [DAMASK ROSE] Rosaceae
(contains a volatile oil)
The petals of the most scented varieties have on their inner surface minute scent glands containing the volatile essence, which are clearly visible under a microscope, while on the petals of the sweet briar rose the scent glands are clearly visible even to the naked eye (Genders 1972, p. 198).

Rose water has a long history – several hundred years – and so, like the essential oil of lavender, has been recommended and used for many different purposes to treat a wide range of maladies ranging from dry or damaged skin and wrinkles to frigidity, from sunburn to mouth ulcers and coughs, relieving stress and comforting the spirit.

Genuine, unadulterated rose water is not the same as commercial rose water, which is produced, at least partially, in the laboratory (see Ch. 5); the aroma of both is almost exactly like a tea rose, although the *damascena* hydrolat is much more perfumed than the product produced in France from the *rose de mai* (Goëb 1998). One needs to know the source of the rose water before using it for therapy and caution needs to be exercised before using it on the eyes, because some regulations insist that ethanol (up to 15%) is added to the rose distillate as a preservative.

The main components of the hydrolats analysed suggest the following properties may apply:

32–66% alcohols	antiinfectious, antiviral, bactericidal, decongestant, stimulating
8–9% esters	antifungal, antiinflammatory, antispasmodic, balancing (to nervous system), calming, cicatrizant, uplifting
5–6% aldehydes	antiinfectious, antiinflammatory, antiviral, calming, circulatory (hypotensor), febrifuge, tonic

Summary of the above properties:
antifungal, **antiinfectious, antiinflammatory, antispasmodic,** *antiviral,* **bactericidal,** *balancing,* **calming, cicatrizant,** *circulatory (hypotensor),* **decongestant,** *febrifuge,* **stimulating, uplifting**

The highlighted properties appear in the text below, and the following have also been suggested:
analgesic, antiirritant, antiseptic, astringent, cooling, digestive, hormone balancer, ophthalmic, regenerative, sedative, soothing, styptic, toning

'The distilled water of Roses is good for the strengthening of the heart, and refreshing of the spirits, and likewise for all things that require a gentle cooling' (Gerard 1964, p. 273).

In modern herbal medicine the flowers of the common red rose dried are given in infusions and sometimes as powder for haemorrhage. A tincture is made from them by pouring 1 pint of boiling water on 1 oz of the dried petals, adding 15 drops of oil of vitriol and 3 or 4 drachms of white sugar. The tincture when strained is of a beautiful red colour. Three or four spoonfuls of the tincture taken two or three times a day are considered good for strengthening the stomach and a pleasant remedy in all haemorrhages.

Culpeper (n.d., p. 298) mentions a syrup made of flowers of the damask rose by infusing them for 24 hours in boiling water, then straining off the liquid and adding twice the weight of refined sugar to it. He says that this syrup is an excellent purge for children and adults of costive habit (constipated), a small quantity to be taken every night to keep the bowels regular.

He also says (p. 299) that a decoction (see glossary) of red roses made with white wine and used is very good for headache and pains in the eyes, ears, throat and gums. Grieve (1998, p. 688) tells us that honey of roses was popular for sore throats and ulcerated mouth and was made by pounding fresh petals in a small quantity of boiling water, filtering, then boiling again with honey.

The water alone can be used as a mouthwash for mouth ulcers (Price & Price 1999). naturesgift.com/hydrosols recommend it as a gargle or throat spray for sore or inflamed throat. Taken internally, it says, the hydrolat is effective against streptococcal and staphylococcal infections – and many others.

Fischer-Rizzi (1990) suggests taking rose hydrolat internally for liver congestion, gall bladder infection, nausea and vomiting. She recommends it externally for conjunctivitis.

Rose water has been used through the millennia for religious ceremonies, as a courtesy to guests, for physical, emotional, and spiritual healing and some recommend it as a douche for frigidity; it seems to act on both the body and the psyche. Rose (1999, p. 171) considers it to be aphrodisiac, easing nervousness and mental strain.

Catty (2001, p. 123) recommends the hydrolat as a hormone balancer, saying it combats PMS, moods, and helps menopausal symptoms in combination with naturopathic treatment; it is also useful against cramps and is mildly astringent.

Regarding its relaxing qualities, Price & Price (1999) find it sedative and calming, and Sanoflore (2000) finds it fortifying and calming. Some people recommend taking a teaspoon of the hydrosol to calm stress and anxiety; others say it can be used as a facial spray to relieve mental strain.

Davis (1988) finds it soothing, recommending its use on cotton pads for irritated eyes, eye infections and conjunctivitis, Nasr (2000, p. 27) echoing her findings.

Skin

Fischer-Rizzi (1990) uses it as a revitalizing massage lotion for the head and scalp and also as a facial tonic. Rose floral water is traditionally used to keep a clear complexion. Its fresh, delicate scent is a pleasure to be enjoyed often (Sanoflore 2000).

By itself, it is an excellent tonic when used in a spray (Goëb 1998) and is suitable for all skin types (Davis 1988). It can also be used by itself as a toner, to moisten a mask, or in place of water in lotions or cosmetics recipes. Rose water stimulates the skin, heightening the blood flow. It controls and balances sebum production, making it useful for both dry and oily skin. It can balance and restore the skin's pH and helps tighten pores (naturesgift.com/hydrosols). It has been found to be effective on couperose and wrinkled skin also.

It is soothing and regenerating, particularly for a dry skin (Bego 1995), when it can be combined with French clay in a mask. Catty (2001, p. 123) also recommends its use on mature, sensitive and devitalized skins, in masks, steam and compresses.

Nasr (2000, p. 27) says that rose water is a cooling astringent and that his mother used to make a paste of rose water and starch to put on sunburnt skin.

Rose is very soothing to devitalized and sun damaged skin (6scent), and is reputed to be useful in the treatment of all sorts of dermatitis, its antibacterial properties helping also to fight acne. It is a good antiseptic (Davis 1988).

innerself.com\magazine\herbs\essential_oils (2001) suggests it can be used with glycerine as a hand lotion.

Culinary

Rose water adds a touch of flair to home cooking and is used in the manufacture of Turkish delight. It used to be (and still is in top restaurants) used in the making of candied borage flowers; the flowers are boiled in rose water and sugar and afterwards sprinkled with icing sugar (Clair 1961, p. 124).

Catty (2001, p. 123) suggests its use in desserts, sorbets and with fruit and it has also been suggested that it be added to alcoholic drinks (innerself.com/magazine/herbs/essential_oils 2001).

Claire (1961, p. 96), offers the following poem:

Good huswives provide, ere an' sickness do come,
Of sundry good things, in her house to have some;
Good aqua composita, and vinegar tart,
Rose-water and treacle to comfort the heart.

Rosmarinus officinalis [ROSEMARY] Lamiaceae

(contains a volatile oil)

> *Distilled simply with a gentle heat it yields a fragrant water called Dew of Rosemary; distilled with water in the usual way in an alembic it affords a water tasting strong of it, but a less agreeable smell; with rectified spirit it makes the fragrant and cephalic liquor called Hungary water. (New English Dispensatory)*

The main components of the hydrolat analysed suggest the following properties may apply:

16–18% alcohols	antiinfectious, antiviral, bactericidal, decongestant, stimulating
54–56% ketones	analgesic, anticoagulant, antiinflammatory, calming, cicatrizant, digestive, expectorant, lipolytic, mucolytic, sedative, stimulant
12–13% esters	antifungal, antiinflammatory, antispasmodic, balancing (to nervous system), calming, cicatrizant, uplifting

Summary of the above properties:

analgesic, *anticoagulant, antifungal, antiinfectious,* **antiinflammatory,** *antispasmodic, antiviral, bactericidal, balancing, calming,* **cicatrizant,** *decongestant,* **digestive,** *expectorant, lipolytic,* **mucolytic,** *sedative,* **stimulant**

The highlighted properties appear in the text below, and the following have also been suggested:

antioxidant, circulatory, diuretic (mild), emmenagogic, (ophthalmic)

Viaud (1983) considers this hydrolat to be emmenagogic and a bladder cleanser.

> *There is a water made from rosemary flowers, which disperseth films in the eyes after this manner: Take of rosemary flowers as many as are sufficient to fill a glass which must be well stopt, and set it in the wall against the South sun, thence will an oyl come, which with a feather anoynt the eyes with. (Dr Lazarus Riverius, 1668, in Clair 1961, p. 221)*

Rosemary hydrolat is considered to be healing and stimulating to the circulation and it is helpful against rheumatism (Price & Price 1999, p. 115). The authors have found that, because of its circulation stimulating properties, it makes an efficient friction rub for hair loss.

Catty (2001, p. 124) gives it as a mental and physical stimulant and as a digestive (may ease hunger and aid detoxification), stimulating to the liver and gall bladder and mildly diuretic (perhaps due to hepatostimulant properties). She says it is also a strong antioxidant and, used during the allergy season, will aid breathing difficulties. She suggests that this hydrolat should be avoided by those with high blood pressure and during pregnancy, but does not say why.

Catty gives the cineole chemotype of rosemary as mucolytic. It is not easy to obtain a pure cineole or pure camphor chemotype of rosemary, most plants containing varying amounts of each. Franchomme & Pénoël (1990) say the camphor essential oil chemotype is mucolytic, but not the cineole chemotype. The authors have put the mucolytic property into this section as the cineole and camphor chemotypes have almost the same constituents, properties and indications.

Skin

Claeys (1992) gives rosemary water as being tonic and refreshing and suitable for mixed and greasy types of skin. It is a stimulating facial spray, invigorating as a morning bath and pleasing as an aftershave spray.

Grosjean (1993a, p. 162) considers it to be a skin regenerator; 6scent suggests it is excellent for restoring elasticity to a sagging skin.

Rose (1999, p. 174) says it revitalizes the skin and can be effective on tired feet; it makes one more mentally alert and also restores energy.

Rosemary water is recommended for a devitalized skin, and for treating acne and blemishes. Blended with a little cider vinegar and added to the final rinse it gives soft, shining hair (naturesgift.com/hydrosols).

Culinary

Catty (1998) tells us it makes a delicious drink and can be used in both savoury and sweet (e.g. ice cream) cooking, while Rose (1999, p. 174) suggests it for meat dishes and sprinkled on steamed vegetables.

Grosjean (1993a, p. 162) says it makes a stimulating drink which could replace coffee.

Rosmarinus officinalis ct. verbenone [ROSEMARY VERBENONE] Lamiaceae

(contains a volatile oil)
decongestant, mucolytic

Ruscus aculeatus [BUTCHER'S BROOM] Liliaceae

circulation (Paris 2000)

Ruta graveolens [RUE] Rutaceae

(contains a volatile oil)
Water serves to extract the virtues of the plant better than spirits of wine. Decoctions and infusions are usually made from the fresh plant, or the oil may be

given in a dose of from 1 to 5 drops. The dried herb – which is a greyish green in colour – has a similar taste and odour, but is less powerful. It is used powdered, for making tea.

insecticide, (ophthalmic)

Grieve (1992, pp. 695–696) tells us that one old book says that rue water sprinkled in the house 'kills all the fleas'.

It was a common belief that an infusion of rue was beneficial for the eyes; Milton mentions how the angel restored Adam's sight by means of euphrasy and rue, and Swan (in Clair 1961, p. 224) says that 'for those who are feeble in their sight, let them distill rue and white roses together, and putting the water thereof into their eies, it will open their windows and let in more light'.

Salvia officinalis [SAGE] Lamiaceae

(contains a volatile oil)

The main components of the hydrolats analysed suggest the following properties may apply:

50–55% eucalyptol	expectorant, mucolytic
37–50% ketones	analgesic, anticoagulant, antiinflammatory, calming, cicatrizant, digestive, expectorant, lipolytic, mucolytic, sedative, stimulant
5–6% alcohols	antiinfectious, antiviral, bactericidal, decongestant, stimulating

Summary of the above properties:

analgesic, *anticoagulant, antiinfectious, antiinflammatory,* **antiviral, bactericidal,** *calming, cicatrizant,* **decongestant, digestive,** *expectorant, lipolytic, mucolytic, sedative,* **stimulant**

The highlighted properties appear in the text below, and the following have also been suggested:

antifungal, antiseptic, astringent, carminative, circulatory, diuretic, emmenagogic, hypotensor

Viaud (1983) regards this hydrolat as an emmenagogue and recommends it for the relief of pelvic congestion.

Catty (2001, pp. 127–128) claims that sage hydrolat 'has never shown itself to be emmenagogic, even after weeks of continuous use', but she advocates avoiding it during the first 3 months of pregnancy. She has found it to be a good hormone balancer, helping to regulate the menstrual cycle and reducing PMS and menopausal symptoms.

In Grieve (1998, pp. 703–704) we learn that:

> *in the United States ... it is in some repute, especially in the form of an infusion . . . as a wash for the cure of affections of the mouth and as a gargle in inflamed sore throat ... also for ulcerated throat ... bleeding gums and to prevent an excessive flow of saliva.*

She goes on to say that if a more stimulating effect to the throat is desirable, the gargle may be made with equal quantities of vinegar and water, ½ pint of hot malt vinegar being poured onto 1 oz of the leaves and adding ½ pint of cold water. Perhaps using vinegar in other recipes may also increase the effect!

For swallowing, sage tea is best, made from 1 oz sage leaves to 1 pint boiling water, taking a wineglassful as often as required. Lemon rind and/or juice, with sugar, added to this tea, then strained, is cooling in fevers and purifying to the blood (Grieve 1998, p. 704).

Greek sage water is a popular first aid remedy ingested (25 ml) for griping pain and bloating. It is a very good carminative and relieves indigestion. The water has a reputation for reducing high blood pressure, cleansing the blood and as a general tonic (Nasr 2000, p. 27). Grosjean (1993a, p. 177) recommends it for poor circulation and says its diuretic properties help to relieve congestion and fluid retention. The authors have found it helpful against rheumatic pains and ulcers (Price & Price 1999, p. 115).

Skin

Claeys (1992) says that sage hydrolat is both astringent and antiseptic; it can be used for greasy and acne type skins. Because of these properties it is useful used on wounds, eczema and other skin conditions. Nasr (2000, p. 27) echoes its antiseptic properties, which make it useful also as a mouthwash and gargle.

Catty (2001, pp. 127–128) suggests that sage hydrolat is, among its other attributes given above, balancing to the menstrual cycle, reducing symptoms of PMS, and may be useful for fertility; it restores vitality, is a strong antioxidant and excellent in anti-ageing treatments. Chronic fatigue can benefit over the long term from the antibacterial, antifungal and antiviral effects of sage hydrolat.

She suggests avoiding it during pregnancy and also with high blood pressure, as 'sage hydrosol will raise blood pressure significantly more than the essential oil; the lower the dose the stronger the effect'. There is no research reference in support of this opinion.

Culinary

The hydrolat has a distinctive flavour and makes a delicious drink; it can be used in cooking with fatty fish or meat (Catty 2001, p. 128).

Salvia sclarea [CLARY] Lamiaceae

(contains a volatile oil)

In Germany, clary has been used as an adulterant to improve a poor wine by making an infusion of clary and elderflowers to add to the wine, giving it a muscatel flavour – hence the German name for clary, which is *Muskateller salbei* (Clair 1961, p. 142).

The main components of the hydrolats analysed suggest the following properties may apply:

11–49% alcohols	antiinfectious, antiviral, bactericidal, decongestant, stimulating
3–76% esters	antifungal, antiinflammatory, antispasmodic, balancing (to nervous system), calming, cicatrizant, uplifting

Summary of the above properties:

antifungal, antiinfectious, **antiinflammatory, antispasmodic,** *antiviral, bactericidal, balancing (to nervous system),* **calming,** *cicatrizant, decongestant,* **stimulating, uplifting**

The highlighted properties appear in the text below, and the following have also been suggested:

analgesic, antiseptic, astringent, hormone balancer

The authors have found that, used as a gargle, clary sage hydrolat can help relieve a sore throat. Because it is a hormone balancer, it is an effective hydrolat for women, easing PMS (even moodiness) and the pain of irregular and troublesome periods – *if* taken daily for the 10 days prior to menstruation; it is also useful taken daily during the last 3 weeks of pregnancy to prepare the uterus for the birth and will help relieve pain during labour. Later, during the menopause, it is an effective aid against hot flushes. It is antidepressant and is effective used for depression and anxiety (Price & Price 1999, p. 115).

Catty (2001 p. 129) adds that it is antispasmodic and a gentle antiinflammatory.

Clary wine was known for its narcotic properties; 'it maketh men drunke, and causeth headache, and therefore some brewers do boyle it with their beere, in steed of hops' (Dodoens, *Herbal*, 1554).

Skin

Claeys (1992) states that clary is astringent and antiseptic; suitable for acneic and greasy skins. It also improves the appearance of mature and inflamed skin (Price & Price 1999, p. 115).

Culinary

The hydrolat has quite a strong and distinctive flavour, but Catty (2001, p. 129) finds it makes a delicious martini or white wine punch and is delicious with desserts.

Sambucus nigra [ELDERFLOWER] Caprifoliaceae

Medicines made from the elder tree are prolific, the bark, roots, leaves, buds and flowers all being used in the making of infusions, tinctures, teas, ointments and powders. Only the flowers are used to make the distilled hydrolat but it is possible that some of the attributes for the other parts of the plant may be applicable to the hydrolat also, for example respiratory problems.

The British pharmacopoeia says that elderflower water must be made from 100 parts of elderflowers distilled with 500 parts of water.

antiasthmatic, antiinflammatory, antiseptic, astringent, calming, circulatory, diuretic (mild), expectorant, laxative, ophthalmic, stimulant, (sudorific)

Viaud (1983) considers the distilled hydrolat to be a major antiasthmatic, Grieve (1998, p. 273) giving the same attributes to a wine made from the berries.

Apparently, our forefathers used the distilled hydrolat for bronchial and pulmonary problems, measles and other eruptive diseases as well as for inflammation of the eyes (Grieve 1998, p. 271).

Catty (2001 p. 130) believes that elderflower hydrolat may be a gentle circulation stimulant, a mild diuretic and a specific for the kidneys. She thinks it may be helpful in a compress for arthritis, rheumatism and muscle or sports injuries. reducing stress.

Grieve (1998, p. 270) tells us that an infusion of the dried flowers will promote expectoration in pleurisy; it is gently laxative and is considered excellent for inducing free perspiration. It is a good old-fashioned recipe for colds and throat trouble, taken hot on going to bed. An almost infallible cure for influenza in its first stage is a strong infusion of a handful each of dried elderflowers and peppermint with 1½ pints of boiling water, simmering it for half an hour. After straining and sweetening it, a cupful should be drunk in bed as hot as possible. Heavy perspiration and refreshing sleep will follow, and the patient will wake up well on the way to recovery and the cold or influenza will probably be banished within 36 hours.

In Grieve's day, tea made from elderflowers was recommended to be taken every morning before breakfast for some weeks as a spring medicine, as it was considered to be an excellent blood purifier.

Skin

Elderflower water is a gentle stimulant and mildly astringent and in the nineteenth century was invaluable for clearing the complexion of freckles and sunburn, and keeping the skin in good condition. Apparently every lady relied on it to keep her skin fair, white and free from blemishes. Grieve (1998, p. 272) says it was recommended after bathing in the sea, and she suggests that if any eruption should appear on the face from the effect of the salt water, it is a good plan to use a mixture composed of elderflower water plus glycerine and borax, and apply it night and morning.

Culinary

Catty (2001, p. 130) tells us that the hydrolat makes a delicious beverage and can be used in ice cubes, punch and added to sweets and desserts.

Santalum album [SANDALWOOD] Santalaceae

(contains a volatile oil)

antiinfectious, antiinflammatory, astringent (mild), balancing, calming

Catty (2001, p. 131) says that sandalwood hydrolat is quite rare and attributes many virtues to it, including its application as a douche for vaginitis and *Candida albicans*, plus the fact that it is mentally balancing and calming.

Skin

Catty believes it to be exceptional in skin care, recommending it in a compress for mature and delicate skin (though she also says it is slightly drying and astringent); she says it may also help rosacea, broken veins, eczema and psoriasis. She considers it to be a great aftershave.

Santolina chamaecyparissus [COTTON LAVENDER] Asteraceae

(contains an essential oil)

vermifuge (Viaud 1983)

Saponaria officinalis [SOAPWORT] Caryophyllaceae

Viaud (1983) considers soapwort hydrolat to be beneficial to eczema, furuncles and diabetes.

Sarothamnus scoparius [BROOM] Papilionaceae

Viaud (1983) recommends this hydrolat for the lungs.

Satureia hortensis [SUMMER SAVORY] Lamiaceae

(contains a volatile oil)

Found to have antibacterial activity against *Bacillus amyloliquefaciens, B. brevis, B. cereus, B. subtilis* var. *niger, Enterobacter aerogenes, Escherischia coli, Klebsiella pneumoniae, Proteus vulgaris, Salmonella enteritidis, S. gallinarum, S. typhimurium, Staphylococcus aureus, Yersinia enterocolitica* (Sağadiç & Özcan 2003).

Satureia montana [WINTER SAVORY] Lamiaceae

(contains a volatile oil)

antibacterial, antifungal, antiinfectious, antiviral, immunostimulant, revitalizing, stomachic

Both Viaud (1983) and Price & Price (1999) have found this hydrolat to be revitalizing. Being antibacterial, antiseptic and antiviral, it is also extremely effective taken with water for severe or viral stomach upsets and food poisoning (personal experience!).

Catty (2001, p. 132) recommends its use for vaginal, urinary, throat and mouth infections; she advocates using it in steam for head or chest infections and as a cleanser for acneic skin. She gives it as also being antifungal and an immune booster.

Scabiosa succisa [SCABIOUS] Dipsacaceae

(antiinflammatory), antiseptic, cicatrizant, (febrifuge)

Culpeper (n.d., p. 324) considered the distilled water of the herb to be a good remedy for green wounds or old sores, cleansing the body inwardly and freeing the skin from sores, scurf pimples, freckles, etc. He said the decoction (see glossary) of the herb was effective as a gargle for a swollen throat and tonsils.

Grieve (1992, p. 722) says that the plant makes a useful tea for coughs, fevers and internal inflammation. The remedy is generally given in combination with others, the infusion being given in wineglassful doses at frequent intervals. Taken internally, it purifies the blood, and used as an external wash it is a good remedy for eruptions of the skin. The warm decoction (see glossary) has also been used as a wash to free the head from scurf, sores and dandruff.

Solidago canadensis [GOLDEN ROD] Asteraceae

analgesic, antiinflammatory, antispasmodic (mild), astringent, diuretic, litholytic, relaxing

Rose (1999, p. 170) considers this hydrolat to be antiinflammatory, astringent, relaxing and a possible diuretic.

Catty (2001, p. 133) considers the hydrolat of Canadian golden rod will help prevent or dissolve kidney stones when taken internally (do not take if suffering from a kidney disease). She has found it to be analgesic and soothing to rheumatic and arthritic pain in a compress; it is a mild antispasmodic.

Its astringent qualities make it useful for varicose veins and broken capillaries and she suggests avoiding it if suffering from low blood pressure as the hydrolat is capable of lowering the blood pressure.

Solidago virgaurea [GOLDEN ROD] Asteraceae

universal repairer, albuminuria, (Viaud 1983)

Spirea ulmaria [MEADOWSWEET] (see ***Filipendula ulmaria***)

Stachys officinalis, Betonica officinalis [BETONY] Lamiaceae

Betony was known and used in Anglo-Saxon days and the *Leech Book of Bald* recommends the drinking of this herb infused in hot, sweet wine, as a cure for lumbago (Clair 1961, p. 122). The dried leaves can be used for a tea (Stuart 1987).

Syzygium aromaticum [CLOVE BUD] Myrtaceae

(contains a volatile oil)

Parkinson notes: 'Garcia [Garcia da Orta, author of a Portugese herbal] saith that the Portugal women distill the cloves while they are fresh, which make a most sweet and delicate water, no lesse useful for sent than profitable for all the passions of the heart' (Claire 1961, p. 54).

Tanacetum vulgare [TANSY] Asteraceae
calming to the psyche (Viaud 1983)

Taraxacum officinale [DANDELION] Asteraceae
No information available

Thuja occidentalis [THUJA] Cupressaceae
(contains a volatile oil)
anticancerous, antitumoral (Viaud 1983)

Thymbra spicata [BLACK THYME] Lamiaceae
(contains a volatile oil)

Found to have antibacterial activity against *Bacillus amyloliquefaciens, B. brevis, B. cereus*, one strain of *Escherischia coli, Proteus vulgaris, Salmonella enteritidis, S. gallinarum*, one strain of *Staphylococcus aureus* and *Yersinia enterocolitica* (Sağadiç & Özcan 2003).

Thymus serpyllum [WILD] Lamiaceae
(contains a volatile oil)

Grieve (1992, p. 814) says that wild thyme has the same properties as common thyme, but to a lesser degree. Formerly several preparations of this plant were sold commercially, and a distilled spirit and water, both of which were very fragrant.
antibacterial, anticancerous, antiseptic, digestive, intestinal antiseptic, (mucolytic)
Viaud (1983) considers serpyllum hydrolat to be anticancerous, antibacterial (Gram negative) and an intestinal antiseptic.

Grieve (1992, p. 814) recommends the infusion for respiratory system disorders, including coughs (also whooping cough), catarrh and sore throats. It should be prepared with 1 oz of dried herb to ½ pint of boiling water, which can be sweetened with sugar or honey – and she suggests doses of 1 tablespoonful or more several times daily. She tells us that the same infusion can be used for a weak digestion, being a good remedy for flatulence.

Wild thyme tea, either drunk by itself or mixed with other plants such as rosemary, etc., is an excellent remedy for headache and other nervous affections (Culpeper n.d., p. 372). He also recommends the infusion for headaches caused by drunkenness, and says it is a certain remedy on going to bed for 'that troublesome complaint the nightmare'.

Thymus vulgaris [COMMON THYME] Lamiaceae
Normally, thyme plants contain an essential oil which consists mainly of the phenols carvacrol and thymol, but when growing in the wild, variations in the essential composition within the plant can occur naturally, so that the main character of the essential oil is not phenolic. Thus thymes may quite naturally contain a majority of alcohols, such as linalool, geraniol and thujanol-4, which renders the oil (and therefore the hydrolat) more gentle and less aggressive on the body. These plants are

found and identified in the wild and cuttings taken so that they can be produced commercially. The clones survive and flourish quite well, except for the thujanol-4 chemotype which does not grow well under cultivation, therefore neither the essential oil nor, consequently, the distilled water are commonly available. The thymes containing phenols are often known as thyme or red thyme and the gentler thymes with alcohols are known as sweet thyme or sometimes yellow thyme; however, the Latin binomial is more precise and leaves no room for error.

Thymus vulgaris **ct. carvacrol, thymol** [THYME] Lamiaceae

(contains a volatile oil)

antifungal, antiseptic, antiviral, circulatory, digestive, germicidal, (respiratory), revitalizing, stimulating, (sudorific)

Viaud (1983) considers the carvacrol chemotype of thyme hydrolat to be an intestinal antiseptic.

Grieve (1998) does not mention the distilled water of phenolic thymes, and although thymol and carvacrol are not present in such a high percentage in the hydrolat, she tells us (p. 811) that an infusion will alleviate sore throats and catarrh, the tea being digestive, relieving wind spasms and colic and also promoting perspiration at the beginning of a cold and in general feverish complaints. This suggests that enough of the phenols must have been extracted to have these digestive, respiratory and sudorific effects.

Price & Price (1999, p. 115) have found the hydrolat to be stimulating and revitalizing, its use in the bath helping with general fatigue.

Rose (1999, p. 174) considers thyme hydrolat to be antiseptic, digestive, stimulating and revitalizing and a boost for the circulation.

Further effects suggested by Catty (2001, p. 137) are that it is immunostimulant, mildly antiviral and antifungal. Its antibacterial effects make it useful on wounds and boils, etc. by means of a compress. She also recommends it as an antiseptic mouthwash for care of mouth ulcers, the teeth and gums, and as a gargle for a sore throat.

Skin

Applied to the skin, it cleans the pores and tends to normalize sebaceous gland activity, having a healing effect on acne. It is also effective on insect bites (Price & Price 1999, p. 115).

Rose (1999, p. 174) recommends it for dermatitis and eczema and Grosjean (1993a, p. 184) considers it revitalizing for the hair, as part of an overall treatment.

Culinary use

Rose (1999, p. 174) suggests its use for lamb and vegetable cookery.

Thymus vulgaris **ct. geraniol, linalool, thujanol-4** [SWEET THYMES]

(contains a volatile oil)

The thujanol chemotype is found only in the wild and is not in plentiful supply, as attempts to grow this plant under cultivation have so far met with little success.

Although these three chemotypes, in the essential oil, may have some slightly different effects, all three, due to their main components being monoterpene alcohols (monoterpenols), are antibacterial, antiinfectious, antiinflammatory, antiviral and neurotonic. It follows that the hydrolats of the same chemotypes may therefore share many of their effects.

The three hydrolat chemotypes are taken together under the name 'sweet thymes', as they are all composed mainly of alcohols. They are all antiseptic, antibacterial, antiinfectious and antiviral. The geraniol and linalool chemotypes, in addition, are antifungal.

The main components of the hydrolat analysed (ct. linalool) suggest the following properties may apply:

91–93% alcohols **antiinfectious,** *antiviral,* **bactericidal,** *decongestant,* **stimulating,** *tonic*

The highlighted properties appear in the text below, and the following have also been suggested:

antifungal, antiseptic, immunostimulant, ophthalmic

The three hydrolats are both useful to clean wounds, preventing infection. Their antibacterial and antiseptic properties make them also an excellent choice for bedsores, the antifungal property (ct. geraniol and linalool) being helpful in *Candida albicans.* All sweet thymes are effective on eye infections (Price & Price 1999, p. 115) and should be diluted 50/50 to use in an eye wash or eye bath.

Catty (2001, p.134) suggests that the geraniol chemotype is immunostimulant and (p. 135) she says that the linalool hydrolat is a digestive and intestinal cleanser and a useful aid in colonics; it also makes a healthy daily tonic.

Skin

The authors have found sweet thyme hydrolats to be effective on acne and other skin infections.

Tilia* × *europaea **(fol.),** ***T. sylvestris*** [LIME LEAF, LINDEN LEAF] Tiliaceae

This hydrolat is taken from the leaves.

antiinflammatory (mild), antiirritant, calming, digestive, relaxing, sedative, stimulating, vasodilator

Viaud (1983) finds the hydrolat of the leaves is stimulating and a vasodilator – a low dose is calming, a high dose being stimulating.

Grieve (1992, p. 486) tells us that lime flowers are used in an infusion, or made into a distilled water, as remedies for indigestion or hysteria, nervous vomiting or palpitations. Prolonged baths prepared with the infused flowers are also good in hysteria.

She goes on to say that if the flowers used for teas are too old they may produce symptoms of narcotic intoxication. One of the authors, S. Price, has not experienced this, but when old, they certainly have no flavour – and unlike the fresh flower tisane, do not help insomnia. Since the discovery of the hydrolat, Price never dries the lime flowers for winter use, using the hydrolat in winter and a tisane of the fresh flowers from her garden in summer.

Rose (1999, pp. 171, 173) suggests using the hydrolat in a spray for shingles, as it is very soothing. She also finds it euphoric, calming, relaxing and sedative, relieving anxiety and depression. She has found it to be excellent for baby care.

Combating headaches and migraines and nervous exhaustion, it is useful internally as well as externally for shingles (Catty 2001, p. 138).

Skin

Dry eczema, itchy skin eruptions, puffy skin (Catty 2001, p. 138).

Culinary use

Delicious combined with other herbal waters or teas and used in savory and sweet dishes of a delicate flavour (Catty 2001, p. 138).

***Tilia sylvestris* (lig.)** [LIME SAPWOOD] Tiliaceae

This hydrolat is taken from the wood.
arthritis, gout, rheumatoid arthritis, (Viaud 1983)

Urtica dioica [NETTLE] Urticaceae

The main components of the hydrolat analysed suggest the following properties may apply:

71% dimethyl sulphide	(see p. 70)
10% ketones	analgesic, anticoagulant, antiinflammatory, calming, cicatrizant, digestive, expectorant, lipolytic, mucolytic, sedative, stimulant

Viaud (1983) recommends nettle hydrolat for the gall bladder and care of the hair and skin.

Valeriana officinalis and ***V. wallichii*** [VALERIAN] Valerianaceae

A distilled water and a syrup appear in the French Codex (Grieve 1992, p. 827).
calming, sedative
Viaud (1983) considers this hydrolat to be calming to the parasympathetic nervous system, Franchomme & Pénoël (1990, p. 286) saying it is sedative and that 2 teaspoons should be administered at night for 30 days. This dosage can be repeated if necessary, after a pause.

Vetiveria zizanioides [VETIVER] Gramineae

Vetiver aromatic water is used locally to the place of manufacture in the preparation of a delicious sherbet.

Viola tricolor ssp. ***arvensis*** [HEARTSEASE] Violaceae

The main components of the hydrolat analysed suggest the following properties may apply:

19% eucalyptol	expectorant, mucolytic
31–33% alcohols	antiinfectious, antiviral, bactericidal, decongestant, stimulating
34–35% ketones	analgesic, anticoagulant, antiinflammatory, calming, cicatrizant, digestive, expectorant, lipolytic, mucolytic, sedative, stimulant

Summary of the above properties:
analgesic, anticoagulant, antiinfectious, antiinflammatory, antiviral, bactericidal, calming, cicatrizant, decongestant, digestive, expectorant, lipolytic, mucolytic, sedative, stimulant

Viscum album [MISTLETOE] Loranthaceae

Viaud (1983) tells us that mistletoe hydrolat is listed as being good for the heart.

Zingiber officinale [GINGER] Zingiberaceae

(contains a volatile oil)

digestive, ophthalmic
Although ginger is well known for its digestive properties, the distilled water of ginger was, in the past, regarded as one of the best remedies for cataract of the eye (Valnet 1980, p. 136).

Ginger hydrolat is recommended for airsickness, carsickness, morning sickness, in fact, any sort of nausea or indigestion can be soothed by ginger's stomachic properties (naturesgift.com/hydrosols).

10

Methods, dosage and recipes

- Reasons for using hydrolats 149
- Hydrolats used in association with other therapeutic products 150
- Uses of distilled waters 151
- Methods: external pathways 152
- Methods: internal pathways 155
- Dispersants 157
- Cautions 158
- Conclusion 158
- Recipes 160
- Recipes for common ailments 160
- Culinary recipes 173
- Making your own hydrolats 177

– *'A nice attention, however, is certainly necessary in the use of them'*, John Farley (1783), Principal Cook at the London Tavern, Dublin, referring to the water and infusions of bay.

Reasons for using hydrolats

Hydrolats have been in continual use certainly for three and a half centuries, perhaps longer, being employed in cooking, for medicine, and for enhancing personal cleanliness (Genders 1977, p. 17). This extensive and continual use of hydrolats over several centuries indicates that they have a pedigree of both worthwhile therapeutic application and safety. For example, the hydrolat obtained from the distillation of *Salvia triloba* is widely used in a number of Middle Eastern countries and there have been no recorded unwanted side effects (Nasr 2000, p. 26).

As hydrolats are ultra mild in action compared with essential oils they are useful for the treatment of the young, the elderly and those in a state of delicate health (Price & Price 1999, p. 113), including babies and convalescents. Hydrolats are especially recommended for young children, for both external and internal use, because of this lack of aggression, and they have long been used as gentle therapeutic agents (Montesinos 1991). The less volatile odorous molecules are integrally dispersed in the distillation water in ionized form, and so irritation of the skin and mucous surfaces is avoided; in addition, this dispersion makes the essential oil compounds more acceptable to the body fluids, which are aqueous in nature.

Hydrolats are impregnated with some of the water soluble (hydrophilic) compounds that are not present in essential oils – for example, soothing, antiinflammatory carboxylic acids are found almost exclusively in hydrolats. Being mildly astringent yet non-drying to the skin, distilled plant waters (true hydrolats) are ideal for severe cases of psoriasis or highly sensitive skin, or for any case where essential oils might be too strong (Keville & Green 1995, p. 90).

Like essential oils, hydrolats can be used both externally and internally, either on their own, in blends, or mixed with other products. They can of course be used individually but (just like essential oils) they may be employed – perhaps to better effect – in mixes of two or three hydrolats together. Many are also useful warmed, as a comforting bedtime drink (Bego 1995, p. 45).

Unlike essential oils, which, if used incorrectly, can present hazards, hydrolats, as stated above, are completely safe and can be used by all, as they are extremely mild by comparison. They are universally useful for all problems where internal use is called for, and are used by some pharmacists.

Hydrolats may be substituted for herbal tinctures where there are physical and/or moral objections to the use of alcohol, for example in the case of religious beliefs, for young children, in alcoholism, and where there are medical objections because alcohol is drying to the skin, or stings.

Hydrolats used in association with other therapeutic products

Everyone knows that oil and water do not mix (although this may now no longer be true – Pashley (2003) removed all dissolved gas from a water–oil mixture, at which point the mix spontaneously formed a cloudy emulsion). However, the distilled waters are an excellent complement to the essential oils and provide an effective overall treatment. They can be used in conjunction with the essential oil of the same name to create a synergistic blend – in effect, putting the plant back together, thus having the benefits of more of the plant. Apart from blending hydrolats with essential oils in a vaporizer, mixtures of reinforced medicated water can be made using the two plant products, giving a stronger, more holistic mix.

Because distilled plant waters (hydrolats) work naturally and synergistically with essential oils, they can be prescribed as a complement to either phytotherapy (Streicher 1996) or aromatherapy. In the context of overall harmonization of the whole body, hydrolats can also be combined with homoeopathy (a mother tincture can be used to reinforce hydrolats which are used medicinally). They can be used in conjunction with other disciplines also, such as osteopathy, naturopathy, acupuncture and so on. Herbalists in France do not use hydrolats on their own to any great extent, but as a complement to other phytotherapeutic treatments both internally and externally, where they are used both singly and as ready prepared mixes for such conditions as eczema, bronchitis, tracheitis and for use in nasal sprays (Montesinos 1991, p. 15).

Hydrolats are often prescribed after taking count of the energy balance and the 'environment' (both internal and external) of the person, according to Chinese medicine. Among conditions treated are disorders of the digestive system (including constipation), rheumatism, migraine (liver), parasites, and disorders of the ear, nose and throat. Another important aspect is the energy state of the active principles as they appear in the hydrolats, in which some of the aromatic principles are completely dispersed in ionized (energized) form, which obviates any irritation of the skin and mucous surfaces: this is beneficial to sufferers of eczema, ulcers and colitis (Viaud 1983).

Some hydrolats are antiviral and antiparasitic and complement the antiseptic, antimicrobial, antifungal actions of the related essential oils. According to Viaud (1983, p. 30), the main effects of the hydrolats are superficial, vascular, serous and sub-diaphragmatic, in contrast to the essential oils, whose main actions are above the diaphragm where they act at a deeper level and have effect also on the lymph and serous fluids.

One school of thought says that it is better to use the whole plant than isolated extracts; others believe that using the essential oil and the hydrolat in synergy is closer to wholeness, the one component complementing and possibly augmenting the action of the other, giving a stronger, more synergistic, holistic mix. In fact, the essential oil components and the water-soluble plant molecules in a hydrolat can work together to give an effect closer to the herbal remedy or to the essential oil, depending on the particular plant and its hydrophilic components; for example melissa essential oil has many water-soluble components and thus its hydrolat is quite powerful. Sometimes the plant has virtually no medicinal effects except for the essential oil; in other cases, especially where the herb contains very little or no essential oil, the effect is due to other plant components.

Uses of distilled waters

Suitably selected hydrolats given in the proper dose are useful for many health problems. Although appropriate and revitalizing for all types of skin, they are, because they are almost free of irritating components such as terpene hydrocarbons, particularly well suited for extremely sensitive skin.

Generally hydrolats are used in the following areas:

- *general*: cooking, cooling spray, ice cubes, pet care, room spray.
- *hair care*: shampoos, conditioners, hair rinses
- *medicinal blends or products*: asthma, bronchitis, colitis, douches, eczema, gargles, mouthwashes, nappy rash, tracheitis, ulcers, wounds, compresses (burns, aches and pains, eyes, etc.)
- *skin care*: creams, facial sprays, skin toners, lotions, aftershave lotions, masks

Because of their subtle effect and lack of irritation hydrolats can be used on open wounds for disinfection and on mucous surfaces, and so are also suitable for vaginal douches. Their gentleness enables them to be used safely on mucous membranes, for example mouthwashes and gargles, and even in inflammation of the eyes; internal use also may safely be recommended where appropriate (Roulier

1990, p. 115). They are often used for the treatment of pain, either local or generalized; for example *Chamaemelum nobile* (Roman chamomile) is said to be active in countering post-zoster pain and several hydrolats relieve the pain of inflamed eyes (Franchomme & Pénoël 1996, p. 86).

Although hydrolats are already dilute by reason of their method of production, they may be further diluted for use. Payne (1999) suggests that 1 teaspoonful (5 ml) of distilled plant water can be diluted in 200 ml of pure water and still be effective (equivalent to 25 ml in 1000 ml). The therapeutic index (Appendices A and B) gives the properties and indications for the use of hydrolats for general physical conditions, skin conditions and emotional states: it is based almost wholly on anecdotal evidence in the absence of any other kind of proof. There is a table giving the principal constituents of hydrolats in Chapter 8.

Methods: external pathways

Baths

Normal bath

Put 50 ml (approximately 2 tablespoonfuls) of the chosen hydrolat or blend of hydrolats into a bath to aid relaxation and promote the soothing effect. As with essential oils, the bath should be run to the desired temperature before adding the hydrolat(s), after which the water should be 'swished' well to disperse thoroughly throughout the bath. For full effect, remain in the bath for at least 10 minutes.

- For a child up to 6 months, 1–2 teaspoonfuls (5–10 ml) of aromatic water can be used in a baby bath.
- For children up to 12 years old, use 15–50 ml, depending on the age of the child.
- Adults can add up to 500–750 ml to a bath of water, though this may be more expensive than 6–8 drops of essential oil dissolved in a suitable medium. Rose (1999, p. 168) recommends a few cupfuls in the bath.

Foot, hand and sitz bath

These are useful for swelling, inflammation or pain (such as rheumatism) and infections or a fungus, such as athlete's foot or *Candida albicans*.

- Put 100–250 ml of hydrolat into a large bowl of warm water for foot and sitz baths, and 50–100 ml into a smaller bowl for hand baths.

Compresses

These can be used successfully for a number of problems: insect bites, arthritic joints, period or stomach pains, headaches, sprains, varicose veins, etc. They are also most effective used on the eyes with cotton wool pads and hydrolats of *Chamaemelum nobile* (Roman chamomile) and/or *Centaurea cyanus* (cornflower). Decide first whether you need a hot or a cold compress: where there is inflammation and heat, a cold one is best; for a dull ache or pain, use a warm one.

Cotton (handkerchiefs or tea towels) is the best medium, being very absorbent. The size of the basin should be chosen according to the size of the area to be treated, for example for a finger compress a cup is big enough. Use only the amount of water plus hydrolat thought necessary to soak into the compress; heat if a warm compress is required. As hydrolats are not at all strong:

- they can be used neat for adults
- dilute 50/50 for children.

Lower the cotton material into the basin until the hydrolat is completely absorbed, squeeze gently to remove excess water and lay on the problem area, holding in place with cling film (if practical). For a cold compress, a sealed plastic bag of crushed ice cubes or a packet of frozen peas held in place with a thin scarf or a stocking is helpful; for a warm one, a woollen scarf, a thermal garment or a warmed heat pack can be placed over the cling film. To keep a compress in place on an arm or leg, a sock or a pair of tights is ideal. Leave the compress in place for at least 1 hour, or overnight for something sceptic.

Douches

- Use 1–3 parts of hydrolat to 4 parts of water.

Eye care

Hydrolats can be used in preparations for eyewashes to soothe inflammation and tiredness, etc.

- Dilute 50/50 with warm water for adults (result should be comfortably warm).
- Dilute 20% of hydrolat in 80% warm water for children.

NB: Ethanol is often added to hydrolats to prolong shelf-life: *please ensure that hydrolats used for the eyes do not contain this alcohol or any other preservative.*

Hair care

Hydrolats can be blended into shampoos, conditioners and rinses for hair and scalp care, both for daily maintenance and to remedy problems such as dandruff, greasy or dry hair, problem scalps, etc.

Nebulizers

Hydrolats are more suited for use in nebulizers than are essential oils, as sometimes the latter can eat into plastic, harming the nebulizer.

Skin care

Hydrolats, which are medicated by nature of their chemical make-up, have long been used in skin care; they are increasingly frequently employed in therapeutic and everyday cosmetics, in particular because they are non-irritating and non-aggressive to the skin and mucous membranes due to their low content of essential oil molecules. Because of their affinity for the skin, they are well suited for skin care preparations, including cleansing, baby care and face and body care (Claeys 1992). They are sometimes added in the aqueous phase of creams and lotions, to make products such as aromatic baths, masks, creams, lotions and gels, etc.

All hydrolats will counteract the drying effects of a long aeroplane flight, as well as those caused by air-conditioned rooms and cars (a spray is the easiest method). They can be used alone as toners, or added to other substances such as aloe vera and are also effective blended into masks (Keville & Green 1995, p. 90).

Blends can be made for all skin types, for skin problems and for daily maintenance of the following skin types: dry, sensitive, greasy, red or blotchy skin, acne, dermatitis, psoriasis, rosacea.

Jaques Palz, Paris, uses five different hydrosol blends in a phytoaromatic skin care range (Streicher 1996), including *Rosmarinus officinalis* (verbenone) and *Thymus vulgaris* (linalool) for dry skin, chamomile (variety not specified) and *Artemisia arborescens* for sensitive skin.

Creams and lotions

The use of vegetable oil alone is not the complete answer to a dry skin, even though it will give a silky feel to the skin. It will, however, help prevent moisture escaping from the skin surface and will give a smoother texture to rough, scaly skin. Water, on the other hand, evaporates too quickly to be of help to a dry skin and causes further dryness (Keville & Green 1995, p. 90). What is needed is a blend of water and oil, which should be well homogenized to keep the skin moist and 'plump'. Moisturising creams made with a higher percentage of water than oil are the most effective, the oil aiding the penetration of the water, which is vital to replace moisture lost daily by the skin.

Bartram (1995, p. 456) cites a formula from Dr A. Vogel which is made up of nine parts distilled witch hazel, five parts St John's wort oil (hypericum), three parts tincture of echinacea and two parts wheat germ oil, homogenized to form a 'salve'. It is designed to treat a wide range of skin conditions, but especially acne.

It is reasonable to suppose that if hydrolats are used in place of de-ionized water in a moisturizing cream or lotion, the benefits of the hydrolat will be added to the overall effect on the skin. In fact, 5% of a selected hydrolat, or mix of hydrolats, can be added to a prepared skin care item, including a toning lotion, when it can be used on cotton wool or in a spray.

As well as for the skin problems noted above, lotions can be made for sunburn, various dermatoses, skin irritation and other skin conditions.

Sprays

Hydrolats can be used undiluted in sprays as a skin or body tonic, for cooling the body, disinfecting rooms, dampening laundry, etc.

Vaporizers

Although the aroma from hydrolats is not as powerful – and sometimes not as nice – as that from an essential oil of the same name, their use is, according to Payne (1999), a good way of supplementing, or even replacing, essential oils. As preventatives, they can be used in this way every day to keep infections at bay over the winter months.

The safest vaporizer is an electric one (thus avoiding a naked flame), especially where children and old people are concerned, although these are more expensive. Provided one takes care to position them well, night-light vaporizers are adequate, especially for use with hydrolats, and a multitude of different sizes and designs are available. The advantage of using hydrolats in a vaporizer is that the containers do not dry out so quickly as when essential oils alone are used, when the heavier molecules of the oil can have an acrid smell as they burn off. There is no need to dilute hydrolats for use in a vaporizer.

Other external uses

Rose (1999) gives many other uses for hydrolats, including cooling a hot flush, disinfecting hands, making pet wipes and spraying into the air in hotel rooms to freshen and sanitize. They can also be used for the pleasure of having pleasant-smelling table or bed linen (B. Payne, personal communication, 2001) or simply to dampen the ironing to give a fresh aroma to laundered garments.

Methods: internal pathways

Hydrolats can be used internally, either for medicinal reasons or for the pleasure of the flavour, added to teas drunk every day. However, it must be emphasized that for internal use only hydrolats of therapeutic quality should be used, as in the case of essential oils (see cautions below). Taken orally, hydrolats pass through the mucous membrane of the digestive tract and from there into the bloodstream, thus reaching and aiding the problem for which they were ingested.

Hydrolats have a higher concentration of volatile elements than teas and so are more efficacious and quicker acting and are easy to use, as only small quantities are needed. The culinary aspect is also appealing, as hydrolats are easily added to foods (e.g. soups, sauces, fruit salads, etc.) to enhance the flavour of the dish – and at the same time, aid health.

For internal use of essential oils it is imperative not only to know which oils are suitable for this method but also to dilute them to a 0.5 % concentration before use. Unlike the oils, it is not always necessary to dilute hydrolats. They can be diluted by up to 50% should it be wished.

For children, hydrolats may be sweetened if necessary to make them more palatable. As stated earlier, they are recommended for young children for both external and internal use because of their lack of aggression.

For indigestion and other digestive disorders such as constipation or diarrhoea, a cup of hydrolat-flavoured water or tea two or three times a day is more pleasant than tablets; urinary tract problems such as cystitis react favourably to this form of treatment. Hydrolats and teas can also be helpful for insomnia and arthritic pain and offer a low-risk method of ingesting plant benefits compared to essential oils.

There is one slight difficulty concerning the internal use of hydrolats, stemming from the prejudice against internal usage of essential oils. Catty (1998a) tells us that hydrolats are a subtle way of introducing the internal consumption of aromatics, as anyone who has tasted and tried them by this method will agree. However, this concept is still intimidating to many people in the UK, probably due to incomplete aromatherapy training. British aromatherapy courses have concentrated on massage; had they also included the knowledge necessary for this direct and efficient method of use, the situation would now be different. It is true that many books which reflect this limited training carry dire warnings on the internal use of essential oils and, in one way, this is no bad thing, considering the poor quality (therapeutically speaking) of most essential oils on the market. However:

> *Hydrosols can change a person's mind on internal use of aromatics in just one sip. Once accustomed to the idea, profound and effective health protocols may be established in conjunction with topical use of essential oils, or with a hydrosol therapy all on its own. I have seen amazing results from these 'natural curative waters'. (Catty 1998a)*

When using hydrolats internally, the recommended dilutions are as follows:

- For a baby of 6–12 months: 5 ml (1 tsp) in 100 ml water (50 ml per litre).
- For children under 10: 10 ml in 100 ml water (100 ml per litre).
- For children of 10–14: 25 ml per year of age in 1 litre of water (250–350 ml per litre).
- For adults: 50–75% hydrolat with 50–25% water (500–750 ml per litre).

Different sources recommend different doses, varying greatly, from 3 *teaspoon*fuls (15 ml) per day, up to 2–3 *tablespoon*fuls (30–45 ml) *twice* per day. However, much depends on the reason for taking hydrolats in the first instance; if for simple daily health maintenance or a chronic problem, 2–3 teaspoonfuls (10–15 ml) twice a day is enough, but if the problem is acute, needing treatment for a short duration of time, it is completely safe to ingest the 2–3 tablespoonfuls suggested, three times a day. Unlike essential oils, the dilution of hydrolats is not crucial; whether or not they are used neat is more a matter of taste than safety.

Frequency and duration of treatment is also dependent both on the system and the age of the person being treated. When a satisfactory outcome has been achieved, the dose should be reduced, but not stopped, until 2 weeks have gone by. Manfredi, cited in Montesinos (1991, p. 43), states that for the treatment of the liver and kidneys, the time of day the hydrolat is taken is as important as the dose: for treatment of the liver it should be taken before supper or going to bed (as the liver works during the night), but for treatment of the kidneys and bladder, it should be taken between 15.00 and 19.00 hours.

Beverages (water and tea)

When making ice cubes, try making them with a hydrolat (or a blend of hydrolats) to make a drink more interesting; use the hydrolat neat, or diluted to the strength desired.

Up to 1 teaspoonful (5 ml) of a hydrolat can be added to tea or coffee (here petitgrain or orange flower water is delicious), or in a morning glass of water where the hydrolats used will assist in regulating and revitalizing the person.

Culinary uses

Hydrolats from herbs and spices give additional flavour to soups and other savoury dishes; the amount to add depends on individual taste, so add a little at a time and taste before adding more. They can also be used in a salad dressing. Peppermint, aniseed, nutmeg, clove and the exotic waters of rose otto, neroli and melissa can be added to fruit juice, cake mixtures, fruit salads, yoghurts, etc.

Gargles and mouthwashes

Hydrolats can be used neat for gargles and mouthwashes in the dilutions given above for internal use. Hydrolats are ideal for this kind of treatment as, unlike essential oils, they dissolve readily in water and, because of their gentleness, the dose is not crucial, as it is when taking essential oils internally.

Hydrolats can also be used for ear, nose and throat (ENT) problems, voice loss, sore throats, and colds which may go onto the chest, when a twice or thrice daily gargle is extremely helpful. They can be used either in a glass of water or in a spray. Put your chosen hydrolat into a glass (a blend of waters such as sandalwood with Roman chamomile, geranium or cypress is soothing). Stir well, take a mouthful, gargle and either swallow it or spit it out (this aromatic water may safely be swallowed for enhanced effect). Stir again and repeat.

The procedure for mouthwashes is exactly the same, except that the liquid is swished around inside the mouth for a few seconds instead of at the back of the throat. For enhanced effect, roll it around for a full minute before spitting out or swallowing.

Rectal use

Hydrolats may be used to good effect 50/50 with water in an enema, where the hydrolat can reach the mucous surfaces of the large intestine.

Vaccinations

Given before and after vaccinations *Laurus nobilis* (bay) acts prophylactically to prevent many of the associated side effects and helps the body deal with the vaccination process (Catty 1998a).

Dispersants

When adding essential oils to hydrolats, a dispersant such as Disper, Solubol or Labrafil can be blended first with the essential oil, to ensure its complete dispersion in the hydrolat.

The two following recipes have been suggested:

- 1 ml essential oil with ½ –1 ml dispersant to 1 litre hydrolat; take 1 teaspoonful (5 ml) in a cup of water 2–3 times per day.
- 15–50 ml essential oil and 5–20 ml dispersant to 1 litre hydrolat; take 15–25 drops of this mix in a cup of water 2–3 times per day.

There is quite a big difference between the two recipes and they show a great disparity between the doses. However, the second recipe may be deliberately stronger, as the dosage taken from it is very low.

Cautions

Genuine or laboratory made hydrolats?

As with essential oils, hydrolats can be genuine, or made in a laboratory. The latter are the ones usually used in cosmetics, but for use by therapists, genuine hydrolats are necessary.

> *Hydrolats, as with other partial plant extracts, will only possess the claimed activity of the plant if the constituents of the plant giving this activity are contained within that fraction of the plant which forms the partial plant extract. Many partial plant extracts, particularly distillates, have the advantage of being virtually colourless, making for ease of incorporation into a range of products. Unfortunately, this has led over the years to the production of distillates from a wide range of plant materials which are not suitable to this form of processing, and therefore little credence can be given to any claimed activity of the plant material or its extract. (Helliwell 1989)*

Hydrolats that have had preservatives added are best not used for culinary or therapeutic purposes: a preservative is often added to natural essential waters to improve the shelf-life. When purchasing hydrolats it may be necessary to obtain a certificate from the supplier to ensure that the proper conditions of harvesting, processing and stocking have been observed.

Hydrolats which have not been well distilled, or which have been mishandled or incorrectly stored, may contain material which decomposes, giving a greenish character; this indicates a change in character of the water. A bad smell precludes use (Montesinos 1991).

It is imperative that the only products used are those obtained during steam distillation and free from colouring matter, stabilizers and preservatives. Products procured from a High Street chemist's shop do not usually conform to this high standard.

Conclusion

Hydrolats have a subtle effect, do not irritate, and so are good for the treatment of internal problems and of mucous membranes (e.g. eye inflammation); however, it is necessary to be aware of hydrolats that have had alcohol or other preservative added (a legal requirement in some countries) – these are not suitable for all therapeutic purposes, especially for the eyes and use on babies and children.

Physically, hydrolats contain some water-soluble molecules known to be therapeutic, in common with essential oils and some compounds found in other types of herbal preparations. It may be that they also carry information and energy somewhat analogous to homoeopathic remedies. They are gentle in use and may safely be used in cases where the use of the more powerful essential oils would be inadvisable. They may be used to complement other forms of treatment and also together with essential oils. Additionally, they have the advantage of being relatively inexpensive.

Making your own hydrolats may not be an easy task, but it is possible and exciting to carry out your own small-scale distillation (see p. 175). Infusions and decoctions, on the other hand, are very easy to make and extremely useful in everyday health care (see p. 194).

RECIPES

The recipes given below cover: common ailments, including baby and child care, circulation, colds and 'flu, detoxification, diarrhoea, digestive, eyes, general health, hair, hypertension, legs, lice, lymph, nervous system, respiratory, rheumatism, skin, slimming, teeth, tonic, urinary problems; culinary recipes, and instructions on making your own hydrolats.

Recipes for common ailments

Aches and pains

(topical - compress and tisane) – **(Shirley Price)**
Aches and pains, whether backache or other muscular pains or rheumatism and arthritis, can benefit from analgesic and antiinflammatory hydrolats.

Mix together equal amounts of:

- *Pinus sylvestris* [PINE]
- *Rosmarinus officinalis* [ROSEMARY]
- *Coriandrum sativum* [CORIANDER]

Compress

The cloth chosen should be the right size to cover the affected area and the amount of hydrolat/s just enough to wet this cloth. Aches and pains benefit from warmth, so heat your hydrolats to a comfortable temperature before wetting the cloth. After lightly squeezing it, place on the affected area and cover with a piece of cling film, followed by a scarf, blanket or other warm material, the size determined by the size of the area treated. Leave for at least an hour.

Tisane

Make any tea or tisane of your choice, and put 1 teaspoon each of the above hydrolats into your cup before filling it up with tea. Drink one or two cups three times a day.

Baby and child care

(bath, ingestion, spray) – **(Suzanne Catty)**
The hydrolat of *Chamaemelum nobile* (Roman chamomile) is ideal for infant and baby care. Sprayed onto nappy rash or added to the diet, this hydrolat has been found excellent for relaxing and soothing and provides relief for many teething symptoms including: gum swelling, diarrhoea, insomnia and crying.

Baby and child care

(bath, ingestion, topical) – **(Nelly Grosjean)**
(Scientific names of plants not specified)

Bath

- 30 ml lavender and chamomile hydrolats
- Makes a soothing and calming bath for children.

Children's health drink

- 5 ml pine hydrolat
- 1 cup warm water
- honey to taste

Infant chills

- mix together pine and lavender hydrolats
- Rub on the chest and back (for very young babies).

Cellulite

(ingestion and application) – **(Shirley Price)**

Cellulite can only be eliminated with perseverance since it requires twice daily application over a number of weeks or months, otherwise it is a waste of time. However, with diligence, cellulite can be helped considerably. The application of essential oils in a carrier is excellent for breaking down the lumpy tissue and the internal use of diuretic hydrolats encourages the release of the broken-down molecules through the kidneys. Sensible eating is also advised!

Hydrolat mix (ingestion):

- 200 ml *Cupressus sempervirens* [CYPRESS]
- 200 ml *Pinus sylvestris* [PINE]
- 600 ml *Juniperus communis* (fruct.) [JUNIPER BERRY]

Essential oil mix (application only):

- 200 ml carrier oil or lotion
- 1 ml (20 drops) *Foeniculum vulgare* (dulce) [SWEET FENNEL]
- 1 ml (20 drops) *Juniperus communis* (fruct.) [JUNIPER BERRY]
- 1 ml (20 drops) *Pelargonium graveolens* [GERANIUM]
- 0.5 ml (10 drops) *Boswellia carteri* [FRANKINCENSE]

Application

Apply the essential oil mix given above and firmly rub it into the area twice daily (a rubber brush is an additional aid).

Ingestion

Take 1 tablespoonful of the mixed hydrolats morning, lunchtime and evening.

Cellulite

(application, spray, topical) – **(Carolyn Marshall)**

The following procedure needs about half an hour a day to carry out, using the two recipes:

Make up a bottle using 50% each of:

- *Fucus vesiculosus* [BLADDERWRACK] hydrolat
- *Juniperus communis* (fruct.) [JUNIPER BERRY] hydrolat

1. Apply in a spray to exfoliated skin (aids absorption).
2. Blend with green clay to a paste and brush onto affected area (bandages can be applied starting at the distal end of the limb, gently lifting and rolling the bandage). Leave for ½ hour, then shower off.
3. Massage the area with petrissage and percussion movements using the recipe below.

- 50 ml *Calendula officinalis* [CALENDULA] fixed oil
- 50 ml *Daucus carota* [CARROT] fixed oil
- 3–4 drops *Citrus limon* [LEMON] essential oil

Chickenpox

(topical, spray) – **(Carolyn Marshall)**

The chickenpox virus is incubated for 12–20 days before symptoms appear. The child then develops a temperature and feels unwell, and small, itchy spots begin to erupt over the chest, trunk and eventually face. These spots will blister and eventually form crusts. The following blend helps soothe and heal the spots and will prevent them from drying and becoming more 'pickable' by the child; this prevents the pox from scarring. Spray over the affected area but make sure to keep away from the eyes.

(Recipe includes essential oils)

- 1 × 50 ml plastic spray bottle
- 25 ml *Mentha × piperita* [PEPPERMINT] hydrolat
- 25 ml *Chamaemelum nobile* [ROMAN CHAMOMILE] hydrolat
- 2 drops *Lavandula angustifolia* [LAVENDER] essential oil
- 2 drops *Pelargonium graveolens* [GERANIUM] essential oil

Shake well each time before use.

Circulation mix

(ingestion) – **(Michelle Paris)**

(recipe contains essential oils)

Hydrolats to 1 litre in total:

- *Cupressus sempervirens* [CYPRESS]
- *Erigeron canadensis* [FLEABANE]
- *Melilotus officinalis* [MELILOT]
- *Ruscus aculeatus* [BUTCHER'S BROOM]

Essential oils to 1 ml in total:

- *Cupressus sempervirens* [CYPRESS]
- *Pistacia lentiscus* [MASTIC TREE]

Quantity to take and frequency not specified (see p. 156).

Colds and 'flu

(ingestion, spray, vaporizer) – **(Barbara Payne)**

Gargle

The best way to prevent a cold going onto the chest is to gargle with hydrolats, making sure to swallow the mixture - do not spit it out.

- 10 ml *Myrtus communis* [MYRTLE]
- 20 ml *Eucalyptus smithii* [GULLY GUM]
- 20 ml *Rosmarinus officinalis* [ROSEMARY]

Internal

Put 3 teaspoons of each of the hydrolats above into a glass and drink it; repeat three or four times a day.

Vaporizer

Top up a vaporizer with the hydrolats of:

- *Rosmarinus officinalis* [ROSEMARY] or *Myrtus communis* [MYRTLE]
  Add 3 drops of *Eucalyptus smithii* [GULLY GUM] essential oil.

This procedure will disinfect the room and the eucalyptus is also an immunostimulant. Sometimes it is possible to get hydrolat of this eucalyptus, which is even better. It is also possible to make a spray using only the hydrolats (which are bronchodilators and antiseptics) for the patient to use to freshen up or cool themselves.

Detoxification

(ingestion) – **(Victoria Edwards)**
10–12 drops of *Achillea millefolium* [YARROW] in a glass of distilled water.

Digestion

CONSTIPATION (ingestion) – **(Shirley Price)**

The easiest and quickest way to treat any digestive problem is to take a remedy internally:

- *Rosmarinus officinalis* [ROSEMARY]
- *Citrus aurantium* var. *amara* (flos) [BITTER ORANGE FLOWER]

1. Make a weak tisane with any tea of your choice and add 2 teaspoonfuls each of the hydrolats above, drinking this 3 or 4 times a day, or/and
2. Put 1 tablespoonful of each hydrolat into a glass and drink before going to bed.

DIARRHOEA DUE TO AN INFECTION (ingestion) – **(Shirley Price)**

The following hydrolats are effective intestinal antiseptics and lavender hydrolat is antibiotic; the three hydrolats can be taken for this kind of diarrhoea to kill the germs.

Use equal quantities of each of:

- *Thymus vulgaris* [THYME]
- *Salvia officinalis* [SAGE]
- *Lavandula officinalis* [LAVENDER]

Take half a small glassful every 2 hours during the day.

GENERAL DIGESTIVE MIX (ingestion) – **(Michelle Paris)**

1 drop each of essential oils of:

- *Rosmarinus officinalis* ct. verbenone (ROSEMARY)
- *Artemisia dracunculus* [TARRAGON]
- *Ocimum basilicum* [BASIL]
- *Lavandula angustifolia* [LAVENDER]

2 ml each of hydrolats of:

- *Lavandula angustifolia* [LAVENDER]
- *Origanum majorana* [MARJORAM]

A digestive mix made entirely of hydrolats may consist of:

- *Laurus nobilis* [BAY]
- *Levisticum officinale* [LOVAGE]
- *Mentha × piperita* [PEPPERMINT]
- *Ocimum basilicum* [BASIL]
- *Peumus boldus* [BOLDO LEAF]
- *Rosmarinus officinalis* ct. verbenone [ROSEMARY VERBENONE]

NAUSEA, DIARRHOEA, SICKNESS (ingestion) – **(Barbara Payne)**

A tablespoonful of equal quantities of fennel and peppermint hydrolats (previously mixed together in a bottle) added to a cup of tea without milk is excellent for queasiness, diarrhoea and sickness.

PROPHYLACTIC TREATMENT

(ingestion) – **(Shirley Price)**

When visiting Mediterranean countries like Egypt, a good precautionary measure against stomach problems is to put one or both of the following hydrolats into each litre bottle of water you drink to keep your stomach healthy. If using both waters, reduce the quantity to 50 ml of each.

- 100 ml *Foeniculum vulgare* var. *dulce* [FENNEL]
  or/and
- 100 ml *Mentha × piperita* [PEPPERMINT]

Shake well and take frequent sips.

STOMACH UPSETS (ingestion) – **(Barbara Payne)**

Make a teapot of Earl Grey tea.

- Add 30 ml of *Mentha × piperita* [PEPPERMINT] hydrolat.
- Serve with a little honey.

The honey will also serve as a healer and antiseptic.

STOMACH UPSETS (severe) and *VIRAL ENTERITIS* (ingestion) – **(Shirley Price)**

Hydrolats are a perfect antidote to any stomach upset. This recipe has been effective in several cases involving diarrhoea and sickness. In the event of not having one of the hydrolats in this recipe, study the properties of hydrolats in Appendix B.

It is possible to use just one hydrolat, but the author has found that, as with essential oils, the effects are enhanced by using a synergistic blend.

- 50 ml *Thymus vulgaris* ct. geraniol [SWEET THYME] (antiviral to enteritis)
- 50 ml *Mentha × piperita* [PEPPERMINT] (antiinflammatory – gastritis, digestive)
- 50 ml *Salvia officinalis* [SAGE] (antiviral to enteritis)
- 50 ml *Pelargonium graveolens* [GERANIUM] (antiinfectious – infectious colitis, astringent)

Mix all the hydrolats together in a bottle. For each dose, put 2 teaspoonfuls into a small glass and half fill with water; drink at regular intervals.

Eye conditions

Warning – Ethanol is often added to distilled plant waters to prolong shelf-life: it is necessary to ensure that all waters used for the eyes are free of this alcohol and/or other preservatives.

Hydrolats can be safely used to help eye problems, as they are mild enough to use on this delicate area (see p. 153).

Culpeper's recipe is as follows: 'Take of Fennel, Eyebright, Roses, white, Celandine, Vervain and Rue, of each a handful, the liver of a Goat chopt small, infuse them well in Eyebright Water, then distil them in an alembic, and you shall have a water which (will) clear the sight beyond comparison.'

CONJUNCTIVITIS, TIRED EYES, INFLAMMATION (compress, drops) – **(Shirley Price)**

I first made up a recipe for the eyes when I developed a dendritic ulcer across my left eye (due to using my facecloth carelessly when I had a herpes on my lip). I did not have the time to go to the hospital every time the ulcer reappeared, and Len suggested I make some eye drops using essential oils. This extremely dilute mix was so successful that I marketed it as Chamomile Eye Drops.

Many years ago, in France, I had forgotten my chamomile eye drops and my friend Claire Montesinos, who distills her own oils and hydrolats not far from our farmhouse, gave me a bottle of 'bleuet' (*Centaurea cyanus* – cornflower water). I first used it by soaking cottonwool pads in it and placing these on my closed eyes for several minutes.

A few years ago, when Len first started this book, we had many hydrolats sent to us for testing and for analysis. One of the first remedies I tried was for both Len's and my own eyes, which were either inflamed or watering or tired through long spells spent at a computer. The following is the recipe I use – in two different ways:

- *Centaurea cyanus* [CORNFLOWER]
- *Chamaemelum nobile* [ROMAN CHAMOMILE]

Compress

- Put 1 tablespoonful of each hydrolat (or 2 tablespoons of one or the other) into a cup.
- Add 1 (or 2) tablespoonfuls of water.
- Soak two cotton wool circles in the mix
- Place a pad on each eye and leave in place for about 10 minutes.

Eye drops

- Put 1 teaspoonful of each hydrolat (or 2 of either one) into a 50 ml bottle
- Fill to the neck with distilled or spring water and shake well
- Put one or two drops into the eye with an eye dropper when needed.

INFLAMMATION OF THE EYES (compress) – **(Claire Montesinos)**

Compress

1 teaspoonful each of the following hydrolats:

- *Plantago major* [PLANTAIN]
- *Chelidonium majus* [GREATER CELANDINE]

- *Chamaemelum nobile* [ROMAN CHAMOMILE]
- *Melilotus officinalis* [MELILOT]
- *Centaurea cyanus* [CORNFLOWER]

Soak cotton pieces in the hydrolats and place on the eyes.

INFLAMMATION OF THE EYES (compress) – **(Price & Price 1999, P. 113)**

Myrtus communis [MYRTLE] and *Chamaemelum nobile* [ROMAN CHAMOMILE] soothe pains due to inflammatory states of the eyes.

SWOLLEN, WATERING EYES, PINK EYE (spray) – **(Kurt Schnaubelt)**

Spray myrtle hydrolat (*Myrtus communis*) directly onto closed eyelids, or into the eye, every hour. The authors would suggest using an eye dropper, rather than a spray, if putting the hydrolat directly into the eye.

TIRED EYES (compress) – **(Barbara Payne)**

Chamaemelum nobile [ROMAN CHAMOMILE] or *Centaurea cyanus* [CORNFLOWER]
Put the cooled hydrolat onto cotton pads and place on the eyes to soothe.
Relax for 10 minutes.

General health

– **(Nelly Grosjean)**
(Scientific names of plants not specified):

Daily drink

30 ml of the following hydrolats (a blend of two or three or all):

- sage, mint, oregano, savory, thyme, eucalyptus, juniper
- 1.5 litres of water

Drink throughout the day.

Infusion

- 5 ml per cup of hot (not boiling) water
- mint, sage, rosemary, oregano, savory, thyme, verbena

'Sugar free' syrup (useful for children)

- mint, verbena
- 30–60 ml per litre of water (+ fructose or honey if required)

Hygienic drink

- 150 ml peppermint hydrolat
- 1 litre of water

Digestive system daily drink

- sage, rosemary, oregano

Tonic bath

- thyme, rosemary, oregano, savory

Hair

GREASY HAIR RINSE – **(Nelly Grosjean)**

- 15 ml of soap (savon de Marseille) grated into a bowl of warm water

Add some lavender water and a few drops of *Lavandula angustifolia* [LAVENDER] essential oil. Wash hair with this, then rinse well.

ALL HAIR PROBLEMS – **(Nelly Grosjean)**

- sage, thyme, lavender, ylang-ylang and cedar

Headache

(compress, ingestion) – **(Shirley Price)**

The hydrolat to use depends on the cause of the headache; for example, a headache due to menstruation is best treated with the hydrolat of *Origanum majorana* [SWEET MARJORAM], that connected with the digestion needs *Mentha* × *piperita* [PEPPERMINT] and one due to stress would react favourably with *Chamaemelum nobile* [ROMAN CHAMOMILE]. Therefore, the most sure way to cure a headache is to make a mixture of the hydrolats below and use it in two ways:

- *Origanum majorana* [SWEET MARJORAM]
- *Mentha* × *piperita* [PEPPERMINT]
- *Chamaemelum nobile* [ROMAN CHAMOMILE]

Compress

Choose a piece of cotton the right size for your forehead and temples and make up enough of the mixed hydrolats to wet it thoroughly. After lightly squeezing the cloth, place on the forehead and cover with a piece of cling film, followed by a small scarf or other warm material. Leave for at least an hour.

Ingestion

Put 45 ml of each hydrolat into a glass and drink it; repeat every 15 minutes until the headache is gone. This method can be used in conjunction with the compress if the headache is severe.

Hypertension, high BP

(bath) – **(Barbara Payne)**

High blood pressure can be regulated in conjunction with your usual medication by using hydrolat of *Pelargonium graveolens* [GERANIUM] in the bath – 30 ml should be enough. Make sure the bath is not too hot.

Legs

(spray) – **(André Rouvière and Marie-Claire Meyer)**

Refreshing to legs:

- 30 ml *Rosmarinus officinalis* [ROSEMARY] hydrolat
- 15 ml *Salvia officinalis* [SAGE] hydrolat

- 15 ml sweet almond carrier oil
- 5 ml glycerine

Lice

(application) – **(Claire Montesinos)**
Mix together equal quantities of each of the following hydrolats (or a mix of any three or four). Rub daily onto the scalp to deter lice.

- *Satureia montana* [SAVORY]
- *Lavandula angustifolia* [LAVENDER]
- *Salvia officinalis* [SAGE]
- *Thymus vulgaris* [THYME]
- *Chamaemelum nobile* [ROMAN CHAMOMILE]
- *Laurus nobilis* [BAY LEAF]

Lymph Glands

(internal) – **(Suzanne Catty)**
In over two dozen cases of long-term palpable swollen lymph nodes in breast tissue, *Laurus nobilis* [BAY LEAF] hydrolat has effected a complete disappearance of the swelling and tenderness within 5 days by dilute internal use.

Menopause

(spray) – **(Barbara Payne)**
For hot sweats and flushes use equal quantities of hydrolats of:

- *Mentha × piperita* [PEPPERMINT]
- *Salvia sclarea* [CLARY]
- *Citrus aurantium* var. *amara* (flos) [BITTER ORANGE FLOWER]

Shake well before spraying each time you feel hot or over burdened.
If put into a pretty perfume spray bottle, no one will know what it is for.
If you keep your hydrolat in the refrigerator when at home, it will be especially cooling for such emergencies.

The hydrolat of *Rosa centifolia* [ROSE] will work just as well as those suggested, but you must be sure to obtain the true hydrolat.

Nervous system

(Nelly Grosjean)
(Scientific names of plants not given)
A course of marjoram, oregano, rosemary, savory – in rotation – for lack of energy.

PMS

(internal) – **(Shirley Price)**
Although symptoms of pre-menstrual syndrome (PMS) can vary from woman to woman, and the condition is hormonal, the most common basic state is stress, because the person knows that the mood swings (often accompanied by

headaches) can affect other people at work and at home; these are sometimes accompanied by weight gain and fluid retention. Adjusting the diet and cutting down or avoiding such items as coffee (the caffeine increases stress and insomnia), salt and chocolate can help (Price 1995), as can avoiding too much coca-cola and alcohol.

Taking hydrolats from 10 days before menstruation is expected to commence, up to the second day of the period itself, will help prevent and reduce any symptoms suffered. Make up a litre bottle to the following recipe and drink a wineglassful two or three times a day, depending on the severity of the symptoms. Alternatively, make a weak tea or tisane of your choice (tannin-free) and add 1 tablespoonful of the same recipe to each cupful, drinking 6–8 cups a day:

- 250 ml *Salvia sclarea* [CLARY SAGE] (oestrogen-like)
- 200 ml *Chamaemelum nobile* [ROMAN CHAMOMILE] (calming, soporific)
- 50 ml of any two (or all three) of the following:
  –*Citrus aurantium* v. *amara* (flos) [NEROLI BIGARADE] (calming and uplifting)
  –*Pelargonium graveolens* [GERANIUM] (decongestant, relaxant)
  –*Rosa damascena* (distilled) [DAMASK ROSE] (general tonic)
- 500 ml spring water

Respiratory problems

BRONCHITIS (ingestion) – **(Suzanne Catty)**

For chronic cases of lung problems, the dose and frequency should be half that for acute cases.

- 30 ml *Eucalyptus globulus* [EUCALYPTUS] hydrolat
- 1 litre water

Sipped throughout the day and sustained over a period, this can clear a case of bronchitis without antibiotics.

Rheumatism

(bath) – **(Shirley Price)**

- 15 ml *Salvia officinalis* [SAGE]
- 15 ml *Rosmarinus officinalis* [ROSEMARY]
- 15 ml *Juniperus communis* [JUNIPER]

Add these hydrolats to a ready prepared bath. Stay in the water for at least 10 minutes.

Viaud (1983) recommends *Thymus vulgaris* [THYME], so this could be used on its own or with one or two of the hydrolats above, to increase the synergistic effects.

Skincare (all topical)

The skin depends on water to maintain good condition; vegetable oils can improve skin texture and help prevent water loss from the skin. Therefore creams and lotions bring together these two qualities to keep skin moisturized and protected, in proportions to suit the type of skin. The author (S. Price) has found that for dry skins a cream consisting of roughly equal parts of oil and water is best, while for other types of skin, lotions incorporating up to 90% water are recommended. Distilled waters are well suited for blending into skin care products, providing not only moisture but also beneficial therapeutic effects.

Most hydrolats are good to use on normal and oily complexions (or on acne), and many are suitable for dry skin. All of them counteract the drying effects encountered on long aeroplane flights, as well as in air-conditioned rooms (Keville & Green 1995, p. 90).

BROKEN CAPILLARIES AND COUPEROSE SKIN – **(Carolyn Marshall)**

33% of each of the following hydrolats:

- *Cupressus sempervirens* [CYPRESS]
- *Cistus ladaniferous* [ROCK ROSE]
- *Pelargonium graveolens* [GERANIUM]

Use blended or alone in a spray.

DEVITALIZED DRY SKIN – **(Carolyn Marshall)**

- 25% *Tilia × europaea* [LINDEN BLOSSOM]
- 25% *Centaurea cyanus* [CORNFLOWER]
- 50% *Rosa damascena* (distilled) [DAMASK ROSE]

1. Blend in a spray and use neat on the skin morning and evening.
2. Add 10% into a cleanser base.
3. Blend with a gel base 50/50 for a hydrating mask.
4. Add to a milk/lotion base with calendula carrier oil to make a great moisturizer. (*Authors' note*: add the carrier oil to the lotion a very little at a time; a lotion will usually accept about 20–25% of oil without separating.)
5. Mix with calamine powder to a paste for a gentle cleansing, desquamating mask.

From time to time exchange one hydrolat for *Hamamelis virginiana* [WITCH HAZEL] or *Cistus ladaniferus* [ROCK ROSE] to stimulate fibroblasts and lock in the moisture.

DRY SKIN – **(Nelly Grosjean)**

Any hydrolats chosen from lavender, rosemary, thyme, wild rose and chamomile (Scientific names of plants not specified)

FACIAL TONICS – **(Claire Montesinos)**

Hydrolats fresh from the refrigerator neat on a cotton pad make effective toners. Use separately or in a blend:

- *Rosa damascena* [DAMASK ROSE]
- *Achillea millefolium* [YARROW]
- *Salvia officinalis* [SAGE]

MATURE/DEHYDRATED SKIN – **(Carolyn Marshall)**

One third each of:

- *Cistus ladaniferus* [ROCK ROSE]
- *Rosa damascena* (distilled) [DAMASK ROSE]
- *Helichrysum italicum* [EVERLASTING]

1. Blend in a spray and use neat on the skin morning and evening.

2. Add 10% into a cleanser base.
3. Blend with gel base 50/40 and add 10% aloe gel as a hydrating mask, leave on for up to 20 minutes then massage the gel into the skin, wiping off any excess.

OILY SKIN – **(Carolyn Marshall)**

- 50% *Juniperus communis* [JUNIPER BERRY] or *Cupressus sempervirens* [CYPRESS]
- 25% *Hamamelis virginiana* [WITCH HAZEL]
- 25% *Pelargonium graveolens* [GERANIUM] or *Citrus aurantium* flos [NEROLI]

1. Blend in a spray and use neat on the skin morning and evening.
2. Add 15% into a cleanser base.
3. Blend with gel base 50/50 and add 0.5% tea tree essential oil to make an effective spot gel.
4. Add to a milk or lotion base with carrot and hazelnut carrier oil to make a moisturizer (see authors' note under recipe for dry skin/devitalized, above).
5. Mix with green clay to a paste for a deep cleansing, desquamating mask to help draw out impurities.

REDNESS OF THE SKIN – **(Henri Viaud)**

- *Cupressus sempervirens* [CYPRESS]
- *Helichrysum italicum* [EVERLASTING]
- *Hamamelis virginiana* [WITCH HAZEL]
- *Matricaria recutita* [GERMAN CHAMOMILE]

REJUVENATOR AND TONIC FOR ALL SKINS – **(Nelly Grosjean)**

(Scientific names of hydrolats not specified)

lavender, thyme, rosemary, sage, carrot, cedar, chamomile

SKIN CONDITIONS AND SCARS – **(Nelly Grosjean)**

(Scientific names of plants not specified)

Hydrolats of cedar, wild rose and lavender.

WRINKLED AND MATURE SKIN – **(Nelly Grosjean)**

(Scientific names of plants not specified)

A wrinkle lotion may be prepared from blends of rosemary, sage, lavender and wild rose hydrolats.

Slimming

(bath, internal) – **(Shirley Price)**

For those who are trying to slim, the following hydrolats can be added to the bath and also into drinking water. This must, of course, be combined with careful eating.

- 15 ml *Foeniculum vulgare* [FENNEL]
- 15 ml *Juniperus communis* [JUNIPER] (twig and berry)
- 15 ml *Carum carvi* [CARAWAY] or 15 ml *Cupressus sempervirens* [CYPRESS] can be added also.

Sore throat

(application, gargle, mouthwash or compress) – **(Shirley Price)**
The best way is to tackle a sore throat as soon as it starts by gargling, but if it has developed and is inflamed before starting treatment, try a mouthwash or compress as well as gargling, as this will double the benefits. When gargling, be sure to swallow the mix – do not spit it out.

Apply the antibacterial, antiinfectious and antiinflammatory hydrolats to the throat area over a basin and rub in well each time; alternatively, and especially if the problem is well developed, apply a compress using the same mix and leave for at least 1 hour.

- 10 ml *Origanum vulgaris* [OREGANO]
- 20 ml *Centaurea cyanus* [CORNFLOWER]
- 20 ml *Chamaemelum nobile* [ROMAN CHAMOMILE]

Teeth

(mouthwash) – **(Shirley Price)**

Infected gums

- 50 ml *Rosmarinus officinalis* [ROSEMARY]
- 30 ml *Mentha* × *piperita* [PEPPERMINT]
- 20 ml *Thymus vulgaris* – any chemotype [THYME]

Mix the hydrolats together.

- Take about 1 teaspoonful into the mouth and swish well.
- Spit out – and repeat two or three times.
- Do this morning and night.

Bleeding gums

- 30 ml *Pelargonium graveolens* [GERANIUM]
- 30 ml *Cupressus sempervirens* [CYPRESS]
- 30 ml *Rosmarinus officinalis* [ROSEMARY]

Use as above.

Thrush

(spray) – **(Carolyn Marshall)**
Candida albicans is a fungal infection affecting the digestive system. It can spread via the bloodstream throughout the body and invade other mucous membranes. Vaginal thrush is particularly uncomfortable but I have found this recipe to be successful. Using a spray directly onto the affected area is instantly soothing and more economical than using the remedy as a wash. It can also be used as a mouthwash or gargle if the mouth is affected.

(This recipe includes essential oils)

- 1 × 50 ml plastic spray
- 25 ml *Melaleuca alternifolia* [TEA TREE] hydrolat
- 25 ml *Lavandula angustifolia* [LAVENDER] hydrolat
- 5 drops *(Melaleuca alternifolia)* [TEA TREE] essential oil

Shake well before use.
If very itchy add 2 drops *Mentha × piperita* [PEPPERMINT].

Urinary infection

(ingestion) – **(Michelle Paris)**
(Recipes contain essential oils)

- 1 litre of *Thymus vulgaris* ct. linalool [SWEET THYME] hydrolat
- 1 ml in total (i.e. 4–5 drops of each) of the following essential oils:
- *Cinnamomum verum* fol. [CINNAMON LEAF]
- *Mentha × piperita* [PEPPERMINT]
- *Origanum compactum* [OREGANO]
- *Rosmarinus* ct. *verbenone* [ROSEMARY VERBENONE]
- *Thymus vulgaris* ct. thymol [RED THYME]

Kidney stones

(ingestion) – **(Shirley Price)**

- 600 ml *Juniperus communis* (berry) [JUNIPER] hydrolat
- 400 ml *Foeniculum vulgare* [FENNEL] hydrolat
- 10–15 drops *Citrus limon* [LEMON] essential oil

Take 1 tbsp in half a glass of water three times daily.

Vaccination

(ingestion) – **(Suzanne Catty)**
Given before and after vaccinations, bay leaf hydrolat acts prophylactically to prevent many of the associated side effects and helps the body deal with the vaccination process:

- 30 ml *Laurus nobilis* [BAY LEAF]

Culinary recipes

Floral waters are used primarily in the cuisines of India, the Middle East, and Eastern Europe. Throughout Turkey, Lebanon, Syria, Egypt, Tunisia and Morocco, pastries, puddings and other sweets are scented with rose or orange-blossom water. It is the custom in India to sprinkle (genuine) rose water on guests arriving at weddings.

Orange-blossom water has been flavouring sweets in Spain from the years of Moorish rule - roughly the 8th to the 15th centuries. In the Middle East, a mixture of boiling orange-flower water and sugar, called white coffee, is often given to children before bedtime to relax and aid in digestion. During the authors' visit to Tunisia, Shirley Price was given orange-flower water to combat a stomach upset and since that time, the authors have not only used it for this purpose but have also added it to coffee and fruit salads. Used sparingly, it can add a mysterious, delicate flavour to desserts, and a tablespoon of either rose water or orange-blossom water is usually enough in most recipes; if overdone, the resulting taste could be unpleasant. In a cup of coffee, one teaspoonful is adequate.

Unfortunately, until aromatherapists became interested in hydrolats, genuine rose hydrolat was (and still can be) difficult to come by unless bought from a known source. Check before buying it in a pharmacy; it may be a prepared water containing synthetics intended for use in cosmetics – not for cooking! Rose water, both true and false, is used in Turkish Delight, one of the oldest known confections and one which is more enjoyable if the rose water used is genuine – which usually makes it expensive. Called *rahat loukoum* ('rest for the throat' in Turkish), this aromatic sweet was legendary in the harems of the Middle East, said to be eaten by women to keep themselves plump.

General tips

When using hydrolats in cooking, care must be taken not to add too much – remember, it is easy to add more, but impossible to take any out.

Try a teaspoonful of orange flower hydrolat in a cup of coffee, or in fruit salad, adding more to this last if a richer flavour is desired. All soups, gravies and sauces can be enhanced by the addition of a *small* amount of hydrolat; the secret, as in all cooking, is to taste each time you add a teaspoonful until the desired flavour is reached.

Common plant names are used in this culinary section.

- 1 tbsp (tablespoon) = 15 ml
- 1 tsp (teaspoon) = 5 ml
- 1 cup = 200 ml

Savouries

VEGETABLE SOUP – **(Shirley Price)**

- 2 medium carrots
- 1 parsnip
- 6–8 florets from a broccoli spear
- ½ Spanish onion or 4–5 shallots
- 1 vegetable stock cube
- 1 litre water
- 1–2 tbsp (15–30 ml) thyme hydrolat – any chemotype
- 1–2 tbsp (15–30 ml) sweet marjoram hydrolat

Scrub carrots but do not peel; peel parsnip and cut into small pieces. Bring the water to the boil with the crumbled vegetable cube. Add all vegetables except broccoli and onions. Add broccoli after 5 minutes and cook until all vegetables are soft. Meanwhile, peel and cut up the onion/shallots. Melt a knob of butter (not margarine) and a dessertspoonful of olive oil in a small frying pan. Fry onions lightly in this. Add onions to soup and liquidize. Add hydrolats – 1 tbsp of each first, then taste, adding more if necessary. Serve, drizzling three very small rings of cream on the surface of each bowl.

Desserts and sweets

AROMATIC WHIPPED CREAM – **(Shirley Price)**

Try adding a teaspoonful of hydrolat to whipping cream before whipping.

The following, used individually, may give you some ideas:

- cinnamon – with apple pie
- peppermint or orange flower – with chocolate mousse or chocolate cake
- rose – with peaches or apricots

For a low-fat topping, add hydrolats to yogurt instead.

ORANGE ROSEMARY SORBET – **(Mindy Green and Kathy Keville)**

- ¼ cup water
- 2 tbsp honey
- 2 cups freshly squeezed orange juice
- ½ tsp finely chopped fresh rosemary leaves
- 2 tbsp rosemary hydrolat

Gently warm water and honey together until the honey melts. Add orange juice, hydrolat and rosemary leaves. Churn in ice-cream maker and serve in chilled bowls for a refreshing fat-free dessert.

TURKISH DELIGHT - **(epicurious.com)**

Said to be fairly easy to make, but quite lengthy
Ingredients (for approximately 80 pieces):

½ cup sugar
4½ cups of water
2 tsp lemon juice
1 ¼ cups cornflour
1¼ tsp cream of tartar
1 ½ tbsp rose water
red food colouring (optional)
1 cup icing sugar
2 large heavy saucepans

Oil a 9 inch (22 cm) square non-stick tin and line it with cling film, oiling this too. In the first saucepan, over a medium heat, combine the sugar, 1½ cups of the water, and the lemon juice. Stir until the sugar dissolves and the mixture boils (when the sugar syrup boils, coat the inside of the saucepan with a brush dipped in cold water to prevent sugar crystals from forming). Simmer gently on a low heat, without stirring, until the mixture reaches the soft-ball stage (240 °F/120 °C if you have a jam thermometer), then remove from the heat.

In the second saucepan, over a medium heat, stir together 1 cup of the cornflour and the cream of tartar. Gradually stir in the remaining 3 cups of water until no lumps remain. Stir constantly, until the mixture boils and is a thick, gluey paste. Slowly pour the hot sugar, water and lemon juice syrup into the cornflour mixture, stirring constantly. Simmer, stirring often to prevent sticking, for about an hour or until the mixture becomes a pale golden colour. Stir in the rose water and tint if desired with food colouring. Pour the mixture into the prepared pan and spread evenly. Cool to room temperature and let stand, uncovered, overnight to set.

Sift the icing sugar and the remaining ¼ cup of cornflour onto a large cutting board. Turn the Turkish delight out and cut into 1-inch squares with an oiled knife. Roll the pieces in the sugar mixture to coat well. Store in an airtight container with sheets of waxed paper, dusted with the sugar mixture, separating every layer.

DATE AND ORANGE-BLOSSOM BAKLAVA – (christmasjoy.com)

Baklava is a Turkish dessert that originated during the Ottoman empire. It consists of chopped nuts such as walnuts, almonds or pistachios, sandwiched between thin layers of filo pastry and coated in syrup. This unusual baklava is filled with dates and scented with orange-blossom water. If possible, use fresh filo, as it is easier to work with without crumbling. Makes 30 servings.

Syrup

- ½ cup sugar
- ¼ cup water
- 1 tbsp fresh lemon juice
- 2 tbsp honey
- 2 tsp orange-blossom water

Filling

- 3 cups pitted dates (2 packets of 10 ounces each)
- ½ cup orange juice
- ½ cup water
- 1 tbsp orange zest
- 1 tsp ground cinnamon

Pastry

- ½ cup sugar
- 2 tsp ground cinnamon
- 24 sheets filo pastry, preferably fresh
- 8 tbs (1 stick) unsalted butter, melted

To make the syrup: in a saucepan over low heat, combine sugar, water, lemon juice and honey, heating and stirring until sugar dissolves. Increase the heat, stirring all the time, and boil for 1 minute. Remove from the heat and add orange-blossom water. Put to one side to cool.

For the filling: place dates, orange juice, ½ cup water, orange zest and cinnamon in a food processor. Using pulse, process until dates are minced. Continue to process until a coarse paste forms. Put filling to one side.

For the pastry: preheat oven to 350°F/175 °C. Mix sugar and cinnamon together. Unroll filo pastry and stack on work surface. Using the bottom of a 10-inch round cake tin (preferably springform) as a guide, cut 24 10-inch rounds from the pastry. Line the bottom of the tin with a circle of parchment paper or foil and brush the bottom and sides with butter. Cover outside of tin (sides and bottom) with foil to prevent leaking. Place two filo rounds into the tin. Brush with melted butter and sprinkle with cinnamon sugar. Repeat the layering four more times for a total of 10 sheets.

Evenly spread half of the filling over the top. Top with two filo circles. Brush with melted butter and sprinkle with cinnamon sugar and repeat for a total of four sheets. Spread with remaining filling.

Layer the remaining 10 circles (two at a time) over the filling, brushing the top of each layer with butter and sprinkling with cinnamon sugar.

Using a sharp knife, score the pastry by cutting through the top layer (without cutting through to the filling) in six parallel lines. Working in the opposite direction, cut five parallel lines on the diagonal to form diamond shapes.

Bake the baklava for 30 minutes, cover with foil and bake for a further 20 minutes or until the top is golden brown. Remove from oven, cool slightly, and then cut through scored lines to bottom of pan. Spoon the cold syrup over the hot baklava and allow to cool.

Making your own hydrolats

Recipes for making hydrolats (essential waters, hydrosols, floral waters - call them what you will) can be found in both old and modern books and papers. You may like to try making your own from the recipes given below – it is quite good fun, if a little frustrating at times! Recipes for making false waters (i.e. by maceration or by adding essential oils to water) are also given.

If you wish to make a large number of hydrolats, it is possible to buy small glass stills from a pharmaceutical supply company (around £400 at the time of writing).

Have a look at what is available in your garden, in the hedgerow, the woods and the fields. Leaves often make a stronger water than flowers. Waters which have not had alcohol or other preservatives added have a limited life, which is why, as Hephrun says (2000a, p. 19), both Cleopatra and Elizabeth I had people preparing their waters for them on a regular basis so that they were fresh. Nowadays, the refrigerator lengthens the life of waters and it is also possible to freeze them in small bottles.

The making of a genuine or true hydrolat will be given first, followed by prepared (false) waters. Remember that a true hydrolat should keep for about a year in cool conditions.

Distilled, true hydrolat

Rose (1992, p. 174) uses a copper teapot to make her hydrolats. A stainless steel one would perhaps be easier to come by, and in the authors' opinion, probably better, as the resulting water would have no copper deposits. On the other hand, the copper can act as a preservative, so the choice is yours. Genders (1986a, p. 178) suggests using a kettle. The method for both is the same.

The authors have not tried it, but it should be possible to make a true hydrolat using a pressure cooker, by removing the safety valve and fitting a rubber tube so that the condensed liquid can be received in a jar.

- 40–60 g plant material – leaves, flowers, etc., or a mix of plants if wished
- 1 litre distilled, deionized or spring water
- 1 large copper, stainless steel or glass teapot, or a large kettle with an old-fashioned spout (not plastic, as the plant matter may affect it) or a pressure cooker.
- 1 small grid or a piece of wire mesh (shaped to form a platform at the base of the teapot or kettle) or some smooth, small pebbles, to prevent plant material touching the base of the vessel used
- 0.5–1 metre of soft, flexible rubber tubing (cut, if too long, to go from the vessel, into and out of the washing-up bowl, into the receiving container).
- 1 washing up bowl or large casserole full of ice and cold water
- 1 large jam jar or other container

First, place the grid, wire mesh or pebbles in the bottom of the chosen vessel to ensure that the plant matter will not 'catch' on the bottom of the vessel when heated. Add the plant material and water to the vessel. Attach rubber tubing to spout of kettle or teapot or top of pressure cooker, ensuring a good seal. Lay the tubing in the ice and water and fit free end into receiving jar.

Bring the water to the boil, then simmer on a low heat until most of the water has boiled off, travelled through the tube (condensing as it passes through the ice bath) and arrived in the container. The time will vary according to the plant matter, but is usually around 30–60 minutes. The resulting liquid is your true hydrolat of whatever flower, herb or plant you started with.

Rose (1992, p. 174) suggests that if your hydrolat does not smell strong enough, you can add a few drops of essential oil. However, the result would then not be a true hydrolat, but a false one, though of good quality. If you want a true hydrolat of a greater strength, it is better to repeat the distillation process as follows:

- Use fresh plant material
- Use the hydrolat you have just collected – not fresh water – adding it to the water left in original vessel.

Hephrun (2000, p. 18) suggests using just the lavender flowers and leaves without the stalks, suggesting that perhaps it is the woody parts which cause it to be not so fragrant. Genders (1986a, p. 178) gives a recipe for lavender water which contains other plants; perhaps, again, this may be to counteract the sometimes 'not so nice' smell of lavender hydrolat:

- Put lavender flowers and cinnamon bark in a still
- When the water is collected add an equal amount of rose water
- Use as an astringent and as a complexion water.

Farley (1783, p. 208), a cook of repute in his time, wrote down his method of producing essential water of lavender:

> *Put a quart of water to every pound of lavender neps. Put them in a cold still, and induce a slow fire under it. Distill it off very slowly, and put it into a pot until you have distilled all your water. Then clean your still well out, and put your lavender water to it, and distill it off as slowly as before. Then put it into bottles and cork it well.*

Macerated plant waters

It is possible to obtain a plant water by maceration, though this is naturally much weaker. In this method, cold water is poured over the plant matter and left for several hours at room temperature (stirring occasionally to improve the end product), before straining. This method is particularly suitable for plants which contain mucilage (a gluey mixture of carbohydrates present in plants such as marshmallow root. However, as macerated waters carry a high percentage of bacteria, the end water should be boiled before use (Wichtl 1994, p. 26).

Hephrun (2000, p. 7) makes toilet waters by this method, i.e. without using any heat. Such waters are not true hydrolats as they are not distilled, and they do not extract as many constituents from the plant. However, the 'waters' obtained are nevertheless completely natural. (The author has amended the following recipe slightly.)

- 30–40 g plant material
- 1 litre distilled or deionized water
- 1 blender
- 1 sieve
- several filter papers
- 1 jug

Place the plant material in the blender with the water. Blend for about a minute until the mass is very green and well macerated. Pass this through an ordinary flour sieve to remove the thick sludge. Filter the resulting liquid into the jug (this may take a long time and it may be necessary to change the filter paper once or twice) to have a relatively clear solution.

Hephrun advises that this water should be used fairly quickly , although it will keep in the fridge for several days; however, the authors suggest that if this method is used, the extract should be brought to the boil before bottling: the water could also be frozen. Like Rose (1992, p. 174), Hephrun suggests that adding essential oils 'may help to give an added zest to the waters . . . and it also gives you the chance of adding your favourite oil to bring out a nice smell'. He suggests adding alcohol to extend its life (which would be an alternative to Wichtl's boiling to reduce the germ count), but once you add alcohol or essential oils, remember you do not have a true water.

A simple 'rose water' can also be made in the early summer by picking about 50 petals from a fragrant variety just as the buds are opening. Cover these with water, allow to stand overnight, and strain (recipe from thetribunenews.com article headline Petal power).

Grieve (1998, p. 814) mentions making a water using wild thyme, where the flowering tops are macerated for 24 hours or so in water and salt, to make a perfumed water. She does not give quantities.

False hydrolats (prepared waters)

Rose (1992, p. 253) suggests a recipe made entirely of essential oil and water, to 'mimic a true hydrosol':

- 40 drops essential oil
- 4 oz (120 ml) of pure distilled water

Shake each time before use.

Rose emphasizes that a water-based product made in this fashion does not possess the qualities of a true distilled water, but others try to make a virtue of these false waters, saying: 'Our floral waters are made from all natural essential oils' (lemelange.com\flower_water).

Keville & Green (1995, p. 100) give a recipe for a skin toner which consists of 10 drops essential oil shaken into 4 oz (120 ml) distilled water and stored in a glass spray bottle: to be shaken well before each use.

Grieve (1992, p. 473) suggests a recipe for a prepared lavender water that can be made at home from the essential oil:

> *Into a quart bottle are put 1 oz. essential oil of Lavender, one drop of Musk and 1½ pint spirits of wine. These three ingredients are well mixed together by*

> *shaking. The mixture is left to settle, shaken again in a few days, then poured into little perfume bottles fitted with air-tight stoppers.*

Genders (1986a, p. 178) gives a recipe for Carmelite water, the hydrolat made by the nuns of the Carmelite abbey of St Just in the 14th century and which was used all over Europe. This hydrolat is distilled from plants with alcohol as part of the liquid used; because of the alcohol, Carmelite water is, strictly speaking, an 'adulterated' water. Genders has translated the measurements of pounds, ounces and pints into grams and litres:

- 500 g lemon balm leaves
- 60 g lemon peel
- 30 g each of nutmeg, cloves, coriander seeds and chopped angelica root
- 500 ml orange blossom or elderflower water
- 1 litre alcohol

Distil the above slowly in a kettle, collecting the toilet water (after it has passed in a tube connected to the spout below some cold water) into a large jar.

Genders also tells us (1972, p. 159) that a fine lavender water may be made by distilling the essential oil together with rectified spirit and rose water, producing a clear limpid water.

True rose water comes, as we know, from distilled rose petals and Hephrun (2000, p. 19) stresses that commercial rose water is usually made from concentrates prepared from absolutes.

A Grieve recipe, which is neither a true hydrolat nor a prepared water, is to mix 2 oz of lavender essential oil with ¾ pint of good brandy. She advises that this 'lavender water' is so strong that it must be diluted with water before it is used.

Yet another recipe, which Grieve tells us comes from an old family book, makes 'a pleasant and efficacious cordial, very useful in languor and weakness of the nerves, lowness of spirits, faintings, etc.':

> *Put into a bottle half a pint of spirit of wine and two drachms of oil of lavender. Mix it with rose-water, five ounces, orange-flower water, two ounces, also two drachms of musk and six ounces of distilled water.*

Balz (1986, p. 72) gives the following suggestions as a basis for waters to be used as perfumes only:

Eau-de-Cologne	3% essential oil(s) plus 70° alcohol to 100%
Eau de toilette	6% essential oil(s) plus 70° alcohol to 100%
Perfume	20% essential oils plus 90° alcohol to 100%, or 20% essential oils plus vegetable oil such as olive, almond or sesame to 100%
Aftershave lotion	add a little glycerine to an eau de toilette to obtain a good aftershave lotion.

11

Case studies

Two case studies from Caroline Hoffman

Hoffman worked in the Middlesex Hospital intensive care unit in London for over 6 years, introducing (and researching) the use of essential oils in this context (Stevenson 1994). There were occasions where the use of essential oils was seen possibly to complicate further an already complex situation (e.g. patients suffering from multiple problems, requiring complicated drug treatment regimens). There were also cases where the use of massage was inappropriate due to the presence of pyrexia or the acuteness or severity of the patient's condition.

Being a nurse and aromatherapist, for a number of years, Hoffman was keen to give her patients what she felt would be the most effective form of treatment – i.e. the administration of essential oils in the form of massage, inhalation, compress, mouth rinses, etc. She was not convinced that by using hydrolats she would get the clinical results hoped for. However, as the following cases show, they proved to be effective. The patient's real names have not been used.

Case study 1

Pseudo name: Sue
Condition: Terminal (multiple organ failure)
Age: 54
Therapist: Caroline Hoffman
Hydrolat used: rose (unspecified)

Sue was in multiple organ failure and death was only a matter of time away. She had been in the intensive care unit for some weeks suffering from complications following cardiac surgery. She had initially been massaged with essential oils, but as her condition deteriorated this approach became inappropriate. Sue's relatives said that she had always loved the smell of roses and had grown them in her garden. A care plan was then created so that she would be soothed with rose hydrolat several times per day and also when she appeared agitated and distressed. This procedure was shown to her husband who administered the flower water to her hands, face and chest. In these situations, with relatives constantly at the bedside, it is likely that the effect was equally comforting for the relatives to be involved in care as it was for Sue. The soft gentleness of the flower water did offer calm to both relatives and patient alike. While not easily able to communicate, the patient was calm and relaxed when the rose water was applied, whereas she often grimaced with other procedures. This was continued for the 5 days leading up to a peaceful death for Sue.

Offering aromatic waters (hydrolats) is often seen as an act of extra kindness by relatives who can see how busy the medical and nursing staff are with the technical care of looking after patients in this extremely demanding environment. For professional staff, to use floral and other hydrolats is also a pleasant and uplifting experience in an atmosphere that can otherwise be overwhelmingly clinical.

Case Study 2

Pseudo name: Jill
Condition: Eczema and mild depression
Age: 40
Therapist: Caroline Hoffman
Hydrolat used: *Lavandula angustifolia*

While working at the Royal London Homoeopathic Hospital, London, I was asked to see a patient who suffered not only from extreme allergies and eczema, but also a state of mild depression which she attributed to years of anxiety about her ability to eat certain foods and use any fragrance products. This offered me a challenge to find a way to offer support without using essential oils.

One of my colleagues had met Jill, a frequent visitor to the hospital ward to get help with her allergies and eczema. Patch testing positively at 1% *Lavandula angustifolia* in vegetable oil for an aromatherapy treatment, it was clear that this approach was not going to be possible, because of the fragrance. Following this, a patch test with lavender hydrolat was tried. A care plan was devised where the lavender water was applied to a small area of eczema on Jill's left cubital fossa over the next week of her stay in hospital. Jill was thrilled at the improvement in her skin over the area that was treated and was given confidence to use the lavender water further.

On Jill's next in-patient visit to the hospital 3 months later, she was pleased to tell the staff that not only had her eczema improved and stopped weeping and reduced in size over the areas that she had tried the flower water, but also she felt less depressed and more hopeful about her future.

Case study from Carolyn Marshall

Pseudo name: Miss Potter
Condition: *Acne rosacea*
Treatment start date: August 2000
Age: 26
Therapist Carolyn Marshall
Aromatic water used: *Pelargonium asperum*

Miss Potter had tried many therapies before coming to see me, including Chinese herbalism, reflexology and homoeopathy – all without success. I was faced with a shy woman with long blonde hair covering her face, head hung low and a face covered in thick make-up. She could not look me in the eye and talking about her condition made it flare up in front of my eyes.

Her skin condition was worse around the forehead, which had many papules and pustules – it was very inflamed and angry looking. The nose area had a typical butterfly pattern over it and was also inflamed and angry and was covered in raised blind lumps. Her chin was quite clear but erupted in whiteheads from time to time, which she picked, so they sometimes became infected. Her cheeks were very dehydrated on the surface and flaky due to the use of very astringent products in the past.

At first I gave my client a full body aromatherapy treatment, using only Bourbon geranium (*Pelargonium graveolens*) essential oil in a carrier, with a separate facial treatment following her usual cleansing routine, where geranium aromatic water was introduced as the toner.

After six visits of having both treatments, it was decided to continue only with the facial treatment as having both was a strain on her pocket.

Facial treatment (17 of these to date)

After cleansing with sweet almond oil, a mask was applied for 20 minutes, using 10 ml of a gel-based mask with 10 ml of the geranium hydrolat. Applying a little almond oil to my hands, I massaged in the mask until it lost its slip, when it was removed with cotton wool moistened with geranium hydrolat. A tiny amount of sweet almond oil was then applied to finish off. (I would have preferred to make a moisturising cream but this would have introduced another product and confused everything.)

The facial treatment was continued monthly for another 3 months, during which time a change could be seen; the inflammation reduced dramatically and the skin became smoother on all areas of the face. The forehead was virtually free of any blemishes and the nose area had calmed down, becoming less raised and angry. There were no pustules or lumps. The flakiness had gone and the skin was generally looking more hydrated and plumped out. The chin however had become a little worse and taken on the characteristics of the original forehead. The condition appeared (strangely enough) to be migrating downwards and it was hoped that it would not continue down her neck. Fortunately, after a few more treatments, the chin, too, began to clear.

Home use

Before treatments began, Miss Potter had been using Clearasil which had over-dried her face. Now, after cleansing with sweet almond oil, Miss Potter uses an atomizer with geranium hydrolat each morning and night, moisturizing with a small amount of sweet almond oil.

Every 4 days she uses the mask used in her treatment, leaving it on for 20 minutes, massaging it in gently for a few minutes and taking off the residue with cotton wool dampened with geranium hydrolat.

Outcome

The difference is remarkable – not only a new skin but a new person as well. The shy, timid, introverted person has changed into a chatty, confident woman who now has short hair brushed off her face, uses less make-up, walks with her head held high and a smile on her face.

There is reduced inflammation generally on the whole face, 90% fewer lumps and raised blind spots, smoother more hydrated skin with no flakiness or dry patches. Typical butterfly pattern of inflammation reduced by 50% in size, pustules reduced to the occasional breakout. Confidence and self-esteem are raised by an immeasurable amount.

Two case studies from Shirley Price

Case study 1

Pseudo name: Ann-Marie
Condition: Cramp during menstruation
Age: 26
Therapist: Shirley Price
Hydrolats used: *Melissa officinalis, Ocimum basilicum, Origanum majorana, Salvia sclarea*

Being retired, I only take on a case when asked by a friend. Ann-Marie was just such a case, being the daughter of a friend in France.

Ann-Marie dreaded her periods each month because of the severe cramps during the first 2 days. Normally, I would have recommended massaging her abdomen with essential oils in a carrier, but her mother said she did not think she would do that. As internal treatment is expected on a visit to a doctor, my first thought was to make up a bottle of essential oils in Disper and water for her to take internally. However, remembering that we needed cases using hydrolats for this book, I made up instead a mix of hydrolats (from local distillation the previous season):

- 25 ml *Melissa officinalis* [MELISSA] (cohobated and undiluted)
- 200 ml *Ocimum basilicum* [BASIL]
- 200 ml *Origanum majorana* [SWEET MARJORAM]
- 100 ml *Salvia sclarea* [CLARY SAGE]
- 400 ml spring water

I advised Ann-Marie to begin taking 1 tbs (15 ml) of this mix in half a glass of water morning and evening up to 10 days before menstruation was due to start (or as near as she could estimate, as they were not absolutely regular), stopping the dose 2 days into the period.

It was not until 3 months later that I could enquire into the results.

First month: the cramp persisted, although not so painful – and no headaches (which she had not told me before that she was suffering from).

Second month: her period was early and she had only been taking the hydrolats for 5 days when her period arrived. She had no headaches, although suffering slightly from cramp the first day. She said she wanted to continue taking the hydrolats, so I mixed another bottle in case she ran out before my next visit.

Third month: no headaches, no cramp.

Fourth and fifth months: still no symptoms and I have given the recipe to a delighted Ann-Marie for one of her friends who has the same problem (the waters are easy to obtain in that part of France).

Case study 2

Names:	Shirley and Len
Condition:	Severe stomach poisoning
Ages:	71 and 74
Therapist:	Shirley Price
Hydrolats used:	
High blood pressure	*Pinus sylvestris, Rosmarinus officinalis* – plus essential oil of *Syzygium aromaticum*
Viral enteritis	*Origanum vulgare, Thymus vulgaris* ct. geraniol, *Rosmarinus officinalis*

Just before leaving Spain, in November, Shirley and Len had enjoyed a delicious meal (at a renowned fish restaurant), consisting only of shellfish: crabs, oysters, mussels, scallops and elephant's feet (these are shaped like a finger, the shell being beautifully opalescent, like abalone).

The next night, Shirley was violently ill – sickness and diarrhoea simultaneously – every 20 minutes all during the night. They had to start the journey home the next day and although feeling weak, managed the journey with frequent stops. By the time they reached their hotel, Shirley was feeling much better, but not well enough to eat anything. Len went down to the restaurant for a meal and Shirley accompanied him, thinking she might have a slice of bread and a glass of water. Just after placing his order, Len said he didn't feel very well. *En route* to the toilet, he faltered and Shirley and a waiter dashed over just in time to stop him falling against the corner of a table as he passed out.

The hotel called a doctor, who gave him an injection, as his blood pressure had gone dangerously low (he takes medication for hypertension). He was not as sick as Shirley, but was very weak. They only had about 100 miles to travel the next day to their house in France, so against everyone's wishes, they left, driving slowly. There was gradual improvement over 3 days.

Reaching the north of France a week later, illness forgotten, they were invited out to a friend's house and were served – steak tartare! Apprehensively, they ate it. The next night, Shirley was again very ill, followed by Len the following night, who fainted and banged his head on the tiled floor. There was no doctor available, but as there were some hydrolats in the house, Shirley gave him a dose of rosemary and pine water undiluted – 1 tbsp (15 ml) of each – with two drops of clove bud essential oil to help raise his blood pressure. It was a worrying time for Shirley but he was much better by the morning.

Christmas came and went, without any digestive problems. They returned to Spain in January for 2 weeks, where they had a buffet lunch on their second day. Shirley only had three prawns (normally she has a dozen) just in case the 'bug' was still in their systems. The next night, just before starting their meal, Shirley was violently sick, repeating her experience of November during the night, but much worse. It was not until nearly daylight that she remembered that, although there were no hydrolats in the apartment, there were some essential oils (she had been too ill to think about treating herself!). She immediately got up and made herself a prepared water with the following essential oils and took two teaspoonfuls (10 ml) of the mix every hour:

- 2 drops *Thymus vulgaris* ct. geraniol [SWEET THYME]
- 2 drops *Cupressus sempervirens* [CYPRESS]
- 2 drops *Origanum vulgare* [OREGANO]
- 2 drops *Mentha × piperita* [PEPPERMINT]
- 8 drops Disper to dissolve the oils
- ½ pint water

As soon as Len awoke, she gave him the same dose, even though he was not feeling ill. Len had a very mild stomach upset the following day and felt 'off' for a couple of days. Shirley took a bit longer to recover.

As soon as they returned to England, they started on a course of the hydrolats of the same names as the essential oils used in Spain, taking a tablespoonful (15 ml) once a day for 3 weeks. A week later Shirley ate some gravadlax without thinking and started to feel ill. However, due to taking the previous daily dose of hydrolats, stepped up to every hour when the symptoms started, she recovered in a matter of hours.

They then began taking the recipe on page 185 every day as a preventative and have had various kinds of fish, smoked and plain, regularly since without ill effect. The ultimate test was in France 2 months later when prawns, crab and mussels had no ill effects. Oysters and elephants' feet have yet to be tested!

12

Decoctions, infusions, teas

- Introduction 187
- Infusions, teas and tisanes 188
- Difference between a hydrolat and an infusion 188
- Tea with added hydrolats 190
- Tisanes, with and without hydrolats 190
- Teas made by the authors 191
- Decoctions 194
- Cautions to observe when drinking medicinal teas 195

Introduction

Macerations, decoctions and infusions (which include teas and tisanes), although obtained with water, are each different in composition from hydrolats, due to the differing methods of preparation. All contain health-giving properties of the plant, some attributes occurring in all of them to some degree:

- *Hydrolat*: steam distillation when only volatile molecules pass into the resultant liquid.
- *Cold maceration*: cold water is poured over the finely chopped plant, left for several hours and strained. Here, only those water-soluble molecules which leave the plant easily are extracted into the liquid.
- *Infusion*: boiling water is poured over plant material and left to macerate for several minutes in the gradually cooling water. Boiling water extracts more water-soluble components, including some of the heavier ones which cannot come over in distillation.
- *Decoction*: cold water is poured over the plant material in a pan, brought to the boil and simmered for around 20 minutes. More molecules are extracted compared with an infusion, resulting in a much stronger liquid.

In all methods, flowers, unless huge, are usually delicate enough to leave whole, but will release their constituents more easily if slightly bruised; small leaves can be used as they are but if large, tough or hard they should be finely chopped; bark, roots, seeds (if large), stems and roots should be crushed and, where necessary, comminuted (cut into small pieces).

Infusions, teas and tisanes

An infusion is made in exactly the same manner as black tea. The amount of plant material used in an infusion varies and when a very small amount is used, the liquid made is referred to as a tea or tisane, as the taste in this instance is the most important factor. Thus teas and tisanes are just weak infusions They can be made from the leaves of the tea plant, or, as stated above, the leaves, flowers or seeds (and occasionally roots) of any other plant. When traditional tea leaves are used the resulting liquid is named tea; there are many varieties of tea leaves originating from China, Japan and India, each with its own flavour; some are fermented and some are not, the latter being without tannin. When an infusion for drinking is made from herbs it is usually referred to as a tisane, although Grieve (1998) often calls this a tea.

All tisanes from plants have their own individual flavour and most are without tannin. There are many on the market today, possibly the most popular being chamomile. It has been estimated that over 1 million cups of chamomile tea are taken every day worldwide (Foster 1996, p. 6).

Teas, infusions and tisanes prescribed by phytotherapists are often enriched by adding a drop of essential oil, which increases their potency. It is possible to add one or even two drops of essential oil, the important thing being that the liquid should be well stirred before drinking (if adding essential oil it is preferable to make the tea in a teapot). However, therapists, unless qualified and insured to do so, cannot officially prescribe essential oils internally; on the other hand, hydrolats can be prescribed because they are much less concentrated and up to a tablespoonful (15 ml) can safely be added to an infusion (whether a tea or a tisane).

Difference between a hydrolat and an infusion

A hydrolat stands intermediate between an infusion and an essential oil and all have active principles in common. Like an infusion, a hydrolat contains the lightest hydrosoluble active principles; in fact, a hydrolat is on average three to four times richer in volatile principles than an infusion of the same plant and so is possibly more efficacious and quicker acting than the tisane; but it would need research to discover which of these preparations is the strongest therapeutically. Tea is certainly a very easy and pleasant method of use; on the other hand, a hydrolat does not contain some of the heavier compounds such as the bitter principles, tannins and heterosides.

Caffeine and tannin

More and more complementary therapists are drinking less and less 'black' tea (e.g. Indian) and more decaffeinated coffee. These two main non-alcoholic drinks of our society became popular because of the energy (stimulation) they provided during a long working day – due to the caffeine content.

In the authors' youth, taking coffee was a once or twice a day occurrence – mid-morning and possibly after a special dinner; most people ate their main meal at midday followed by a cup of tea and had 'supper' or 'high tea' in the evening (much better for the digestion!), when tea or cocoa would be the usual drink.

'All poisonous or toxic plants are useful at certain times and coffee's stimulant qualities can halt comatose or reverse other poisons' (Davies 1985, p. 1). However, it is a more well-known fact that excessive caffeine can cause irritability, insomnia, muscle spasm (Smith 1989, p. 140) as it interferes with natural metabolic processes and is responsible for a wide range of disorders (Bartram 1995, pp. 80–81), which in turn may lower the body's resistance to infection. Davies tells us (p. 1) that 'most dangerous of all, it can cause heart palpitations and tachycardia'. She tells the following story (a précis by the author):

A woman, working at an NHS hospital, found herself getting quite drastic heart palpitations and feared the worst. Several tests were carried out and a thorough case history was taken. . . . Her condition deteriorated to the point where she feared heart attacks. While waiting for results of further complicated tests, her friend (a herbal practitioner who had accompanied her for moral support) noticed that during the course of an hour, she had drunk five cups of coffee from the vending machine.

When the herbalist suggested that coffee should be cut out, the advice fell on deaf ears. With difficulty, she eventually convinced her friend to cut out coffee, resulting in a clean bill of health after a very short time, with complete elimination of any heart palpitations.

The increase in the daily intake of coffee in the UK began about 40–50 years ago, coinciding with travel becoming more widely available, generally to the USA and continental Europe, where coffee is the main drink, especially at the beginning of the day; so much so, that hotels now offer tea as the 'alternative' choice.

Not many people realize that 'black' tea, with its astringent tannin content (this can be good or bad – see below), contains twice as much caffeine as coffee. Coffee also contains tannin, so replacing coffee with 'black' tea may not help. To compound the issue, most people take milk in their tea, which means that they are taking in about ten times as much tannin and caffeine as those who drink it without milk. This is because, when milk is taken, more tea is needed in the initial brew to make it strong enough to resist the effect of the milk, which has a powerfully weakening effect on the taste of the tea.

If using a traditional tea bag to make a cup of weak tea, simply dip it quickly twice into a cup of boiling water; there will still be enough strength in the tea bag to be used by someone else – who takes milk! This observation comes from personal experience, as the authors drink all teas without milk (including normal 'black' tea, although very dilute, if a guest somewhere), when the taste of the tea is appreciated so much more.

Whenever teaching or attending exhibitions on complementary therapies, the authors have noted that many aromatherapists and other complementary therapists drink herbal teas (tisanes) because they are aware of the negative properties of 'black' tea and coffee. Sadly, many so-called herbal drinks, especially in the USA, contain artificial colouring and synthetic flavouring, for example raspberry *leaf* tea, which is, in many brands, a strong red colour with an artificial raspberry *fruit* flavour. As aromatherapists dedicated to persuading therapists to use genuine, non-adulterated essential oils, these artificial 'tisanes' are not for us. French and German tisanes are more often made from the actual plant, with no additions, for example chamomile, peppermint, lime blossom, vervain, etc. Commercial tisanes from these countries (and from quality suppliers in the UK and the USA) are usually genuine herb teas whose properties can be drawn out by boiling water, much as the essential oil and aromatic water are drawn out of the plant by distillation. For this reason, genuine tisanes have a place in this book.

Storage

Always buy loose or dried herbs in small quantities; if a supplier will not let you have less than 250 g of loose herbs, do without, unless you are given specific storage instructions. They should not be kept in paper bags alone, but in airtight, light-proof containers, then stored in a cool, dark and dry place away from other products which have a strong aroma.

Tisanes are best made with plants in season; those we have tried successfully (some for medical reasons) include red poppy, hyssop, lime blossom, willow herb and melissa. The authors have also dried the flower heads so that the tea could then be drunk at any time during the year. They have a drying machine which they use every year to dry peaches, apricots, tomatoes, etc. when in season, so they experimented with lime blossom from their garden, putting them afterwards into labelled dark glass jars to exclude air and light.

To ring the changes – or if the infusion is to be drunk for medicinal purposes – a choice of herbs or spices can be added to any tea without tannin. Once, in an Indian restaurant the authors were given the restaurateur's own mix and found it delicious – so good that they bought the fennel seeds, cinnamon sticks and star anise that she had added to the teapot, so that they could make it at home.

Tea with added hydrolats

Black tea

To make ordinary 'black' tea weak and healthier, with or without the addition of hydrolats, it is best to use a teapot of strong tea, pouring only 10 ml – no more! – into the bottom of a cup and using hot water to fill up the cup. Thonnat (2001) writes on caring for your heart that:

> *To make a weak tea it is better to leave the tea to infuse normally, then dilute it with a little water rather than just let it infuse for a very short while, when there is a risk of having more caffeine and less of the tannin.*

The main benefit of using weak, black tea with hydrolats is for the aesthetic appearance, as the tea, however weak, adds a little colour. Although the taste of tea with added hydrolats will be slightly different from one containing essential oils, it can be as effective; because hydrolats are much weaker than essential oil, a larger quantity (1–2 tsp, 5–10 ml) in a cup of herbal or tannin- and caffeine-free tea is needed to give the desired effect.

Tisanes, with and without hydrolats

When making tisanes, with or without the addition of hydrolats, the strength is a matter of individual taste.

Fresh herbs

The quantity needed to make a good 'brew' varies with each type of plant used and the palate of the drinker; also, some plants yield a stronger flavour than others. Trial and error is the best way to find out. Start with one sprig, or two petals or leaves in a cup and add boiling water, leaving it for a few moments before testing. Once it is known how much is needed for a cupful, it can be estimated how much is needed for a teapot.

Dried herbs

Tea from dried herbs is best made in a teapot, in exactly the same way as black tea, the quantity used depending on the taste required; one advantage is that a mixture of several herbs can be used, either to enrich the flavour or to make a comprehensive drink for your particular health problem.

If a tisane is to be drunk regularly, whether made from a tea bag or fresh or dried herbs, make it in a teapot; the tisane remaining can be left in the pot to develop a richer flavour. It becomes much stronger by standing, as does normal black tea, and can then be used to make further cups of tea. This strong tisane can also be used for compresses, diluted for an eyebath or used in cooking.

Addition of hydrolats

1–2 tsp of the hydrolat of your choice (mixed or single) should be added to your cup of tea or tisane, however and whenever this has been prepared – it is not easy to estimate how much hydrolat to put into a teapotful, especially if the latter is going to be left to gather strength for the next usage.

Teas made by the authors

Following are some teas made from the fresh plant:

RED POPPY

A French neighbour told me how good this was for sleeplessness, which I had experienced the previous two nights. Having drunk a cup made from the petals of one flower head, I slept very well. I have since used it several times and also recommended it to clients, with considerable success.

LIME BLOSSOM

We have two lime blossom trees in our garden and as the tea is known to be calming and if I am under a lot of stress at blossom time, I drink several cups a day using two sprigs of flowers each time.

WILLOW HERB

The sweet and pleasant tisane made from this plant is good for digestive problems (Schauenberg & Paris 1990, p. 151) and we have used it successfully for indigestion.

MELISSA

Fresh melissa leaves make a wonderful tea which has the reputation of extending life expectancy; it is said that a Welsh prince, Llewelyn, who lived to the ripe old age of 108, drank balm tea every morning and evening. Balm tea, drunk with lemon juice and sugar, is to this day used in country districts as a remedy for feverish colds (Clair 1961, p. 114). It has the best flavour when made from the fresh herb; the taste and effect of tea made from dried melissa is not the same.

Teas the authors drink a great deal include Chinese and Japanese green tea, and Rooibos, a tea from South Africa. This last is delicious and, apart from the rich refreshing flavour, has so many health-giving properties that it deserves a mention in its own right.

Rooibos tea

Rooibos tea is useful for:

- indigestion, drunk hot
- slimming when drunk regularly together with a sensible diet (Rooibos Tea Control Board, South Africa). Note: Thonnat (2001, p. 219) insists that tisanes purporting to assist slimming are part of folklore
- sinus problems and asthma, when drunk cold
- hay fever, drunk hot or cold – the tea is an antihistamine (Davies 1985, p. 130)
- skin rashes (including eczema) – applied cold with cotton wool
- tired or red eyes, using cold tea bags.

Taste and reuse of Rooibos and other herb teas

As previously mentioned, the leaves of most herb teas can be used more than once and Rooibos is no exception. 'Rooibos tea is also very economical as the leaves or bags can be used more than once (Rooibos Tea Control Board, South Africa).' The colour of herb tisanes usually deepens, as the properties tend to continue to enter the cold residue.

Honey in teas

When drinking aromatic waters or aromatic teas, honey can be used as a sweetener should the taste of the drink not appeal to your taste. A squeeze of lemon or orange juice can also alter the flavour.

The authors prefer all teas without sugar or honey, as these tend to detract from the flavour. However, for those who prefer sweet drinks, honey is certainly a better and healthier option than sugar. It is more often used as a food and it is easily digested, containing mainly glucose and levulose, which are easily accepted by the digestive system; this may be due in part to the many enzymes which it possesses. Other sugars such as beet and cane have to be broken down into glucose and levulose for absorption by the body (Davies 1985, p. 48).

Infusion recipes

The following recipe uses a higher quantity of plant material than normal for tisanes: the resulting liquid can be diluted.

- 20–60 g plant material (about 1–6 tablespoons, depending on the density); more than one plant can be used
- 1 pint boiling water

Cut or break the plant material into small pieces if necessary. Put into a jug. Boil the water and pour immediately over the plant material. Allow to stand for 10 minutes if using as a drink, 20 minutes if using topically, for a stronger infusion. Strain before use.

If an even stronger infusion is required for topical use, the amount of plant material can be doubled but still using the same amount of water.

Grieve (1998, p. 543) tells us that an infusion of peppermint (dried) made in a similar way to the above and taken in wineglassful doses regularly at the onset of a cold or early indication of influenza, 'will, in most cases, effect a cure'. On page 708, she tells us that an infusion of St John's wort, also to the above recipe and taken in doses of 1–2 tablespoonfuls at night, will be found effective for children suffering from incontinence and chronic catarrh of the lungs, bowels or urinary passages.

According to Genders (1986b, p. 178), an infusion of the aerial part of scarlet pimpernel in boiling water left for 15 minutes, then strained, is effective on blemished skin and after exposure to the sun.

The infusion of chamomile is a mild sedative, much used in France and Germany. Charles Estienne in Maison Rustique (translation by Richard Surflet) says that:

> *cammomill is singular good to mollifie, resolve, rarify and loosen, and in this respect there is no remedie better for lassitudes or wearisomnes without just onward causes than bathes made with leaves and flowers thereof. (Clair 1961, p. 138)*

Grieve (1992, pp. 703–704) tells us that an infusion made with sage simply by pouring 1 pint of boiling water on to 1 oz of the dried herb, can be used as a gargle or mouthwash for infections of the mouth and inflamed sore throat, relaxing the throat and tonsils. The same infusion can be used as a gargle for bleeding gums and to prevent an excessive flow of saliva. When a more stimulating effect to the throat is desirable, the gargle may be made of equal quantities of vinegar and water, ½ pint of hot malt vinegar being poured on the leaves, adding ½ pint of cold water. If the same infusion is used for internal use, the dose is from a wineglassful to half a teacupful, as often as required.

Grieve continues by saying that the old-fashioned way of making a infusion or tea with sage is more elaborate, and 'the result is a pleasant drink, cooling in fevers, and also a cleanser and purifier of the blood'. The recipe she gives is:

- ½ oz (15 g) fresh sage leaves
- 1 oz (30 g) sugar
- juice of 1 lemon, or ¼ oz (7 g) of grated lemon rind
- 1 quart (1 litre) boiling water

Put the first three ingredients into a jug and add the boiling water. Allow to infuse for half an hour, then strain. (The Jamaicans 'sweeten' sage tea with lime juice instead of lemon.)

Aromatherapists without a qualification in the internal use of essential oils would hesitate before using sage on account of the thujone content. However, the hydrolat contains extremely little by comparison, and it is quite safe to use in teas and tisanes.

Grieve considers sage tea (and the infusion) to be a valuable aid in the 'delirium of fevers' and 'the nervous excitement frequently accompanying brain and nervous diseases', which suggests it is calming; it has considerable reputation as a remedy, given in small and oft-repeated doses. Grieve attributes many qualities to it:

- relieves nervous headaches (a cup of the strong infusion)
- valuable against colds in the head as well as sore throat
- a stimulant tonic in debility of the stomach and weakness of the digestion generally
- beneficial in biliousness and liver complaints
- helpful for kidney troubles
- reduces pains in the joints
- useful as an emmenagogue.

An infusion of sage taken regularly for a month before childbirth will considerably reduce labour pains (Valnet 1982, p. 182).

A strong infusion, without the lemon and sugar, is an excellent lotion for ulcers and to heal raw abrasions of the skin.

A decoction of the leaves and branches of Sage made and drunk, saith Dioscorides, provokes urine and causeth the hair to become black. It stayeth the bleeding of wounds and cleaneth ulcers and sores. . . . Gargles are made with Sage, Rosemary, Honeysuckles and Plantains, boiled in wine or water with some honey or alum put thereto, to wash sore mouths and throats, as need requireth. It is very good for stitch or pains in the sides coming of wind, if the place be fomented warn with the decoction in wine and the herb also, after boiling, be lain thereto. (Culpeper, n.d., p. 312)

It is said that sage tea should not be drunk every day for a long period of time, because nuns who did this over a period of many years became ill.

Decoctions

When a decoction is made the heavier water-soluble components, which do not appear in hydrolats or tisanes, are extracted, which significantly alters the taste, making it not so pleasant as an infusion. The procedure is particularly suitable for woods, roots and bark, especially if they contain tannins (Wichtl 1994, p. 26).

The plant is put into cold water, brought to the boil and simmered for 10–20 minutes. Imagine using this method for teas or tisanes and you will have an idea of how it changes the taste. Bartram (1995, p. 141) tells us that the vessel used should be made of stainless steel, glass, earthenware or ceramic material and that the liquid should be reduced by one-quarter.

Whatever kind of pan is used, it should have a tight-fitting lid, to save losing any of the precious essential oil vapour, if the plant contains any – if you lose some of the steam, you will also lose some of the components. Using a slow cooker is a good idea; with this, not only is no vapour lost, but it saves watching the pan, to prevent it going dry.

- 1 large pan with a tight fitting lid or a slow cooker
- 1 litre distilled, deionized or spring water
- 40–60 g plant material

Put plant matter and water into pan. Cover with tight-fitting lid and bring to the boil. Simmer for 10–20 min. Allow to cool. Bottle and keep in fridge.

If using a slow cooker, use the highest setting and set the time for 1–2 hours.

Cautions to observe when drinking medicinal teas

If you have a heart condition, it is wise to be careful with certain medicinal teas. They may do you enough good for the condition for which you are using them to make you put off seeing the doctor. However, they may be masking a possible condition against which plants are of little avail (Thonnat 2001, p. 219). He continues by saying that certain plants are not inoffensive, for example *séné* (senna), *bourdaine* (black alder tree), boldo, hyssop, *fougère* (fern), which are advised for constipation, irritate the intestinal mucus. Sage tea should be taken for a week or two only because of the potentially toxic effects of thujone (Mabey 1988, p. 72).

APPENDIX A

Therapeutic index

Sources for the properties of the distilled plant waters are shown so that the reader can have the fullest possible information for judging the value of the information given. Very little scientifically based information is available, and the information given here has been judged to be the best available for inclusion in this book. Surprisingly, many aromatherapy writers give only the common name of the plant and do not specify the Latin binomial, nor do some of them specify what part of the plant the water is from (leaf, berry, root, etc.). Therefore, the pertinent scientific name and other details have been added where it has been thought necessary and appropriate.

ANALGESIC

Abies balsamea [CANADA BALSAM]	
Artemisia dracunculus [TARRAGON]	(Viaud 1983)
Chamaemelum nobile [ROMAN CHAMOMILE]	post zoster pain (Franchomme & Pénoël 1996,p. 86)
Hamamelis virginiana [WITCH HAZEL]	rheumatic pain (Catty 2001, p. 96)
Laurus nobilis [BAY LEAF]	(Franchomme & Pénoël 1990, p. 281)
Melissa officinalis [LEMON BALM]	migraine (Kresanek 1982, p. 130)
Picea mariana [BLACK SPRUCE]	(Rose 1999, p. 172)
Portulaca sativa [GOLDEN PURSLANE]	(Grieve 1992, p. 660)
Solidago canadensis [GOLDEN ROD]	(Rose 1999, p. 170)

ANTHELMINTIC

Chenopodium album [FAT HEN]	taenia, intestinal (tapeworm) (Viaud 1983)
Peumus boldus [BOLDO LEAF]	ascaris, intestinal (Franchomme & Pénoël 1990, p. 274)
Thymus vulgaris ct. linalool [SWEET THYME]	ascaris, intestinal (Franchomme & Pénoël 1990, p. 274)

ANTIALLERGIC

Agaricus campestris [FIELD MUSHROOM]	(Viaud 1983)
Chamaemelum nobile [ROMAN CHAMOMILE]	cutaneous (Bego 1995)
Myrtus communis [MYRTLE]	(Schnaubelt 1999), asthma (Catty 2001, p. 115)
Sambucus nigra [ELDERFLOWER]	major antiasthmatic (Viaud 1983)

ANTIBACTERIAL

Citrus aurantium var. *sinensis* (flos) [SWEET ORANGE FLOWER]	collibacillus (Viaud 1983)
Cuminum cyminum [CUMIN]	(Sağadiç & Özcan 2003)
Laurus nobilis [BAY LEAF]	(Baudoux 1996a, p. 108)
Mentha × *sylvestris* [HORSEMINT]	bactericide (Viaud 1983)
Origanum vulgare [OREGANO]	(Rose 1999, p. 173; Sağadiç & Özcan 2003)
Pimpinella anisum [ANISEED]	(Sağadiç & Özcan 2003)
Satureia hortensis [SUMMER SAVORY]	(Sağadiç & Özcan 2003)
Satureia montana [WINTER SAVORY]	(Catty 2001, p. 132)
Thymbra spicata [BLACK THYME]	(Sağadiç & Özcan 2003)
Thymus serpyllym [WILD THYME]	(Viaud 1983)

ANTICANCER

Apium graveolens [WILD CELERY]	(Viaud 1983)
Artemisia dracunculus [TARRAGON]	(Viaud 1983)
Buxus sempervirens [BOX]	(Viaud 1983)
Galega officinalis [GOAT'S RUE]	breast abscess, pancreas, (Viaud 1983)
Harpagophytum procumbens [DEVIL'S CLAW]	(Viaud 1983)
Hypericum perforatum [ST JOHN'S WORT]	(Viaud 1983)
Mentha × sylvestris [HORSEMINT]	(Viaud 1983)
Petroselinum sativum [PARSLEY]	(Viaud 1983)
Thuja occidentalis [THUJA]	antitumoral (Viaud 1983)
Thymus serpyllum [WILD THYME]	(Viaud 1983)

ANTIDIABETIC

Eucalyptus globulus [TASMANIAN BLUE GUM]	(Viaud 1983)
Galega officinalis [GOAT'S RUE]	(Viaud 1983)
Helichrysum italicum [EVERLASTING]	(Viaud 1983)
Juglans regia [WALNUT]	(Viaud 1983)
Robinia pseudoacacia [ACACIA]	(Viaud 1983)
Saponaria officinalis [SOAPWORT]	(Viaud 1983)

ANTIFUNGAL

Hamamelis virginiana [WITCH HAZEL]	(Rose 1999, p. 174)
Melaleuca alternifolia [TEA TREE]	(Catty 2001, p. 109)
Origanum vulgaris [OREGANO]	(Rose 1999, p. 173)
Satureia montana [WINTER SAVORY]	(Catty 2001, p. 132)

ANTIINFECTIOUS

Centaurea cyanus [CORNFLOWER]	all infectious diseases (Grieve 1998, p. 224)
Chamaemelum nobile [ROMAN CHAMOMILE]	urinary tract infections
Laurus nobilis [BAY LEAF]	(Franchomme & Pénoël 1990, p. 281)
Origanum vulgaris [OREGANO]	(Catty 2001, p. 118)
Thymus vulgaris [THYME]	(Catty 2001, p. 137)

ANTIINFLAMMATORY

Achillea millefolium [YARROW]	(Rose 1999, p. 171)
Aloysia triphylla [LEMON VERBENA]	(Catty 2001, p. 107)
Artemisia arborescens [GREAT MUGWORT]	(Rose 1999, p. 170)
Chamaemelum nobile [ROMAN CHAMOMILE]	cutaneous (Goëb 1998; Bego 1995; Rose 1999, p. 170; Catty 2001, p. 83)
Daucus carota (sem.) [CARROT SEED]	(Catty 2001, pp. 89–90)
Hamamelis virginiana [WITCH HAZEL]	(Korting et al 1993; Rose 1999, p. 174; Catty 2001, p. 96)
Ledum groenlandicum [GREENLAND MOSS]	(Catty 2001, p. 106)
Matricaria recutita [GERMAN CHAMOMILE]	(Rose 1999, p. 170; Catty 2001, p. 108; naturesgift.com/hydrosols)
Melissa officinalis [LEMON BALM]	(Catty 2001, p. 111)
Mentha × piperita [PEPPERMINT]	relieves itching, redness (Rose 1999, p. 174)
Rosa damascena [DAMASK ROSE]	
Solidago canadensis [GOLDEN ROD]	(Rose 1999, p. 170; Catty 2001, p. 133)

ANTIOXIDANT

Hamamelis virginiana [WITCH HAZEL]	(Catty 2001, p. 96)
Melissa officinalis [LEMON BALM]	(Catty 2001, p. 111)
Rosmarinus officinalis [ROSEMARY]	
Salvia officinalis [SAGE]	

ANTIPARASITIC

Artemisia vulgaris [MUGWORT]	(Catty 2001, p. 77)
Chamaemelum nobile [ROMAN CHAMOMILE]	lice (C. Montesinos, personal communication, 2001)
Laurus nobilis [BAY LEAF]	lice (C. Montesinos, personal communication, 2001)
Lavandula angustifolia [LAVENDER]	lice (C. Montesinos, personal communication, 2001)
Salvia officinalis [SAGE]	lice (C. Montesinos, personal communication, 2001)
Satureia montana [WINTER SAVORY]	lice (C. Montesinos, personal communication, 2001)
Thymus vulgaris [THYME]	lice (C. Montesinos, personal communication, 2001)

ANTIRHEUMATIC

Thymus vulgaris [THYME]	(Viaud 1983)

ANTISEPTIC

Achillea millefolium [YARROW]	(Keville & Green 1995; Rose 1999, p. 171)
Arbutus uva ursi [BEARBERRY]	(Viaud 1983)
Calendula officinalis [MARIGOLD]	*staphylococcus* (Viaud 1983)
Cedrus atlantica [ATLAS CEDAR]	(Grosjean 1993b, p. 57)
Centaurea cyanus [CORNFLOWER]	plague, infectious diseases (Grieve, 1998, p. 224)
Citrus aurantium var. *amara* (flos) [BITTER ORANGE FLOWER]	antiseptic (Catty 2001, p. 86)
Foeniculum vulgare var. *dulce* (sem.) [FENNEL]	(Viaud 1983; Rose 1999, p. 173)
Hamamelis virginiana [WITCH HAZEL]	(Rose 1999, p. 174; Catty 2001, p. 96)
Lavandula angustifolia [LAVENDER]	(Baudoux 1996a), intestinal (Fischer-Rizzi 1990, p. 58)
Laurus nobilis [BAY LEAF]	intestinal (Viaud 1983), (Baudoux 1996a, p. 108)
Matricaria recutita [GERMAN CHAMOMILE]	(Catty 2001, p. 108)
Melaleuca alternifolia [TEA TREE]	(Catty 2001, p. 109)
Mentha × *piperita* [PEPPERMINT]	(Viaud 1983)
Myrtus communis [MYRTLE]	(Schnaubelt 1999), sore throats, coughs, bronchitis, (Catty 2001, p. 115)
Origanum vulgare [OREGANO]	(Rose 1999, p. 173; Catty 2001, p. 118)
Pinus sylvestris [SCOTS PINE]	(Catty 2001, p. 121)
Salvia sclarea [CLARY]	(Claeys 1992)
Satureia montana [WINTER SAVORY]	(Catty 2001, p. 132)
Thymus serpyllum [WILD THYME]	intestinal (Viaud 1983); (Grieve 1992, pp. 814–815)
Thymus vulgaris [THYME]	(Rose 1999, p. 174), intestinal (Viaud 1983)

ANTISPASMODIC

Artemisia dracunculus [TARRAGON]	digestive spasm (Catty 2001, p. 76)
Artemisia arborescens [GREAT MUGWORT]	(Rose 1999, p. 170)
Chamaemelum nobile [ROMAN CHAMOMILE]	intestinal spasm, (Franchomme & Pénoël 1996, p. 86)
Citrus aurantium var. *sinensis* (flos) [SWEET ORANGE FLOWER]	(Nasr 2000, p. 26)
Citrus aurantium var. *amara* (flos) [BITTER ORANGE FLOWER]	digestive (Catty 2001, p. 86)
Laurus nobilis [BAY LEAF]	(Viaud 1983)
Melilotus officinalis [COMMON MELILOT]	(Viaud 1983)
Mentha sylvestris [HORSEMINT]	(Viaud 1983)
Mentha pulegium [PENNYROYAL]	antidote to spasmodic, nervous and hysterical affections (Grieve 1992, p. 626)
Solidago canadensis [GOLDEN ROD]	(Rose 1999, p. 170; Catty 2001, p. 133)
Thymus serpyllum [WILD THYME]	(Grieve 1992, pp. 814–815)

ANTITOXIC

Galega officinalis [GOAT'S RUE]	breast abscess, pancreas, (Viaud 1983)

ANTIVIRAL

Cistus ladaniferus [ROCK ROSE]	(Baudoux 1996a; Franchomme & Pénoël 1990, p. 286)
Lavandula × intermedia ct. borneol [LAVANDIN]	(Rose 1999, p. 170)
Melaleuca alternifolia [TEA TREE]	(Catty, 2001, p. 109)
Melissa officinalis [LEMON BALM]	(Catty 2001, p. 111), viricide in water (Rose 1999, p. 173)
Origanum vulgare [OREGANO]	(Rose 1999, p. 173)
Thymus vulgaris ct. thujanol-4 [SWEET THYME]	(Baudoux 1996a)

ARTHRITIS

Artemisia arborescens [GREAT MUGWORT]	(Rose 1999, p. 170)
Tilia sylvestris (lig.) [LIME SAPWOOD]	articular rheumatism, gout (Viaud 1983)

ASTHMA

Myrtus communis [MYRTLE]	(Catty 2001, p. 115)
Sambucus nigra [ELDERFLOWER]	(Viaud 1983)

ASTRINGENT

Achillea millefolium [YARROW]	(Keville & Green 1995)
Centaurea cyanus [CORNFLOWER]	
Cistus ladaniferus [ROCK ROSE]	(Catty 2001, p. 84)
Cupressus sempervirens [CYPRESS]	(Catty 2001, p. 88)
Hamamelis virginiana [WITCH HAZEL]	(Bartram 1995; Keville & Green 1995; Winter 1999, p. 458; Sanoflore 2000; Catty 2001, p. 96)
Salvia officinalis [SAGE]	(Claeys 1992)
Salvia sclarea [CLARY]	(Rose 1999, p. 172)
Solidago canadensis [GOLDEN ROD]	(Rose 1999, p. 170)

BOILS

Thymus vulgarus [THYME]	

BRONCHITIS

Eucalyptus globulus [TASMANIAN BLUE GUM]	(Catty 1998a)
Eucalyptus polybractea [BLUE LEAVED MALLEE]	(Catty 1998a)
Inula graveolens [ELECAMPANE]	(Catty 1998a)
Melaleuca alternifolia [TEA TREE]	(Catty 1998a)
Myrtus communis [MYRTLE]	coughs, (Catty 2001, p. 115)
Origanum vulgare [OREGANO]	(Catty 1998a)
Rosmarinus officinalis ct. verbenone [ROSEMARY VERBENONE]	(Catty 1998a)
Satureia montana [WINTER SAVORY]	coughs, (Catty 2001, p. 115)

BRUISES

Centaurea cyanus [CORNFLOWER]	(Catty 2001, p. 81)

CALMING, RELAXING

Aloysia triphylla [LEMON VERBENA]	aids sleep (Rose 1999, p. 173), soothing (Paris 2000), mental relaxant (Catty 2001, p. 107), insomnia (Grosjean 1993a, p. 66)
Chamaemelum nobile [ROMAN CHAMOMILE]	calming, tired eyes (Sanaflore 2000), soothing (Paris 2000)
Citrus aurantium var. *amara* (flos) [BITTER ORANGE FLOWER]	in the bath for excited children (Grieve 1992, p. 602), nervous stressed persons (Goëb 1998; sabia.com 1997–1999; Catty 2001, p. 85)
Citrus aurantium var. *sinensis* (flos) [SWEET ORANGE FLOWER]	cardiac calmative, SAD (Viaud 1983), calming nervine (Nasr 2000, p. 26), nervous depression (Baudoux 1996a)
Crataegus monogyna, [HAWTHORN]	soothing (Paris 2000)
Crataegeus oxyacantha [HAWTHORN]	cardiac (Viaud 1983), antidepressive (Viaud 1983), sleep inducing (Baudoux 1996a)

Helichrysum italicum [EVERLASTING]	soothes irritations, calms heart (Rose 1999, p. 172)
Inula graveolens [ELECAMPANE]	(Baudoux 1996a)
Lavandula angustifolia [LAVENDER]	soothing (Paris 2000)
Matricaria recutita [GERMAN CHAMOMILE]	(Catty 2001, p. 108)
Melissa officinalis [LEMON BALM]	(naturesgift.com/hydrosols), insomnia, sedating (Rose 1999, p. 173)
Mentha × piperita [PEPPERMINT]	hot flushes (Rose 1999, p. 174), cooling, calms stings and rashes, soothes itches
Mentha pulegium [PENNYROYAL]	spasmodic, nervous and hysterical affections (Grieve 1992, p. 626)
Ocimum basilicum [BASIL]	nausea (Rose 1999, p. 172)
Origanum majorana [SWEET MARJORAM]	soothing (Paris 2000)
Origanum vulgare [OREGANO]	calmative to CNS (Viaud 1983)
Ormenis mixta [MOROCCAN CHAMOMILE]	soothing (Paris 2000)
Pelargonium graveolens [GERANIUM]	cooling, hot flushes (Rose 1999, p. 174)
Pimento officinalis [PIMENTO]	hysteria (Grieve 1992, p. 20)
Pinus sylvestris [SCOTS PINE]	balsamic (Viaud 1983)
Sambucus nigra [ELDERFLOWER]	(Catty 2001, p. 130)
Solidago canadensis [GOLDEN ROD]	(Rose 1999, p. 170)
Tanacetum vulgare [TANSY]	calming to the psyche (Viaud 1983)
Thymus serpyllum [WILD THYME]	
Tilia × europea [LIME LEAF]	insomnia (Grosjean 1993a, p. 66), hysteria, palpitations (Grieve 1992, p. 486), cardiac, nerves (Baudoux 1996a)
Tilia sylvestris [LIME LEAF]	(Viaud 1983)

CARMINATIVE

Anethum graveolens [DILL]	flatulence, hiccups
Apium graveolens [WILD CELERY]	(Viaud 1983)
Artemisia dracunculus [TARRAGON]	gas, colic (Catty 2001, p. 76)
Carum carvi [CARAWAY]	flatulent colic of infants (Grieve, 1998, p. 158)
Citrus aurantium var. *sinensis* (flos) [SWEET ORANGE FLOWER]	(Nasr 2000, p. 26)
Coriandrum sativum [CORIANDER]	(Grieve 1992, p. 222)
Crocus sativus [SAFFRON]	(Grieve 1992, p. 700)
Foeniculum vulgare var. *dulce* (sem.) [FENNEL]	(Grieve 1992, p. 296)
Helichrysum italicum [EVERLASTING]	aerophagy (Viaud 1983)
Laurus nobilis [BAY LEAF]	(Viaud 1983)
Mentha spicata [SPEARMINT]	hiccups, flatulence (Grieve 1992, p. 536)
Ocimum basilicum [SWEET BASIL]	digestive (Viaud 1983)
Petroselinum sativum [PARSLEY]	(Culpeper, n.d., p. 258)
Pimento officinalis [PIMENTO]	(Grieve 1992, p. 20)
Salvia officinalis [SAGE]	(Nasr 2000, p. 27)
Thymus serpyllum [WILD THYME]	(Grieve 1992, pp. 814–185)

CATARRH

Thymus serpyllum [WILD THYME]	(Grieve 1992, pp. 814–185)

CHICKENPOX

Mentha × piperita [PEPPERMINT]	(C. Marshall, personal communication, 12 July 1998)
Chamaemelum nobile [ROMAN CHAMOMILE]	(C. Marshall, personal communication, 12 July 1998)

CICATRIZANT see also **SCARS**

Chamaemelum nobile [ROMAN CHAMOMILE]	purifying, (Claeys 1992)
Cistus ladaniferus [ROCK ROSE]	(Baudoux 1996a; Catty 2001, p. 84)
Cupressus sempervirens [CYPRESS]	(Grosjean 1993b, p. 87)
Helichrysum italicum [EVERLASTING]	(Rose 1999, p. 172; Catty 2001)

Laurus nobilis [BAY LEAF]	(Baudoux 1996a)
Lavandula angustifolia [LAVENDER]	(Claeys 1992; Grosjean 1993b, p. 87)
Rosa canina [WILD ROSE]	(Grosjean 1993b, p. 87)
Scabiosa succisa [SCABIOUS]	(Culpeper n.d., p. 324; Grieve 1992, p. 722)

CIRCULATION see also **VARICOSE VEINS**

Achillea millefolium [YARROW]	increases circulation
Artemisia vulgaris [MUGWORT]	peripheral circulatory stimulant (Catty 2001, p. 77)
Cupressus sempervirens [CYPRESS]	(Viaud 1983; Paris 2000; Catty 2001, p. 89) haemorrhoids, venous congestion, varicose veins (Baudoux 1996a)
Erigeron canadensis [FLEABANE]	(Viaud 1983, Paris 2000)
Hamamelis virginiana [WITCH HAZEL]	haemorrhoids
Juniperus communis [JUNIPER]	(Grosjean 1993b, p. 54), circulation stimulant (Rose 1999, p. 173)
Juniperus communis (fruct.) [JUNIPER BERRY]	(Catty 2001, p. 101)
Laurus nobilis [BAY LEAF]	lymphatic system (Catty 2001, p. 103)
Melilotus officinalis [COMMON MELILOT]	(Paris 2000), anticoagulant, embolism, phlebitis (Viaud 1983), good for those who swoon and to preserve them from apoplexy (Culpeper, n.d., p. 232)
Mentha × piperita [PEPPERMINT]	heavy legs (Grosjean 1993b, p. 87)
Origanum onites [FRENCH MARJORAM]	stimulant, cardiovascular system (Aydin et al 1996)
Petroselinum sativum [PARSLEY]	red cell regenerator (Viaud 1983)
Pistacia lentiscus [PISTACHIO]	reticulo-endothelial decongestant (Viaud 1983)
Robinia pseudoacacia [ACACIA]	capillary problems (skin), arterial circulatory system (Viaud 1983)
Ruscus aculeatus [BUTCHER'S BROOM]	(Paris 2000)
Salvia officinalis [SAGE]	menopausal circulation, weak arteries, veins (Grosjean 1993b, pp. 34, 54), circulatory stimulant (Catty 2001, p. 127), cellulite (Grosjean 1993a, p. 65)
Sambucus nigra [ELDERFLOWER]	(Grosjean 1993b, p. 54)
Thymus vulgarus ct. thujanol-4 [SWEET THYME]	increases circulation
Thymus vulgarus [THYME]	increases circulation (Rose 1999, p. 174)
Tilia × europaea [LIME LEAF]	vasodilator (Viaud 1983)

COLDS AND 'FLU

Eucalyptus smithii [GULLY GUM]	(Payne 1999)
Filipendula ulmaria [MEADOWSWEET]	
Myrtus communis [MYRTLE]	(Payne 1999)
Rosmarinus officinalis [ROSEMARY]	(Payne 1999)

COLIC

Carum carvi [CARAWAY]	flatulent colic of infants (Grieve, 1998, p. 158)

COUGHS

Hamamelis virginiana [WITCH HAZEL]	sore throats (Catty 2001, p. 96)
Myrtus communis [MYRTLE]	(Catty 2001, p. 115), sore throats (Rose 1999, p. 173)

CYSTITIS

Eupatorium cannabinum [HEMP AGRIMONY]	chronic cystitis

DIGESTIVE

Artemisia arborescens [TREE WORMWOOD]	stomachic
Artemisia dracunculus [TARRAGON]	stomach problems (Paris 2000)
Chamaemelum nobile [ROMAN CHAMOMILE]	stomach, intestinal disorders (Fischer-Rizzi 1990, p. 58)
Citrus aurantium var. *amara* (flos) [BITTER ORANGE FLOWER]	stimulating bile, relieve heartburn (Catty 2001, p. 86)

Foeniculum vulgare var. *dulce* (sem.) [FENNEL]	stomach ache (Rose 1999, p. 173)
Laurus nobilis [BAY LEAF]	(Viaud 1983; Rose 1999, p. 172; Paris 2000)
Levisticum officinale [LOVAGE]	(Paris 2000)
Melissa officinalis [LEMON BALM]	intestinal antispasmodic (colitis, Crohn's disease) (Catty 2001, p. 111), digestive (Baudoux 1996a)
Mentha × piperita [PEPPERMINT]	eupeptic (Viaud 1983; Baudoux 1996a; Rose 1999, p. 174; Paris 2000)
Ocimum basilicum [SWEET BASIL]	carminative (Viaud 1983, Paris 2000)
Origanum majorana [SWEET MARJORAM]	stomach and intestinal cramp (Fischer-Rizzi 1990, p. 58)
Peumus boldus [BOLDO LEAF]	eupeptic (Paris 2000)
Rosmarinus officinalis [ROSEMARY]	(Grosjean 1993a, p. 64)
Rosmarinus officinalis ct. verbenone [ROSEMARY VERBENONE]	stomachic (Paris 2000)
Salvia officinalis [SAGE]	(Grosjean 1993a, p. 64)
Thymus serpyllum [WILD THYME]	(Viaud 1983), weak digestion (Grieve 1992, pp. 814–815)
Thymus vulgaris [THYME]	(Rose 1999, p. 174)
Tilia × europaea [LIME LEAF]	indigestion, nervous vomiting (Grieve 1992, p. 486)
Zingiber officinale [GINGER]	(naturesgift.com)

DIURETIC

Apium graveolens [WILD CELERY]	(Viaud 1983)
Cedrus atlantica [ATLAS CEDAR]	(Catty 2001, p. 80)
Cupressus sempervirens [CYPRESS]	(Catty 2001, p. 88)
Hamamelis virginiana [WITCH HAZEL]	(Catty 2001, p. 96)
Hieracium pilosella [MOUSE EAR]	(Viaud 1983)
Juniperus communis [JUNIPER]	(Viaud 1983)
Juniperus communis (fruct.) [JUNIPER BERRY]	(Rose 1999, p. 173; Catty 2001, p. 101)
Pinus sylvestris [SCOTS PINE]	(Viaud 1983)
Sambucus nigra [ELDERFLOWER]	(Catty 2001, p. 130)
Solidago canadensis [GOLDEN ROD]	(Rose 1999, p. 170; Catty 2001, p. 133)

EMMENAGOGUE

Rosmarinus officinalis [ROSEMARY]	(Viaud 1983)
Salvia officinalis [SAGE]	pelvic congestion (Viaud 1983)
Thymus serpyllum [WILD THYME]	(Grieve 1992, pp. 814–815)

ENDOMETRIOSIS

Cistus ladaniferus [ROCK ROSE]	(Catty 2001, p. 84)

ENERGIZING, UPLIFTING

Aloysia triphylla [LEMON VERBENA]	stimulating (Rose 1999, p. 173)
Artemisia abrotanum [SOUTHERNWOOD]	(Viaud 1983)
Artemisia arborescens [TREE WORMWOOD]	
Artemisia vulgaris [MUGWORT]	vibrational healing (Catty 2001, p. 77)
Gentiana lutea [YELLOW GENTIAN]	(Viaud 1983)
Juniperus communis (fruct.) [JUNIPER BERRY]	(Rose 1999, p. 173)
Melissa officinalis [LEMON BALM]	antidepressant (naturesgift.com/hydrosols)
Mentha × piperita [PEPPERMINT]	(Rose 1999, p. 174)
Mentha sylvestris [HORSEMINT]	euphoric (Viaud 1983)
Myrtus communis [MYRTLE]	relieves fatigue, reviving (Rose 1999, p. 173)
Origanum vulgare [OREGANO]	(Grosjean 1993b, p. 56)
Pelargonium graveolens [GERANIUM]	stimulates adrenal cortex, antidepressant (Rose 1999, p. 174)
Rosmarinus officinalis [ROSEMARY]	mental and physical stimulant (Grosjean 1993b, p. 56; Catty 2001, p. 124), restores energy, alertness, for tired feet (Rose 1999, p. 174)
Salvia sclarea [CLARY]	euphoric, antidepressant (Catty 2001, p. 129)

Satureia montana [WINTER SAVORY]	revitalizing (Viaud 1983; Grosjean 1993b, p. 56)
Thymus vulgaris ct. thujanol-4 [SWEET THYME]	for fatigue
Thymus vulgaris [THYME]	stimulating, revitalizing (Price & Price 1999, p. 115; Rose 1999, p. 174)

EXPECTORANT

Inula graveolens [ELECAMPANE]	(Catty 2001, p. 99)

EYES

NB: Ethanol is often added to distilled plant waters to prolong shelf-life: please ensure that waters used in the eyes do not contain alcohol or other preservatives.

Calendula officinalis [MARIGOLD]	antiinflammatory, sore eyes (Grieve 1992, p. 518)
Centaurea cyanus [CORNFLOWER]	soothing (Grosjean 1993b, pp. 95, 114; Payne 1999), calming (C. Montesinos, personal communication, 2001), swollen eyes (Rouvière & Meyer, 1989, p. 106)
Chamaemelum nobile [ROMAN CHAMOMILE]	antiallergic for eye inflammation due to conjunctivitis (Bego 1995; Goëb 1998; Catty 2001, p. 83), soothing (Payne 1999), calming (Montesinos 2001), decongestant, soothing (Grosjean 1993b, pp. 87, 95, 114), conjunctivitis (Baudoux 1996b, p. 101), analgesic, antiviral, post zoster pain, conjunctivitis (Franchomme & Pénoël 1990, pp. 287, 303)
Chelidonium majus [GREATER CELANDINE]	calming (C. Montesinos, personal communication, 2001)
Cistus ladaniferus [ROCK ROSE]	wateriness of the eyes (Baudoux 1996b, p. 101)
Citrus aurantium (flos) [ORANGE FLOWER]	dryness of the eyes - compress (Baudoux 1996b, p. 101)
Eucalyptus globulus [TASMANIAN BLUE GUM]	conjunctivitis (Franchomme & Pénoël 1990, p. 287)
Euphrasia officinalis [EYEBRIGHT]	opthalmic (Culpeper n.d., p. 134)
Filipendula ulmaria [MEADOWSWEET]	'The distilled water of the floures dropped into the eies taketh away the burning and itching thereof and cleareth the sight' (Gerard in Woodward 1964, p. 245), inflammations of the eyes (Culpeper, n.d., p. 230)
Foeniculum vulgare var. *dulce* (sem.) [FENNEL]	eye cleansing (Rose 1999, p. 173)
Hypericum perforatum [ST JOHN'S WORT]	conjunctivitis (Franchomme & Pénoël 1990, p. 303)
Inula graveolens [ELECAMPANE]	conjunctivitis (Baudoux 1996b, p. 101)
Iris pseudacorus [IRIS]	remedy for weak eyes (Culpeper, 1652, cited in Grieve 1992, p. 439)
Laurus nobilis [BAY LEAF]	eye infections (Baudoux 1996b, p. 101)
Lavandula angustifolia [LAVENDER]	cleanse eye make-up (Rouvière & Meyer, 1989, p. 106), wateriness of the eyes (Baudoux 1996b, p. 101)
Lavandula latifolia ct. cineole [SPIKE LAVENDER]	conjunctivitis (Franchomme & Pénoël 1990, p. 287)
Linaria vulgaris [TOADFLAX]	inflamed eyes (Grieve 1992, p. 816)
Melilotus officinalis [MELILOT]	calming (C. Montesinos, personal communication, 2001)
Melissa officinalis [LEMON BALM]	soothing, conjunctivitis, blepharitis (Viaud 1983, Baudoux 1996a)
Mentha × piperita [PEPPERMINT]	dryness of the eyes (Baudoux 1996b, p. 101)
Myrtus communis [MYRTLE]	antiinflammatory, conjunctivitis, irritated, tired eyes (Keville & Green 1995; Franchomme & Pénoël 1996, pp. 86, 287, 303; Schnaubelt 1999; Catty 2001, p. 115), eye infections (Baudoux 1996b, p. 101), external eye wash (Rose 1999, p. 173)
Plantago major [PLANTAIN]	calming (C. Montesinos, personal communication, 2001)
Rosa damascena [DAMASK ROSE]	antiinflammatory, conjunctivitis, irritated eyes (Fischer-Rizzi 1990, p. 58), swollen eyes (Rouvière & Meyer, 1989, p. 106) [also *Rosa alba, Rosa canina, Rosa rubra* (Culpeper n.d., pp. 298–302)]
Thymus vulgaris ct. thujanol-4 [SWEET THYME]	(Price & Price 1999, p. 115)

FEET

Mentha × piperita [PEPPERMINT]	foot friction, relieves, refreshes (Grosjean 1993b, p. 42)

FEVER

Filipendula ulmaria [MEADOWSWEET]	

FRIGIDITY

Origanum vulgare [OREGANO]	impotence (Grosjean 1993b, p. 57)
Satureia hortensis [SAVORY]	impotence (Grosjean 1993b, p. 57)

GALACTOGOGIC

Foeniculum vulgare var. *dulce* (sem.) [FENNEL]	(Viaud 1983)

GINGIVITIS

Helichrysum italicum [EVERLASTING]	receding gums (Catty 1998a)
Laurus nobilis [BAY LEAF]	alveolitis, stomatitis, (Baudoux 1996b, p. 96)
Lavandula angustifolia [LAVENDER]	alveolitis, stomatitis, (Baudoux 1996b, p. 96)
Mentha × piperita [PEPPERMINT]	alveolitis, stomatitis, (Baudoux 1996b, p. 96)

GOUT

Tilia sylvestris (lig.) [LIME SAPWOOD]	(Viaud 1983)

GYNAECOLOGICAL

Aloysia triphylla [LEMON VERBENA]	relieves PMS symptoms (Catty 2001, p. 107)
Cistus ladaniferus [ROCK ROSE]	fibroma (Baudoux 1996b, p. 85)
Cistus ladaniferus ct. pinene [ROCK ROSE]	fibroma (Franchomme & Pénoël 1990, p. 279)
Eucalyptus polybractea [BLUE LEAVED MALLEE]	leucorrhoea (Baudoux 1996b, p. 79), condyloma (Baudoux 1996b, p. 86), uterine dysplasia (Baudoux 1996b, p. 87)
Inula graveolens [ELECAMPANE]	candidiasis (Baudoux 1996b, p. 80), vaginitis (Baudoux 1996b, p. 82)
Laurus nobilis [BAY LEAF]	leucorrhoea (Baudoux 1996b, p. 79), vaginitis (Baudoux 1996b, p. 82)
Lavandula angustifolia [LAVENDER]	leucorrhoea (Baudoux 1996b, p. 79), candidiasis (Baudoux 1996b, p. 80), vaginitis (Baudoux 1996b, p. 82), fibroma (Baudoux 1996b, p. 85), uterine dysplasia (Baudoux 1996b, p. 87)
Origanum vulgare [OREGANO]	(Grosjean 1993b, p. 55)
Pelargonium graveolens [GERANIUM]	cools hot flushes, hormonal imbalance (Rose 1999, p. 174)
Pinus sylvestris [PINE]	(Grosjean 1993b, p. 55)
Rosa damascena [DAMASK ROSE]	fibroma (Baudoux 1996b, p. 85)
Salvia officinalis [SAGE]	painful periods, emmenagogue (Baudoux 1996a); (Grosjean 1993b, p. 55)
Salvia sclarea [CLARY]	PMS, hot flushes (Rose 1999, p. 172)
Thymus vulgaris ct. thujanol-4 [SWEET THYME]	candidiasis (Baudoux 1996b, p. 80), chlamydia (Baudoux 1996b, p. 81), condyloma (Baudoux 1996b, p. 86)

HAIR AND SCALP

Buxus sempervirens [BOX]	tonic, (Montesinos 1991)
Cedrus atlantica [ATLAS CEDAR]	makes soft, silky, aids regrowth, after sun (Grosjean 1993b, pp. 87, 95, 114), hair loss, scalp itch, dandruff (Catty 2001, p. 80)
Chamaemelum nobile [ROMAN CHAMOMILE]	blond hair rinse (Grosjean 1993b, pp. 87, 95, 114)
Lavandula angustifolia [LAVENDER]	in shampoo for greasy hair (Rouvière & Meyer, 1989, p. 114), tonic, (Montesinos 1991)
Mentha sylvestris [HORSEMINT]	scurf or dandruff of the head used with vinegar (Culpeper n.d., p. 236)

Ocimum basilicum [BASIL]	hair loss, stimulating (Rose 1999, p. 172)
Rosa damascena [DAMASK ROSE]	scalp stimulant (Fischer-Rizzi 1990, p. 58)
Rosmarinus officinalis [ROSEMARY]	scalp stimulant (Rouvière & Meyer, 1989, p. 119)
Salvia officinalis [SAGE]	scalp stimulant with rosemary (Rouvière & Meyer, 1989, p. 119)
Thymus vulgaris [THYME]	tonic (Montesinos 1991), makes soft, silky, after sun (Grosjean 1993b, pp. 87, 114)
Urtica dioica [NETTLE]	tonic (Viaud 1983, Montesinos 1991)

HEART

Viscum album [MISTLETOE]	(Viaud 1983)

HEPATIC

Acacia decurrens [MIMOSA]	hepatic cleanser, gall bladder drainer (Viaud 1983)
Agaricus campestris [FIELD MUSHROOM]	hepatic drainer (Viaud 1983)
Helichrysum italicum [EVERLASTING]	liver and gall bladder healer (Rose 1999, p. 172)
Inula graveolens [ELECAMPANE]	hepatic stimulant (Catty 2001, p. 99)
Lactuca hortensis [LETTUCE]	hepatic depurative (Viaud 1983)
Lactuca virosa [WILD LETTUCE]	hepatic depurative (Viaud 1983)
Ledum groenlandicum [GREENLAND MOSS]	liver cleanser (Catty 2001, p. 106)
Mentha × piperita [PEPPERMINT]	(Baudoux 1996a)
Origanum majorana [SWEET MARJORAM]	depurative, liver, gall bladder (Viaud 1983; Fischer-Rizzi 1990, p. 58)
Peumus boldus [BOLDO LEAF]	liver decongestant (Viaud 1983)
Rosa damascena [DAMASK ROSE]	liver congestion, gall bladder infection (Fischer-Rizzi 1990, p. 58)
Rosmarinus officinalis [ROSEMARY]	stimulate gall bladder (Catty 2001, p. 124), gall bladder cleanser (Viaud 1983)
Rosmarinus officinalis ct. verbenone [ROSEMARY VERBENONE]	hepatic drainage, regeneration (Baudoux 1996a)
Solidago virgaurea [GOLDEN ROD]	albuminuria, phosphates (Viaud 1983)
Thymus vulgaris ct. thujanol-4 [SWEET THYME]	liver regeneration (Baudoux 1996a)
Urtica dioica [NETTLE]	gall bladder (Viaud 1983)

HORMONAL

Salvia sclarea [CLARY]	balancer (Catty 2001, p. 129)

HYPOTENSOR: HIGH BLOOD PRESSURE

In conjunction with usual medication

Calendula officinalis [MARIGOLD]	Viaud (1983)
Crataegus monogyna [HAWTHORN]	(Fischer-Rizzi 1990, p. 58)
Olea europaea [OLIVE]	antihypertension, cardiac protector (Viaud 1983)
Pelargonium graveolens [GERANIUM]	(Payne 1999)

IMMUNOSTIMULANT

Abies balsamea [CANADA BALSAM]	
Cistus ladaniferus [ROCK ROSE]	immune system booster (Catty 2001, p. 84)
Pinus sylvestris [SCOTS PINE]	(Catty 2001, p. 121)
Satureia montana [WINTER SAVORY]	(Catty 2001, p. 132)
Thymus vulgaris ct. thujanol-4 [SWEET THYME]	(Catty 2001, p. 136)

INSOMNIA

Citrus aurantium var. *amara* (fol.) [PETITGRAIN]	soporific (Franchomme & Pénoël 1990, p. 286)
Tilia × europea [LIME LEAF]	(Grosjean 1993a, p. 66)
Valeriana wallichii [VALERIAN]	soporific (Franchomme & Pénoël 1990, p. 286)

LEGS

- *Rosmarinus officinalis* [ROSEMARY] — refreshing (Rouvière & Meyer, 1989, p. 114)
- *Salvia officinalis* [SAGE] — refreshing (Rouvière & Meyer, 1989, p. 114)

LIPOLYTIC

- *Phytolacca decandra* [POKE ROOT] — adiposity (Viaud 1983)

LITHOLYTIC

- *Hieracium pilosella* [MOUSE EAR] — urinary stones (Viaud 1983)
- *Petroselinum sativum* [PARSLEY] — renal (Viaud 1983)
- *Solidago canadensis* [GOLDEN ROD] — renal (Catty 2001, p. 133)

LYMPH

- *Laurus nobilis* [BAY LEAF] — swollen lymph nodes (breast tissue), vaccination side-effects (Catty 1998)

MENOPAUSE

- *Citrus aurantium* var. *amara* (flos) [BITTER ORANGE FLOWER] — (Payne 1999)
- *Rosa centifolia* [CABBAGE ROSE] — (Payne 1999)

MIGRAINE

- *Chamaemelum nobile* [ROMAN CHAMOMILE] — eases migraine (naturesgift.com/ hydrosols)
- *Melissa officinalis* [LEMON BALM] — antimigraine (Kresanek 1982, p. 130)

MOUTHWASH ETC.

- *Aloysia triphylla* [LEMON VERBENA] — (Catty 2001, p. 107)
- *Elettaria cardamomum* [CARDAMOM] — gingivitis, breath-freshener
- *Helichrysum italicum* [EVERLASTING] — gingivitis (Catty 2001, p. 97)
- *Laurus nobilis* [BAY LEAF] — (Catty 2001, p. 103)
- *Lavandula angustifolia* [LAVENDER] — gargle (hoarseness, loss of voice)
- *Levisticum officinale* [LOVAGE] — gargle for quinsy (Culpeper n.d., p. 219)
- *Melaleuca alternifolia* [TEA TREE] — sore throat, gingivitis (Catty, 2001, p. 109)
- *Mentha sylvestris* [HORSEMINT] — stinking breath, proceeding from corruption of the teeth (Culpeper n.d., p. 236)
- *Mentha* × *piperita* [PEPPERMINT] — mouth ulcers (Baudoux 1996b, p. 98)
- *Origanum vulgare* [OREGANO] — (Catty 2001, p. 118)
- *Plantago major* [PLANTAIN] — ulcerated mouth (Salmon's *Herbal*, 1710, in Grieve 1992, p. 642)
- *Thymus vulgaris* [THYME] — teeth and gums
- *Thymus vulgaris* ct. thujanol-4 [SWEET THYME] — mouth ulcers (Baudoux 1996b, p. 98)

MUCOLYTIC

- *Abies balsamea* [BALSAM FIR] — coughs
- *Eucalyptus dives* [BROAD LEAVED PEPPERMINT] — nasal (Franchomme & Pénoël 1990, p. 302)
- *Inula graveolens* [ELECAMPANE] — (Catty 2001, p. 99)
- *Mentha pulegium* [PENNYROYAL] — nasal (Franchomme & Pénoël 1990, p. 302)
- *Rosmarinus officinalis* ct. verbenone [ROSEMARY VERBENONE] — nasal (Franchomme & Pénoël 1990, p. 302)

PHARYNGITIS

- *Eucalyptus polybractea* [BLUE LEAVED MALLEE] — (Baudoux 1996b, p. 16)
- *Myrtus communis* [MYRTLE] — (Baudoux 1996b, p. 16)
- *Thymus vulgaris* ct. linalool [SWEET THYME] — sore throat, tonsillitis (Franchomme & Pénoël 1990, p. 274)
- *Thymus vulgaris* ct. thujanol-4 [SWEET THYME] — (Baudoux 1996b, p. 16)
- *Thymus vulgaris* ct. thymol [THYME] — sore throat, tonsillitis (Franchomme & Pénoël 1990, p. 274)

RENAL CLEANSER

Arbutus uva ursi [BEARBERRY]	(Viaud 1983)
Arctostaphyllos (unspecified) [BEARBERRY]	renal drainage (Baudoux 1996a)
Juniperus communis [JUNIPER]	kidney deflocculant (Viaud 1983)

RESPIRATORY

Eucalyptus globulus [TASMANIAN BLUE GUM]	(Viaud 1983; Grosjean 1993a, p. 66)
Eucalyptus polybractea [BLUE LEAVED MALLEE]	bronchial mucosa (Baudoux 1996a)
Eupatorium cannabinum [HEMP AGRIMONY]	pulmonary
Galega officinalis [GOAT'S RUE]	respiratory mucous membranes (Viaud 1983)
Helichrysum italicum [EVERLASTING]	pulmonary depurative (Viaud 1983)
Hyssopus officinalis [HYSSOP]	Viaud (1983) advises the use of low dose to clear the lungs
Inula graveolens [ELECAMPANE]	strong respiratory tonic; powerful mucolytic and expectorant, bronchitis, cough (Catty 2001, p. 99), bronchial support (Baudoux 1996a)
Pinus sylvestris [SCOTS PINE]	(Grosjean 1993a, p. 66; Catty 2001, p. 121)
Sarothamnus scoparius [BROOM]	lungs (Viaud 1983)
Thymus vulgaris [THYME]	(Grosjean 1993a, p. 66)

RHEUMATISM

Juniperus communis [JUNIPER]	(Grosjean 1993a, pp. 55, 66)
Pinus sylvestris [PINE]	(Grosjean 1993a, pp. 55, 66)
Thymus vulgaris [THYME]	(Grosjean 1993a, pp. 55, 66)
Tilia sylvestris (lig.) [LIME SAPWOOD]	(Viaud 1983)

SEDATIVE

Cistus ladaniferus [ROCK ROSE]	induces deep relaxation (Franchomme & Pénoël 1990, p. 300)
Matricaria recutita [GERMAN CHAMOMILE]	(Catty 2001, p. 108)
Prunus laurocerasus [CHERRY LAUREL]	
Valeriana wallichii [VALERIAN]	(Franchomme & Pénoël 1990, p. 286)

SHINGLES

Tilia × *europa* [LIME LEAF]	(Rose 1999, p. 171)

SKIN CARE

Aloysia triphylla [LEMON VERBENA]	revitalizing, normal skin (Rose 1999, p. 173; Catty 2001, p. 107)
Cedrus atlantica [ATLAS CEDAR]	weeping, cracked skin (Catty 2001, p. 80)
Cupressus sempervirens [CYPRESS]	red blotches
Fumaria officinalis [FUMITORY]	cleansing agent (Kresanek 1982, p. 90)
Hamamelis virginiana [WITCH HAZEL]	red blotches
Helichrysum italicum [EVERLASTING]	red blotches
Lavandula angustifolia [LAVENDER]	add to deep cleansing (clay) masks, calming lotion for greasy skin (Rouvière & Meyer 1989, pp. 94–96), universal toner (Rose 1999, p. 170) cleansing, healing, all skin types; (Rouvière & Meyer 1989, pp. 91–92; Baudoux 1996a)
Levisticum officinale [LOVAGE]	drains fluid (Viaud 1983)
Matricaria recutita [GERMAN CHAMOMILE]	red blotches, inflamed skin (naturesgift.com/hydrosols)
Melaleuca alternifolia [TEA TREE]	infections (Catty, 2001, p. 109)
Melissa officinalis [LEMON BALM]	externally and internally for *Herpes simplex* (Catty 2001, p. 111)
Mentha × *piperita* [PEPPERMINT]	tonic, refreshing (Baudoux 1996a)
Pelargonium graveolens [GERANIUM]	cell regenerator (Rose 1999, p. 174)
Potentilla anserina [SILVERWEED]	facial tonic (Grieve 1992, p. 741)

Rosa damascena [DAMASK ROSE]	all skin types (Rose 1999, p. 171), broken veins, wrinkles, sensitive skin, dermatitis, sunburn (Bego 1995; Goëb 1998; Sanoflore 2000; 6scent; naturesgift.com/hydrosols; Nasr 2000, p. 27)
Rosmarinus officinalis [ROSEMARY]	revitalizes skin (Rose 1999, p. 174)
Thymus serpyllum [WILD THYME]	skin problems
Thymus vulgaris [THYME]	add to deep cleansing (clay) masks (Rouviére & Meyer 1989, p.94)
Tilia × europaea [LIME LEAF]	cleansing all skin types
Urtica dioica [NETTLE]	(Viaud 1983)

– Acne

Achillea millefolium [YARROW]	(Catty 1998a; Rose 1999, p. 171)
Cedrus atlantica [ATLAS CEDAR]	(Grosjean 1993b, p. 87)
Daucus carota (sem.) [CARROT SEED]	(Catty 2001, pp. 89–90)
Eucalyptus globulus [TASMANIAN BLUE GUM]	(Rose 1999, p. 172)
Inula graveolens [ELECAMPANE]	calms acne (Catty 2001, p. 99)
Juniperus communis [JUNIPER]	(Viaud 1983)
Lavandula angustifolia [LAVENDER]	(Grosjean 1993b, p. 87), teenage acne (Baudoux 1996b, p. 44)
Lavandula × intermedia ct. borneol [LAVANDIN]	(Rose 1999, p. 170)
Mentha × piperita [PEPPERMINT]	teenage acne (Baudoux 1996b, p. 44; Rose 1999, p. 174)
Rosmarinus officinalis [ROSEMARY]	teenage acne (Baudoux 1996b, p. 44)
Salvia officinalis [SAGE]	antiseptic, healing for oily, acneic skin (Baudoux 1996a)
Thymus vulgaris [THYME]	(Grosjean 1993b, p. 87; Rose 1999, p. 174)

– Aftershave

Cistus ladaniferus [ROCK ROSE]	(Catty 2001, p. 84)
Daucus carota (sem.) [CARROT SEED]	(Catty 2001, p. 90)
Hamamelis virginiana [WITCH HAZEL]	(Keville & Green 1995)
Lavandula angustifolia [LAVENDER]	soothing, (Rouviére & Meyer 1989, p. 121; Grosjean 1993b, pp. 87, 95, 114)
Laurus nobilis [BAY]	(Rose 1999, p. 172)
Mentha spicata [SPEARMINT]	(Rouviére & Meyer, 1989, p. 121)
Origanum majorana [SWEET MARJORAM]	
Rosmarinus officinalis [ROSEMARY]	soothing (Grosjean 1993b, pp. 87, 95, 114)

– Bedsores, Scars

Chamaemelum nobile [ROMAN CHAMOMILE]	(Baudoux 1996b, p. 49)
Laurus nobilis [BAY]	(Baudoux 1996b, p. 49)
Rosa damascena [DAMASK ROSE]	(Baudoux 1996b, p. 49)
Thymus vulgaris ct. thujanol-4 [SWEET THYME]	(Baudoux 1996b, p. 49)

– Cellulite

Achillea millefolium [YARROW]	(Rose 1999, p. 171)

– Dry Skin

Chamaemelum nobile [ROMAN CHAMOMILE]	dry, irritated skins (Claeys 1992; Grosjean 1993b, p. 87; Battaglia 1995, p. 425; Sanaflore 2000)
Citrus aurantium [ORANGE FLOWER]	calms, rebalances dry skins (Rose 1999, p. 171; Sanoflore 2000)
Lavandula angustifolia [LAVENDER]	(Grosjean 1993b, pp. 57, 87), softening (Rouvière & Meyer, 1989, p. 101)
Mentha spicata [SPEARMINT]	toner (Rouvière & Meyer 1989, p. 99)
Pelargonium graveolens [GERANIUM]	balances oil glands (Rose 1999, p. 174; Catty 2001, p. 109)
Rosa canina [WILD ROSE]	(Grosjean 1993b, pp. 57, 87)
Rosmarinus officinalis [ROSEMARY]	(Grosjean 1993b, pp. 57, 87) cleanser, toner (Rouvière & Meyer 1989, p. 97)

Salvia officinalis [SAGE]	cleanser, toner (Rouvière & Meyer 1989, p. 99)
Salvia sclarea [CLARY]	(Grosjean 1993b, p. 57). Note: given for oily skin by Rose (1999, p. 172)
Thymus vulgaris [THYME]	(Grosjean 1993b, p. 87)
Thymus vulgaris ct. linalool [SWEET THYME]	

– Eczema

Calendula officinalis [MARIGOLD]	(Viaud 1983)
Daucus carota (sem.) [CARROT SEED]	(Catty 2001, pp. 89–90)
Hamamelis virginiana [WITCH HAZEL]	(Catty 2001, p. 96)
Lavandula angustifolia [LAVENDER]	(Keville & Green 1995)
Saponaria officinalis [SOAPWORT]	furuncles (Viaud 1983)
Thymus vulgaris [THYME]	(Rose 1999, p. 174)
Thymus vulgaris ct. thujanol-4 [SWEET THYME]	(Baudoux 1996a)

– Freckles

Anagallis arvensis [SCARLET PIMPERNEL]	(Stuart 1987, p. 151)
Anemone hepatica [AMERICAN LIVERWORT]	(Stuart 1987, p. 152)
Polygonatum multiflorum [SOLOMON'S SEAL]	(Culpeper, n.d. p. 339; Claire 1961, p. 240)
Sambucus nigra [ELDERFLOWER]	skin blemishes (Grieve 1992, p. 272)

– Herpes

Lavandula × intermedia ct. borneol [LAVANDIN]	(Rose 1999, p. 173)
Melissa officinalis [LEMON BALM]	(Rose 1999, p. 173)

– Oily

Achillea millefolium [YARROW]	(Keville & Green 1995)
Aloysia triphylla [LEMON VERBENA]	(Keville & Green 1995)
Cedrus atlantica [ATLAS CEDAR]	cleanse spots, (Grosjean 1993b, p. 57)
Citrus aurantium var. *amara* (flos) [BITTER ORANGE FLOWER]	toner, (Goëb 1998), skin of nervous, stressed people (Bego 1995)
Cupressus sempervirens [CYPRESS]	cleanse spots,
Hamamelis virginiana [WITCH HAZEL]	astringent for oily, couperose skin (Keville & Green 1995), astringent, teenage skin (Catty 2001, p. 96)
Inula graveolens [ELECAMPANE]	oily skin of hepatic origin (Baudoux 1996a; Catty 2001, p. 99)
Juniperus communis [JUNIPER]	(Viaud 1983)
Juniperus communis (fruct) [JUNIPER BERRY]	(Rose 1999, p. 173)
Lavandula angustifolia [LAVENDER]	(Grosjean 1993b, p. 57; Sanoflore 2000)
Pelargonium graveolens [GERANIUM]	balances oil glands (Rose 1999, p. 174; Catty 2001, p. 109)
Rosmarinus officinalis ct. verbenone [ROSEMARY VERBENONE]	cleansing (Baudoux 1996a)
Salvia officinalis [SAGE]	(Rouvière & Meyer 1989, p. 93)
Salvia sclarea [CLARY]	acneic, greasy skin (Claeys 1992)
Thymus vulgaris [THYME]	

– Psoriasis

Cedrus atlantica [ATLAS CEDAR]	(Catty 2001, p. 80)
Chamaemelum nobile [ROMAN CHAMOMILE]	(Baudoux 1996b, p. 52)
Daucus carota (sem.) [CARROT SEED]	(Catty 2001, pp. 89–90)
Lavandula angustifolia [LAVENDER]	(Keville & Green 1995)
Rosa damascena [DAMASK ROSE]	(Baudoux 1996b, p. 52)
Rosmarinus officinalis ct. verbenone [ROSEMARY VERBENONE]	(Baudoux 1996b, p. 52)

– Scars

Cedrus atlantica [ATLAS CEDAR]	(Grosjean 1993b, p. 95)
Hamamelis virginiana [WITCH HAZEL]	(Catty 2001, p. 96)

Lavandula angustifolia [LAVENDER] (Grosjean 1993b, p. 95)
Rosa canina [WILD ROSE] (Grosjean 1993b, p. 95)

– Sensitive: Redness: Irritation

Artemisia arborescens [TREE WORMWOOD]
Centaurea cyanus [CORNFLOWER] dry, inflamed skin, bruises (Rose 1999, p. 170)
Chamaemelum nobile [ROMAN CHAMOMILE] irritated skin (Grosjean 1993b, pp. 87; Rose 1999, p. 170)
Citrus aurantium var. *amara* (flos) [BITTER ORANGE BLOSSOM] couperose, dry or sensitive skin; soothes (Keville & Green 1995, Baudoux 1996a)
Cupressus sempervirens [CYPRESS] venous circulation, couperose skin, varicose veins, heavy legs (Baudoux 1996a), redness (AGORA), couperose (Rouvière & Meyer 1989, p. 105)
Hamamelis virginiana [WITCH HAZEL] redness (AGORA)
Helichrysum italicum [EVERLASTING] rosacea, broken veins, inflamed skin (naturesgift.com/hydrosols), redness (AGORA)
Lavandula angustifolia [LAVENDER] irritated skin (Grosjean 1993b, p. 87), soothing, couperose (Rouvière & Meyer 1989, pp. 94, 105)
Matricaria recutita [GERMAN CHAMOMILE] sensitive skin, inflamed (Keville & Green 1995), redness (AGORA; Rose 1999, p. 170)
Melissa officinalis [LEMON BALM] sensitive skin (Keville & Green 1995)
Myrtus communis [MYRTLE] allergic reactions (Keville & Green 1995), irritations (Rose 1999, p. 173)
Robinia pseudoacacia [FALSE ACACIA] capillary problems (skin) (Viaud 1983)
Rosa damascena [DAMASK ROSE] mildly astringent for couperose skin, suitable for all skin types; for irritated eyes (Keville & Green 1995)
Rosmarinus officinalis [ROSEMARY] sluggish, sallow, devitalized skin that needs stimulation and regeneration (Keville & Green 1995)

– Sun: Sunburn

Anemone hepatica [AMERICAN LIVERWORT] (Stuart 1987, p. 152)
Cedrus atlantica [ATLAS CEDAR] after sun (Grosjean 1993b, pp. 87, 95)
Hamamelis virginiana [WITCH HAZEL] heals cracked or blistered skin (Catty 2001, p. 96), sunburn, insect bites (Ody 1997)
Lavandula angustifolia [LAVENDER] irritations (Grosjean 1993b, p. 87; Keville & Green 1995; naturesgift.com/hydrosols)
Matricaria recutita [GERMAN CHAMOMILE] (Catty 2001, p. 108; naturesgift.com/hydrosols)
Mentha × piperita [PEPPERMINT] cooling after sun (Grosjean 1993b, p. 87)
Pelargonium graveolens [GERANIUM] (naturesgift.com/hydrosols), sunstroke
Rosmarinus officinalis [ROSEMARY] after sun (Grosjean 1993b, p. 87)
Sambucus nigra [ELDERFLOWER] (Grieve 1992, p. 272)
Thymus vulgaris [THYME] after sun (Grosjean 1993b, pp. 87, 95)

– Wrinkled and mature skin

Achillea millefolium [YARROW] (C. Montesinos, personal communication, 2001)
Chamaemelum nobile [ROMAN CHAMOMILE] antiwrinkle (Grosjean 1993b, p. 57), rejuvenating tonic (Grosjean 1993b, pp. 87, 95, 114)
Cistus ladaniferus [ROCK ROSE] astringent, antiwrinkle (Baudoux 1996a; Catty 2001, p. 84)
Citrus aurantium var. *amara* (flos) [BITTER ORANGE FLOWER] mature skin (innerself.com/magazine/herbs/essential_oils 2001), wrinkled skin (sabia.com 1997–1999), for nervous stressed persons with drawn features (Goëb 1998)
Cupressus sempervirens [CYPRESS] rejuvenating tonic (Grosjean 1993b, pp. 87, 95, 114)
Daucus carota (sem.) [CARROT SEED] (naturesgift.com/hydrosols), rejuvenating (Grosjean 1993b, pp. 87, 95)
Hamamelis virginiana [WITCH HAZEL] mature, damaged skin (Catty 2001, p. 96)
Helichrysum italicum [EVERLASTING] rejuvenating (damaged, mature skin), inflamed skin (Keville & Green 1995)

Lavandula angustifolia [LAVENDER]	antiwrinkle (Grosjean 1993b, p. 57), rejuvenating tonic (Grosjean 1993b, pp. 87, 95, 114)
Rosa canina [WILD ROSE]	rejuvenating tonic (Grosjean 1993b, pp. 87, 114)
Rosa damascena [DAMASK ROSE]	antiwrinkle for many skins (Baudoux 1996a; C. Montesinos, personal communication, 2001)
Rosmarinus officinalis [ROSEMARY]	antiwrinkle (Grosjean 1993b, p. 57), rejuvenating tonic (Grosjean 1993b, pp. 87, 95, 114)
Salvia officinalis [SAGE]	rejuvenating tonic (Grosjean 1993b, pp. 87, 95, 114; C. Montesinos personal communication, 2001)
Thymus vulgaris [THYME]	rejuvenating tonic (Grosjean 1993b, pp. 87, 95, 114)

SLIMMING

Foeniculum vulgare var. *dulce* (sem.) [FENNEL]	slimming drink
Juniperus communis [JUNIPER]	slimming drink (Grosjean 1993b, p. 36)

STOMACH

Artemisia dracunculus [TARRAGON]	(Paris 2000)
Eucalyptus polybractea [BLUE LEAVED MALLEE]	stomach ulcer (Baudoux 1996b, p. 29)
Lavandula angustifolia [LAVENDER]	(Paris 2000)
Mentha × *piperita* [PEPPERMINT]	(Payne 1999)
Myrtus communis [MYRTLE]	stomach ulcer (Baudoux 1996b, p. 29)
Ocimum basilicum [BASIL]	(Paris 2000)
Rosemary officinalis ct. verbenone [ROSEMARY VERBENONE]	(Paris 2000)
Thymus vulgaris ct. thujanol-4 [SWEET THYME]	stomach ulcer (Baudoux 1996b, p. 29)

STYPTIC, ANTIHAEMORRHAGIC

Cupressus sempervirens [CYPRESS]	(Catty 2001, p. 88)
Cistus ladaniferus [ROCK ROSE]	(Baudoux 1996a, 1996b, p. 64; Catty 2001, p. 84)
Erigeron canadensis [FLEABANE]	(uterine, nasal) (Viaud 1983)
Hamamelis virginiana [WITCH HAZEL]	haemostatic (small wounds), veterinary medicine (Bartram 1995, Lower 1999)
Lavandula angustifolia [LAVENDER]	(Baudoux 1996b, p. 64)
Rosa damascena [DAMASK ROSE]	(Baudoux 1996b, p. 64)

SWOLLEN LYMPH GLANDS

Laurus nobilis [BAY LEAF]	(Catty 1998)

THRUSH

Lavandula angustifolia [LAVENDER]	*Candida albicans* (C. Marshall, personal communication, 12 July 1998)
Melaleuca alternifolia [TEA TREE]	*Candida albicans* (C. Marshall, personal communication, 12 July 1998)

THYROID

Aloysia triphylla [LEMON VERBENA]	thyroid stimulant (Catty 2001, p. 107)
Fucus vesiculosus [BLADDERWRACK]	thyroid stimulant

URINARY

Thymus vulgaris ct. linalol [SWEET THYME]	urinary infections (Paris 2000)

VACCINATIONS

Laurus nobilis [BAY LEAF]	prophylactic to side-effects (Catty 1998a)

VARICOSE VEINS see also **CIRCULATION**

Achillea millefolium [YARROW]	
Cupressus sempervirens [CYPRESS]	(Viaud 1983) haemorrhoids, venous congestion (Baudoux 1996a)
Hamamelis virginiana [WITCH HAZEL]	haemorrhoids (Mabey 1988; Grieve 1992, p. 851; Rose 1999, p. 174; Catty 2001, p. 96)

VERMIFUGE

Lactuca hortensis [LETTUCE]	(Viaud 1983)
Santolina chamaecyparissus [COTTON LAVENDER]	(Viaud 1983)

VOMITING

Rosa damascena [DAMASK ROSE]	nausea (Fischer-Rizzi 1990, p. 58)
Tilia × *europaea* [LIME LEAF]	nervous (Grieve 1992, p. 486)

WORMS

– Enterobiasis (oxyuriasis, Threadworms)

Chamaemelum nobile [ROMAN CHAMOMILE]	(Baudoux 1996b, p. 34)
Thymus vulgaris ct. thujanol-4 [SWEET THYME]	(Baudoux 1996b, p. 34)

– Ascariasis: Giardiasis (Lambliasis)

Chamaemelum nobile [ROMAN CHAMOMILE]	(Baudoux 1996b, p. 34)
Satureia montana [WINTER SAVORY]	(Baudoux 1996b, p. 34)
Thymus vulgaris ct. thujanol-4 [SWEET THYME]	(Baudoux 1996b, p. 34)

WOUNDS

Lavandula angustifolia [LAVENDER]	newly pierced ears, cuts, helps to heal
Thymus vulgaris [THYME]	

APPENDIX B

Therapeutic properties of hydrolats: Quick reference

Therapeutic references have been gathered from almost all available books on aromatherapy to include in this book and it is impossible not to be struck by randomness of choice of hydrolat. It must be remembered that at its present stage of development aromatherapy is still largely an art arising out of folklore and tradition, and this applies particularly to the hydrolats, which have not been much used in the last half century.

Plant hydrolat	*Properties*
Abies balsamea [CANADA BALSAM]	analgesic immunostimulant mucolytic, antitussive
Acacia decurrens [MIMOSA]	hepatic depurative (Viaud 1983)
Achillea millefolium [YARROW]	anticellulite (Rose 1999, p. 171) antiinflammatory (Rose 1999, p. 171) antiseptic – acneic skin (Catty 1998a) antiseptic (Keville & Green 1995; Rose 1999, p. 171) astringent (Keville & Green 1995) circulatory varicose veins wrinkled, mature skin (C. Montesinos, personal communication, 2001)
Agaricus campestris [FIELD MUSHROOM]	antiallergic (Viaud 1983) hepatic (Viaud 1983)
Aloysia triphylla [LEMON VERBENA]	aids sleep (Rose 1999, p. 173) antiinflammatory (Catty 2001, p. 107) astringent (mild) (Keville & Green 1995) mouthwash (Catty 2001, p. 107) PMS (Catty 2001, p. 107) relaxing (Paris 2000; Catty 2001, p. 107) revitalizing, normal skin (Rose 1999, p. 173; Catty 2001, p. 107) soporific (Grosjean 1993a, p. 66) stimulant (Rose 1999, p. 173) thyroid stimulant (Catty 2001, p. 107)
Anagallis arvensis [SCARLET PIMPERNEL]	freckles (Stuart 1987 p. 151)
Anemone hepatica [AMERICAN LIVERWORT]	antiinflammatory (sunburn) (Stuart 1987, p. 152) freckles, sunburn (Stuart 1987, p. 152)
Anethum graveolens [DILL]	flatulence, hiccups
Angelica archangelica [ANGELICA]	digestive, sedative (Catty 1998a, p. 76)
Apium graveolens [WILD CELERY]	anticancer (Viaud 1983)

	carminative (Viaud 1983)
	diuretic (Viaud 1983)
Arbutus uva ursi [BEARBERRY]	antiseptic (Viaud 1983)
	renal depurative (Viaud 1983)
Arctostaphyllos (unspecified) [BEARBERRY]	renal depurative (Baudoux 1996a)
Artemisia arborescens [GREAT MUGWORT]	antiinflammatory (Rose 1999, p. 170)
	antispasmodic (Rose 1999, p. 170)
	energizing, uplifting
	stomachic
	sensitive skin
Artemisia abrotanum [SOUTHERNWOOD]	energizing, uplifting (Viaud 1983)
Artemisia dracunculus [TARRAGON]	analgesic (Viaud 1983)
	anticancerous (Viaud 1983)
	arthritis (Rose 1999, p. 170)
	carminative (Catty 2001, p. 76)
	colic (Catty 2001, p. 76)
	digestive spasm (Catty 2001, p. 76)
	stomachic (Paris 2000)
Artemisia vulgaris [MUGWORT]	antiparasitic (Catty 2001, p. 77)
	circulatory stimulant (Catty 2001, p. 77)
	energetic, vibrational healing (Catty 2001, p. 77)
Buxus sempervirens [BOX]	anticancer (Viaud 1983)
	tonic (hair and scalp) (Montesinos 1991)
Calendula officinalis [CALENDULA]	antibacterial (Viaud 1983)
	eczema (Viaud 1983)
	hypotensor Viaud (1983)
	ophthalmic (inflamed eyes) (Grieve 1992, p. 518)
Carum carvi [CARAWAY]	carminative (Grieve 1998, p. 158)
Cedrus atlantica [ATLAS CEDAR]	anti acne (Grosjean 1993b, p. 87)
	antidandruff (Catty 2001, p. 80)
	antirritant (Catty 2001, p. 80)
	antiseptic (Grosjean 1993b, p. 57)
	cicatrizant (Grosjean 1993b, p. 95; Catty 2001, p. 80)
	diuretic (Catty 2001, p. 80)
	psoriasis (Catty 2001, p. 80)
Centaurea cyanus [CORNFLOWER]	antiinfectious (Grieve 1998, p. 224)
	antiinflammatory (Rose 1999, p. 170)
	antiseptic, antiinfectious (Grieve 1998, p. 224)
	astringent
	bruises (Catty 2001, p. 81)
	ophthalmic (Rouvière & Meyer 1989, p. 106; Grosjean 1993b, pp. 95, 114; Payne 1999; C. Montesinos, personal communication, 2001)
Chamaemelum nobile [ROMAN CHAMOMILE]	analgesic (Franchomme & Pénoël 1996, p. 86)
	anthelmintic (Baudoux 1996b, p. 34)
	antiinfectious, urinary tract infections
	antimigraine (www.naturesgift.com/hydrosols)
	antiparasitic (C. Montesinos, personal communication 2001)
	antispasmodic (Franchomme & Pénoël 1996, p. 86)
	calming (Paris 2000; Sanaflore 2000)
	cicatrizant (Claeys 1992; Baudoux 1996b, p. 49)
	cutaneous antiallergic (Bego 1995)
	cutaneous antiinflammatory (Bego 1995; Goëb 1998; Rose 1999, p. 170; Catty 2001, p. 83)
	dry skin (Claeys 1992; Grosjean 1993b, p. 87; Battaglia 1995, p. 425; Sanaflore 2000)

	ophthalmic (Franchomme & Pénoël 1990, pp. 287, 303; Grosjean 1993b, pp. 87, 95, 114; Bego 1995; Baudoux 1996b, p. 101; Goëb 1998; Payne 1999; Catty 2001, p. 83; C. Montesinos, personal communication 2001)
	psoriasis (Baudoux 1996b, p. 52)
	regenerating (Grosjean 1993b, pp. 57, 87, 95, 114)
	soothing (skin) (Grosjean 1993b, p. 87; Rose 1999, p. 170)
	stomachic, intestinal disorders (Fischer-Rizzi 1990, p. 58)
Chelidonium majus [GREATER CELANDINE]	ophthalmic (calming) (C. Montesinos, personal communication, 2001)
Chenopodium album [FAT HEN]	anthelmintic (Viaud 1983)
Cistus ladaniferus [ROCK ROSE]	antiviral (Franchomme & Pénoël 1990, p. 286; Baudoux 1996a)
	antihaemorrhagic (Baudoux 1996a; Baudoux 1996b, p. 64)
	astringent (Baudoux 1996a; Catty 2001, p. 84)
	cicatrizant (Baudoux 1996a; Catty 2001, p. 84)
	fibroma (Franchomme & Pénoël 1990, p. 279; Baudoux 1996b, p. 85)
	immunostimulant (Catty 2001, p. 84)
	ophthalmic (watering eyes) (Baudoux 1996b, p. 101)
	sedative (Franchomme & Pénoël 1990, p. 300)
	soothing (skin) (Catty 2001, p. 84)
	styptic (Catty 2001, p. 84)
Citrus aurantium var. *amara* (flos) [BITTER ORANGE FLOWER]	antiseptic (Catty 2001, p. 86)
	antispasmodic (Catty 2001, p. 86)
	calming (Grieve 1992, p. 602; Goëb 1998; sabia.com 1997–1999; Paris 2000; Catty 2001, p. 85)
	digestive, choleretic, eupeptic (Catty 2001, p. 86)
	dry skin (Rose 1999, p. 171; Sanoflore 2000)
	ophthalmic (dryness) (Baudoux 1996b, p. 101)
	soothing and calming (skin) (Keville & Green 1995, Baudoux 1996a)
	soporific (Franchomme & Pénoël 1990, p. 286)
Citrus aurantium var. amara (fol.) [PETITGRAIN]	insomnia (Franchomme & Pénoël 1990, p. 286)
Citrus aurantium var. *sinensis* (flos) [SWEET ORANGE FLOWER]	antiseptic (Viaud 1983)
	antispasmodic (Nasr 2000, p. 26)
	cardiac calmative, SAD (Viaud 1983), calming nervine (Baudoux 1996a; Nasr 2000, p. 26)
	carminative (Nasr 2000, p. 26)
Coriandrum sativum [CORIANDER]	carminative (Grieve 1992, p. 222)
Cotyledon umbilicus [KIDNEYWORT]	antiinflammatory (digestive system, facial spots), kidney stones, gout, sciatica (Culpeper n.d., p. 206)
Crataegus monogyna [HAWTHORN]	hypotensor (Fischer-Rizzi 1990, p. 58)
	relaxing (Paris 2000)
Crataegus oxyacantha [HAWTHORN]	antidepressive (Viaud 1983)
	cardiac calmative (Viaud 1983)
	soporific (Baudoux 1996a)
Cuminum cyminum [CUMIN]	antibacterial (Sağadiç & Özcan 2003)
Cupressus sempervirens [CYPRESS]	antiseptic
	astringent (Catty 2001, p. 88)
	cicatrizant (Grosjean 1993b, p. 87)
	circulatory (Viaud 1983; Paris 2000; Catty 2001, p. 89)
	diuretic (Catty 2001, p. 88)
	regenerating (skin) (Grosjean 1993b, pp. 87, 95, 114)
	styptic (Catty 2001, p. 88)
	venous congestion, varicose veins (Baudoux 1996a)

Daucus carota (sem.) [CARROT SEED]	anti acne (Catty 2001, pp. 89–90)
	antiinflammatory (Catty 2001, pp. 89–90)
	eczema (Catty 2001, pp. 89–90)
	psoriasis (Catty 2001, pp. 89–90)
	regenerating tonic (Grosjean 1993b, pp. 87, 95)
	soothing (skin) (Catty 2001, p. 90)
Dictamnus albus [BURNING BUSH, DITTANY]	used as a cosmetic
Echinaceae purpurea [PURPLE CONEFLOWER]	immumostimulant (Price, use on clients)
Elettaria cardamomum [CARDAMOM]	calms digestive system, relaxing (Catty 2001, p. 91)
Erigeron canadensis [FLEABANE]	antihaemorrhagic (Viaud 1983)
	circulatory (Viaud 1983, Paris 2000)
Eucalyptus dives [BROAD LEAVED PEPPERMINT]	mucolytic (Franchomme & Pénoël 1990 p. 302)
Eucalyptus globulus [TASMANIAN BLUE GUM]	anti acne (Rose 1999, p. 172)*Eucalyptus globulus*
	antidiabetic (Viaud 1983)
	bronchitis (Catty 1998)
	mucolytic (bronchial) (Viaud 1983; Grosjean 1993a, p. 66)
	ophthalmic (conjunctivitis) (Franchomme & Pénoël 1990, p. 287)
Eucalyptus polybractea [BLUE LEAVED MALLEE]	bronchitis (Catty 1998)
	condyloma (Baudoux 1996b, p. 86)
	leucorrhoea (Baudoux 1996b, p. 79)
	mucolytic (bronchial) (Baudoux 1996a)
	stomach ulcer (Baudoux 1996b, p. 29)
	uterine dysplasia (Baudoux 1996b, p. 87)
Eupatorium cannabinum [HEMP AGRIMONY]	chronic cystitis antiinflammatory
	pulmonary depurative
Euphrasia officinalis [EYEBRIGHT]	opthalmic (Culpeper n.d. p. 134)
Filipendula ulmaria [MEADOWSWEET]	febrifuge
	ophthalmic (inflammation) (Gerard in Woodward 1964, p. 245; Culpeper n.d., p. 230)
Foeniculum vulgare var. *dulce* (sem.) [FENNEL]	antiseptic (Viaud 1983; Rose 1999, p. 173)
	carminative (Grieve 1992, p. 296)
	digestive, stomachic (Rose 1999, p. 173)
	galactogen (Viaud 1983)
	ophthalmic (Rose 1999, p. 173)
Fragaria vesca [STRAWBERRY]	uplifting (Gerard 1964 p. 237)
Fucus vesiculosus [BLADDERWRACK]	thyroid stimulant
Fumaria officinalis [FUMITORY]	cleansing, purifying (Grieve 1998 p. 330, Kresanek 1982, p. 90)
Galega officinalis [GOAT'S RUE]	anticancer – breast abscess, pancreas, antitoxins (Viaud 1983)
	antidiabetic (Viaud 1983)
	antitoxic (Viaud 1983)
	pancreatic (Viaud 1983)
	respiratory mucous membranes (Viaud 1983)
Gentiana lutea [YELLOW GENTIAN]	energizing, uplifting (Viaud 1983)
Hamamelis virginiana [WITCH HAZEL]	analgesic (rheumatic pain) (Catty 2001, p. 96)
	antifungal (Rose 1999, p. 174)
	antiinflammatory (Korting et al 1993; Rose 1999, p. 174; Catty 2001, p. 96)
	antioxidant (Catty 2001, p. 96)
	antiseptic (Rose 1999, p. 174; Catty 2001, p. 96)
	astringent (Bartram 1995; Keville & Green 1995; Winter 1999, p. 458; Sanoflore 2000; Catty 2001, p. 96
	cicatrizant (Catty 2001, p. 96)
	circulatory, haemorrhoids (Mabey 1988; Grieve 1992, p. 851; Rose 1999, p. 174; Catty 2001, p. 96)

	diuretic (Catty 2001, p. 96)
	eczema (Catty 2001, p. 96)
	haemostatic (Bartram 1995, Lower 1999)
Harpagophytum procumbens [DEVIL'S CLAW]	anticancerous (Viaud 1983)
Helichrysum italicum [EVERLASTING]	antidiabetic (Viaud 1983)
	antiinflammatory (naturesgift.com/hydrosols; Catty 1998a)
	cardiac calmative (Rose 1999, p. 172)
	carminative, aerophagy (Viaud 1983)
	cicatrizant (Keville & Green 1995; Rose 1999, p. 172; Catty 2001)
	hepatic (Rose 1999, p. 172)
	pulmonary depurative (Viaud 1983)
	soothing (Keville & Green 1995; Rose 1999, p. 172)
	regenerative (skin) (Keville & Green 1995)
Hieracium pilosella [MOUSE EAR]	diuretic (Viaud 1983)
	litholytic (urinary stones) (Viaud 1983)
Hypericum perforatum [ST JOHN'S WORT]	anticancerous (Viaud 1983)
	ophthalmic (conjunctivitis) (Franchomme & Pénoël 1990, p. 303)
Hyssopus officinalis [HYSSOP]	lung depurative (Viaud 1983)
Inula graveolens [ELECAMPANE]	bronchitis (Catty 1998a)
	calms acne (Catty 2001, p. 99)
	candidiasis (Baudoux 1996b, p. 80)
	cardiac (Baudoux 1996a)
	expectorant (Catty 2001, p. 99)
	hepatic stimulant (Catty 2001, p. 99)
	mucolytic, expectorant (Baudoux 1996a; Catty 2001, p. 99)
	ophthalmic (conjunctivitis) (Baudoux 1996b, p. 101)
	vaginitis (Baudoux 1996b, p. 82)
Iris pseudacorus [IRIS]	ophthalmic (weak eyes) (Culpeper, 1652, cited in Grieve 1992, p. 439)
Juglans regia [WALNUT]	antidiabetic (Viaud 1983)
Juniperus communis [JUNIPER]	antirheumatic (Grosjean 1993a, pp. 55, 66)
	astringent (Viaud 1983)
	circulatory (Grosjean 1993b, p. 54; Rose 1999, p. 173)
	diuretic (Viaud 1983)
	renal depurative (Viaud 1983)
Juniperus communis (fruct.) [JUNIPER BERRY]	astringent (Rose 1999, p. 173)
	circulatory (Catty 2001, p. 101)
	diuretic (Rose 1999, p. 173; Catty 2001, p. 101)
	energizing, uplifting (Rose 1999, p. 173)
Lactuca hortensis [LETTUCE]	anthelmintic (Viaud 1983)
	hepatic depurative (Viaud 1983)
Lactuca virosa [WILD LETTUCE]	hepatic depurative (Viaud 1983)
Lamium album [DEAD NETTLE]	uplifting, refreshing (Gerard 1964, p. 158)
Laurus nobilis [BAY LEAF]	analgesic (Franchomme & Pénoël 1990; p. 281)
	antibacterial (Baudoux 1996a, p. 108)
	antifungal *Candida albicans* (C. Marshall, personal communication, 1998)
	antiinfectious, (Franchomme & Pénoël 1990, p. 281)
	antiinflammatory (Baudoux 1996b, p. 96)
	antiparasitic (lice) (C. Montesinos, personal communication, 2001)
	antispasmodic (Viaud 1983)
	carminative (Viaud 1983)
	cicatrizant (Baudoux 1996a, 1996b, p. 49)
	digestive (Viaud 1983; Rose 1999, p. 172; Paris 2000)

Plant	Uses
	intestinal antiseptic (Viaud 1983) leucorrhoea (Baudoux 1996b, p. 79) lymphatic (Catty 2001, p. 103) ophthalmic (infections) (Baudoux 1996b, p. 101) soothing (skin) (Rose 1999, p. 172) vaginitis (Baudoux 1996b, p. 82)
Lavandula angustifolia [LAVENDER]	anti acne (Grosjean 1993b, p. 87; Baudoux 1996b, p. 44) antiinflammatory (Baudoux 1996b, p. 96) antihaemorrhagic (Baudoux 1996b, p. 64) antiparasitic (lice) (C. Montesinos, personal communication, 2001) antiseptic (Fischer-Rizzi 1990, p. 58; Baudoux 1996a) candidiasis (Baudoux 1996b, p. 80) cicatrizant (Rouvière & Meyer 1989, pp. 91–92; Claeys 1992; Grosjean 1993b, pp. 87, 95; Baudoux 1996a) dry skin (Rouvière & Meyer 1989, p. 101; Grosjean 1993b, pp. 57, 87) eczema (Keville & Green 1995) fibroma (Baudoux 1996b, p. 85) leucorrhoea (Baudoux 1996b, p. 79) ophthalmic (wateriness) (Baudoux 1996b, p. 101) (Rouvière & Meyer, 1989, p. 106) psoriasis (Keville & Green 1995) regenerating (Grosjean 1993b, pp. 57, 87, 95, 114) relaxing, soothing (Paris 2000) soothing (skin) (Rouvière & Meyer, 1989, p. 121; Grosjean 1993b, pp. 87, 95, 114) stomachic (Paris 2000) tonic (scalp) (Montesinos 1991) uterine dysplasia (Baudoux 1996b, p. 87) vaginitis (Baudoux 1996b, p. 82)
Lavandula × *intermedia* ct. borneol [LAVANDIN]	anti acne (Rose 1999, p. 170) antiviral (herpes) (Rose 1999, p. 170)
Lavandula latifolia ct. cineole [SPIKE LAVENDER]	ophthalmic (conjunctivitis) (Franchomme & Pénoël 1990, p. 287)
Ledum groenlandicum [GREENLAND MOSS]	antiinflammatory (Catty 2001, p. 106; Culpeper. n.d., p. 219) hepatic depurative (Catty 2001, p. 106)
Levisticum officinale [LOVAGE]	digestive (Paris 2000)
Linaria vulgaris [TOADFLAX]	ophthalmic (inflammation) (Grieve 1992, p. 816)
Matricaria recutita [GERMAN CHAMOMILE]	antiinflammatory (Keville & Green 1995; Rose 1999, p. 170; Catty 2001, p. 108; naturesgift.com/hydrosols) antiseptic (Catty 2001, p. 108) sedative (Catty 2001, p. 108)
Melaleuca alternifolia [TEA TREE]	antifungal (Catty 2001, p. 109) antiseptic (Catty 2001, p. 109) antiviral (Catty 2001, p. 109) bronchitis (Catty 1998a) *Candida albicans* (C. Marshall, personal communication, 1998)
Melilotus officinalis [COMMON MELILOT]	anticoagulant, embolism, phlebitis (Viaud 1983) antispasmodic (Viaud 1983) apoplexy (Culpeper, n.d., p. 232) circulatory (Paris 2000) ophthalmic (calming) (C. Montesinos, personal communication, 2001)
Melissa officinalis [LEMON BALM]	analgesic (Kresanek 1982, p. 130)

	antidepressant (naturesgift.com/hydrosols) antiinflammatory (Catty 2001, p. 111) antimigraine (Kresanek 1982, p. 130) antioxidant (Catty 2001, p. 111) antiviral (herpes) (Rose 1999, p. 173) antiviral (Rose 1999, p. 173; Catty 2001, p. 111) digestive (Baudoux 1996a; Catty 2001, p. 111) ophthalmic (conjunctivitis, blepharitis) (Viaud 1983, Baudoux 1996a) relaxing (naturesgift.com/hydrosols) soporific (Rose 1999, p. 173)
Mentha × piperita [PEPPERMINT]	anti acne (Baudoux 1996b, p. 44; Rose 1999, p. 174) antiinflammatory (Baudoux 1996b, p. 96; Rose 1999, p. 174) antipruritic (Rose 1999, p. 174) antiseptic (Viaud 1983) circulatory, heavy legs (Grosjean 1993b, p. 87) cooling (Rose 1999, p. 174) energizing, uplifting (Rose 1999, p. 174) eupeptic (Viaud 1983; Baudoux 1996a; Rose 1999, p. 174; Paris 2000) hepatic (Baudoux 1996a) ophthalmic (dryness) (Baudoux 1996b, p. 101) stomachic (Payne 1999)
Mentha pulegium [PENNYROYAL]	antispasmodic, antihysteria (Grieve 1992, p. 626) mucolytic (nasal) (Franchomme & Pénoël 1990, p. 302)
Mentha spicata [SPEARMINT]	hiccoughs, carminative (Grieve 1992, p. 536) soothing (skin) (Rouvière & Meyer, 1989, p. 121) tonic (skin) (Rouvière & Meyer, 1989, p. 99)
Mentha sylvestris [HORSEMINT]	anticancer (Viaud 1983) antidandruff (Culpeper, n.d., p. 236) antispasmodic (Viaud 1983) bactericide (Viaud 1983) euphoric (Viaud 1983)
Myrtus communis [MYRTLE]	antiallergic (Schnaubelt 1999; Catty 2001, p. 115) antiseptic (Schnaubelt 1999) asthma (Catty 2001, p. 115) antitussive, bronchitis (Catty 2001, p. 115) energizing, reviving (Rose 1999, p. 173) eye infections (Baudoux 1996b, p. 101; Rose 1999, p. 173) ophthalmic (inflammation, conjunctivitis) (Franchomme & Pénoël 1996, pp. 86, 287, 303; Schnaubelt 1999; Catty 2001, p. 115) soothing (Keville & Green 1995; Rose 1999, p. 173) stomach ulcer (Baudoux 1996b, p. 29)
Ocimum basilicum [BASIL]	calms nausea (Rose 1999, p. 172) carminative (Viaud 1983, Paris 2000) digestive (Viaud 1983, Paris 2000) stimulant (scalp) (Rose 1999, p. 172) stomachic (Paris 2000)
Olea europaea [OLIVE]	antihypertension (Viaud 1983) cardiac protector (Viaud 1983)
Origanum majorana [SWEET MARJORAM]	antispasmodic (stomach, intestine) (Fischer-Rizzi 1990, p. 58) hepatic depurative (Viaud 1983; Fischer-Rizzi 1990, p. 58) soothing (skin)
Origanum onites [FRENCH MARJORAM]	cardiovascular stimulant (Aydin et al 1996)

Origanum vulgare [OREGANO]	antibacterial (Rose 1999, p. 173; Sağadiç & Özcan 2003)
	antifungal (Rose 1999, p. 173)
	antiinfectious (Catty 2001, p. 118)
	antiseptic (Rose 1999, p. 173; Catty 2001, p. 118)
	antiviral (Rose 1999, p. 173)
	bronchitis (Catty 1998a)
	calmative to CNS (Viaud 1983)
	energizing (Grosjean 1993b, p. 56)
	gynaecological problems (Grosjean 1993b, p. 55)
	sexual tonic, frigidity, impotence (Grosjean 1993b, p. 57)
Ormenis mixta [MOROCCAN CHAMOMILE]	relaxing (Paris 2000)
Pelargonium graveolens [GERANIUM]	antidepressant (Rose 1999, p. 174)
	cellular regenerative (Rose 1999, p. 174)
	cooling (hot flushes) (Rose 1999, p. 174)
	hypotensor (Payne 1999)
	normalizer (skin) (Rose 1999, p. 174; Catty 2001, p. 109)
	stimulating (adrenal cortex) (Rose 1999, p. 174)
Petroselinum sativum [PARSLEY]	anticancerous (Viaud 1983)
	carminative (Culpeper, n.d., p. 258)
	litholytic (renal) (Viaud 1983)
	red cell regenerator (Viaud 1983)
Peumus boldus [BOLDO LEAF]	anthelmintic (Franchomme & Pénoël 1990, p. 274)
	eupeptic (Paris 2000)
	hepatic depurative (Viaud 1983)
Phytolacca decandra [POKE ROOT]	lipolytic (Viaud 1983)
Picea mariana [BLACK SPRUCE]	analgesic (Rose 1999, p. 172)
Pimento officinalis [PIMENTO]	antihysteria (Grieve 1992, p. 20)
	carminative (Grieve 1992, p. 20)
Pimpinella anisum [ANISEED]	antibacterial (Sağadiç & Özcan 2003)
Pimpinella magna [SAXIFRAGE, GREATER BURNETT]	antispasmodic (Culpeper n.d., p. 320)
Pinus sylvestris [SCOTS PINE]	antirheumatic (Grosjean 1993a, pp. 55, 66)
	antiseptic (Catty 2001, p. 121)
	balsamic (Viaud 1983)
	diuretic (Viaud 1983)
	gynaecological problems (Grosjean 1993b, p. 55)
	immunostimulant (Catty 2001, p. 121)
	respiratory (Grosjean 1993a, p. 66; Catty 2001, p. 121)
Pistacia lentiscus [PISTACHIO]	reticulo-endothelial decongestant (Viaud 1983)
Plantago major [PLANTAIN]	cleansing (sores and ulcers) (Salmon's Herbal 1710)
	ophthalmic (calming) (C. Montesinos, personal communication, 2001)
Polygonatum multiflorum (SOLOMON'S SEAL)	freckles (Culpeper, n.d. p. 339, Claire 1961 p. 240)
Portulaca sativa [GOLDEN PURSLANE]	analgesic – toothache (Grieve 1992, p. 660)
Potentilla anserina [SILVERWEED]	facial tonic, freckles, pimples (Grieve 1992 p. 741)
Prunus laurocerasus [CHERRY LAUREL]	sedative
Robinia pseudoacacia [FALSE ACACIA]	antidiabetic (Viaud 1983)
	circulatory, capillary problems (skin), arterial circulatory system (Viaud 1983)
Rosa canina [WILD ROSE]	cicatrizant (Grosjean 1993b, pp. 87, 95)
	normalizer (dry skin) (Grosjean 1993b, pp. 57, 87)
	regenerating (Grosjean 1993b, pp. 87, 114)
Rosa damascena [DAMASK ROSE]	antihaemorrhagic (Baudoux 1996b, p. 64)
	antiinflammatory, skin regenerative (Bego 1995; Goëb 1998; Nasr 2000, p. 27; Sanoflore 2000; 6scent; naturesgift.com/hydrosols)
	astringent (Keville & Green 1995; Baudoux 1996a;

	C. Montesinos, personal communication 2001) cicatrizant (Baudoux 1996b, p. 49) fibroma (Baudoux 1996b, p. 85) nausea, vomiting (Fischer-Rizzi 1990, p. 58) ophthalmic (inflammation, conjunctivitis) (Rouvière & Meyer 1989, p. 106; Fischer-Rizzi 1990, p. 58) [also *Rosa alba, Rosa canina, Rosa rubra* (Culpeper, n.d., pp. 298–302)] psoriasis (Baudoux 1996b, p. 52) stimulant (scalp) (Fischer-Rizzi 1990, p. 58)
Rosmarinus officinalis [ROSEMARY VERBENONE]	anti acne (teenage) (Baudoux 1996b, p. 44) antioxidant depurative (gall bladder) (Viaud 1983) digestive (Grosjean 1993a, p. 64) emmenagogic (Viaud 1983) mental and physical stimulant (Catty 2001, p. 124; Grosjean 1993b, p. 56), energizing, tired feet (Rose 1999, p. 174) normalizer (dry skin) (Grosjean 1993b, pp. 57, 87; Rouvière & Meyer 1989, p. 97) regenerating (Grosjean 1993b, pp. 57, 87, 95, 114) soothing (skin) (Grosjean 1993b, pp. 87, 95, 114) stimulant (gall bladder) (Catty 2001, p. 124) stimulant (scalp) (Rouvière & Meyer 1989, p. 119) stimulant (skin) (Keville & Green 1995)
Rosmarinus officinalis ct. verbenone [ROSEMARY VERBENONE]	bronchitis (Catty 1998a) mucolytic (nasal) (Franchomme & Pénoël 1990, p. 302) psoriasis (Baudoux 1996b, p. 52) stomachic (Paris 2000)
Ruscus aculeatus [BUTCHER'S BROOM]	circulatory (Paris 2000)
Salvia officinalis [SAGE]	anti acne (Baudoux 1996a) antioxidant antiparasitic (lice) (C. Montesinos, personal communication, 2001) antiseptic (Baudoux 1996a) astringent (Claeys 1992) carminative (Nasr 2000, p. 27) cellulite (Grosjean 1993a, p. 65) cicatrizant (Baudoux 1996a) circulatory (Grosjean 1993b, pp. 34, 54; Catty 2001, p. 127) cleanser (dry skin), tonic (Rouvière & Meyer 1989, pp. 97, 99) digestive (Grosjean 1993a, p. 64) emmenagogic, pelvic congestion (Viaud 1983) emmenagogue (Baudoux 1996a) gynaecological (Grosjean 1993b, p. 55) painful periods (Baudoux 1996a) regenerative (Grosjean 1993b, pp. 87, 95, 114; C. Montesinos, personal communication, 2001) stimulant (scalp) (Rouvière & Meyer, 1989, p. 119)
Salvia sclarea [CLARY]	antiseptic (Claeys 1992) astringent (Rose 1999, p. 172) dry skin (Grosjean 1993b, p. 57) Note: given for oily skin by Rose (1999 p. 172) euphoric, antidepressant (Catty 2001, p. 129) hormone balancer (Catty 2001, p. 129) PMS, hot flushes (Rose 1999, p. 172)

Sambucus nigra [ELDERFLOWER]	antiallergic – major antiasthmatic (Viaud 1983)
	antiinflammatory (sunburn) (Grieve 1992, p. 272)
	calming (Catty 2001, p. 130)
	circulatory (Grosjean 1993b, p. 54)
	diuretic (Catty 2001, p. 130)
Santolina chamaecyparissus [COTTON LAVENDER]	vermifuge (Viaud 1983)
Saponaria officinalis [SOAPWORT]	antidiabetic (Viaud 1983)
	eczema (Viaud 1983)
	furuncles (Viaud 1983)
Sarathamnus scoparius [BROOM]	respiratory, lungs (Viaud 1983)
Satureia hortensis [SUMMER SAVORY]	antibacterial (Sağadiç & Özcan 2003)
	sexual tonic, frigidity, importance (Grosjean 1993b, p. 57)
Satureia montana [WINTER SAVORY]	anthelmintic (Baudoux 1996b, p. 34)
	antibacterial (Catty 2001, p. 132)
	antifungal (Catty 2001, p. 132)
	antiparasitic (lice) (C. Montesinos, personal communication, 2001)
	antiseptic (Catty 2001, p. 132)
	coughs, bronchitis (Catty 2001, p. 115)
	immunostimulant (Catty 2001, p. 132)
	revitalizing, energizing (Viaud 1983; Grosjean 1993b, p. 56)
Scabiosa succisa [SCABIOUS]	cicatrizant (Grieve 1992, p. 722)
Solidago canadensis [GOLDEN ROD]	analgesic (Rose 1999, p. 170)
	antiinflammatory (Rose 1999, p. 170; Catty 2001, p. 133)
	antispasmodic (Rose 1999, p. 170; Catty 2001, p. 133)
	astringent (Rose 1999, p. 170)
	calming (Rose 1999, p. 170)
	diuretic (Rose 1999, p. 170; Catty 2001, p. 133)
	litholytic (Catty 2001, p. 133)
Tanacetum vulgare [TANSY]	calming to the psyche (Viaud 1983)
Thuja occidentalis [THUJA]	antitumoral (Viaud 1983)
Thymbra spicata [BLACK THYME]	antibacterial (Sağadiç & Özcan 2003)
Thymus serpyllum [WILD THYME]	antibacterial (Viaud 1983)
	anticancerous (Viaud 1983)
	antiseptic (Grieve 1992, pp. 814–815), (intestinal) (Viaud 1983)
	antispasmodic (Grieve 1992, pp. 814–815)
	calming
	carminative (Grieve 1992, pp. 814–815)
	catarrh (Grieve 1992, pp. 814–815)
	digestive (Viaud 1983; Grieve 1992, pp. 814–815)
	diuretic (Grieve 1992, pp. 814–815)
	emmenagogic (Grieve 1992, pp. 814–815)
Thymus vulgaris [THYME]	anti acne (Grosjean 1993b, p. 87; Rose 1999, p. 174)
	antiinfectious (Catty 2001, p. 137)
	antiparasitic (lice) (C. Montesinos, personal communication, 2001)
	antirheumatic (Grosjean 1993a, pp. 55, 66)
	antirheumatic (Viaud 1983)
	antiseptic (intestinal) (Viaud 1983)
	antiseptic (Rose 1999, p. 174)
	boils
	cicatrizant
	circulatory (Rose 1999, p. 174)
	digestive (Rose 1999, p. 174)
	dry skin (Grosjean 1993b, p. 87)

	eczema (Rose 1999, p. 174)
	insect bites (Rose 1999, p. 174)
	regenerating (Grosjean 1993b, pp. 87, 95, 114)
	respiratory (Grosjean 1993a, p. 66)
	stimulating, revitalizing (Price & Price 1999; Rose 1999, p. 174)
	tonic (scalp) (Montesinos 1991)
Thymus vulgaris ct. linalool [SWEET THYME]	anthelmintic (Franchomme & Pénoël 1990, p. 274)
	antiinfectious (urinary) (Paris 2000)
	dry skin
Thymus vulgaris ct. thujanol-4 [SWEET THYME]	anthelmintic (Baudoux 1996b, p. 34)
	antifungal (Baudoux 1996a)
	antiseptic (Baudoux 1996a)
	antiviral (Baudoux 1996a)
	candidiasis (Baudoux 1996b, p. 80)
	chlamydia (Baudoux 1996b, p. 81)
	cicatrizant (Baudoux 1996b, p. 49)
	circulatory
	condyloma (Baudoux 1996b, p. 86)
	eczema (Baudoux 1996a)
	energizing
	hepatic (Baudoux 1996a)
	immunostimulant (Catty 2001, p. 136)
	ophthalmic (Price & Price 1999)
	stomach ulcer (Baudoux 1996b, p. 29)
Tilia × *europaea* (fol.) [LIME LEAF]	antihysteria, palpitations (Grieve 1992, p. 486)
	antiviral (shingles) (Rose 1999, p. 171)
	cardiac and nerve calmant (Baudoux 1996a)
	digestive, nervous vomiting (Grieve 1992, p. 486)
	soporific (Grosjean 1993a, p. 66)
Tilia sylvestris [LIME LEAF]	calming (Viaud 1983)
Tilia sylvestris (lig.) [LIME SAPWOOD]	arthritis, articular rheumatism, gout (Viaud 1983)
Urtica dioica [NETTLE]	choleretic (Viaud 1983)
	tonic (scalp) (Viaud 1983, Montesinos 1991)
Valeriana wallichii [INDIAN VALERIAN]	sedative (Franchomme & Pénoël 1990, p. 286)
	soporific (Franchomme & Pénoël 1990, p. 286)
Viscum album [MISTLETOE]	cardiotonic (Viaud 1983)
Zingiber officinale [GINGER]	digestive (naturesgift.com)

APPENDIX C

Plant list: scientific and common names

Abies balsamea	[BALSAM FIR, BALM OF GILEAD]	Pinaceae
Acacia decurrens	[MIMOSA, GREEN WATTLE]	Mimosaceae
Achillea millefolium	[YARROW]	Asteraceae
Agaricus campestris	[FIELD MUSHROOM]	Agariceae
Aloysia triphylla (Lippia citriodora)	[LEMON VERBENA]	Verbenaceae
Anagallis arvensis	[SCARLET PIMPERNEL]	Primulaceae
Anemone hepatica	[AMERICAN LIVERWORT]	Ranunculaceae
Anethum graveolens	[DILL WEED]	Apiaceae
Angelica archangelica	[ANGELICA]	Apiaceae
Apium graveolens	[WILD CELERY, SMALLAGE]	Apiaceae
Arbutus uva ursi (*Arctostaphylos uva-ursi*)	[BEARBERRY, MOUNTAIN BOX]	Ericaceae
Arctium lappa	[GREATER BURDOCK, BEGGAR'S BUTTONS]	Asteraceae
Arnica montana	[ARNICA]	Asteraceae
Artemisia abrotanum	[SOUTHERNWOOD, LAD'S LOVE]	Asteraceae
Artemisia absinthium	[WORMWOOD]	Asteraceae
Artemisia arborescens	[TREE WORMWOOD]	Asteraceae
Artemisia dracunculus	[TARRAGON]	Asteraceae
Artemisia vulgaris	[MUGWORT, FELON HERB]	Asteraceae
Asperula odorata	[WOODRUFF]	Rubiaceae
Balsamita suaveolens	[COSTMARY, ALECOST, BALSAM HERB]	Asteraceae
Betula alba and *Betula pendula*	[WHITE BIRCH AND SILVER BIRCH]	Betulaceae
Borago officinalis	[BORAGE]	Boraginaceae
Buxus sempervirens	[BOX]	Buxaceae
Calendula officinalis	[MARIGOLD, POT MARIGOLD]	Asteraceae
Carum carvi	[CARAWAY]	Apiaceae
Cedrus atlantica	[ATLAS CEDAR]	Abietaceae
Centaurea cyanus	[CORNFLOWER, BLUEBOTTLE, BATCHELOR'S BUTTON]	Asteraceae
Chamaemelum nobile	[ROMAN CHAMOMILE]	Asteraceae
Chenopodium album	[FAT HEN, WHITE GOOSEFOOT]	Chenopodiaceae
Chelidonium majus	[GREATER CELANDINE]	Papaveraceae
Chrysanthemum parthenium	[FEVERFEW]	Asteraceae
Cinnamomum verum	[CINNAMON]	Lauraceae
Cistus ladaniferus	[ROCK ROSE, LAUDANUM]	Cistaceae
Citrus aurantium var. *amara* (flos)	[BITTER ORANGE FLOWER]	Rutaceae
Citrus aurantium var. *amara* (fol.)	[PETITGRAIN]	Rutaceae
Citrus aurantium var. *sinensis* (flos)	[SWEET ORANGE FLOWER]	Rutaceae
Citrus limon	[LEMON]	Rutaceae
Cnicus benedictus (*Carbenia benedicta*)	[HOLY THISTLE, BLESSED THISTLE]	Asteraceae
Convallaria majalis	[LILY OF THE VALLEY]	Liliaceae
Coriandrum sativum	[CORIANDER]	Apiaceae

Cotinus coggygria	[SMOKE TREE]	Anacardiaceae
Cotyledon umbilicus	[KIDNEYWORT]	Crassulaceae
Crataegus monogyna, C. oxyacantha	[HAWTHORN]	Rosaceae
Crocus sativus	[SAFFRON]	Iridaceae
Cuminum cyminum	[CUMIN]	Apiaceae
Cupressus sempervirens	[CYPRESS]	Cupressaceae
Daucus carota (sem.)	[CARROT SEED]	Apiaceae
Dictamnus albus	[BURNING BUSH, DITTANY]	Rutaceae
Echinaceae purpurea	[PURPLE CONEFLOWER]	Asteraceae
Eletteria cardamomum	[CARDAMOM]	Zingeriberaceae
Equisetum arvense	[COMMON HORSETAIL]	Equisetaceae
Erigeron canadensis	[FLEABANE]	Asteraceae
Eucalyptus dives	[BROAD LEAVED PEPPERMINT]	Myrtaceae
Eucalyptus globulus	[TASMANIAN BLUE GUM]	Myrtaceae
Eucalyptus polybractea	[BLUE LEAVED MALLEE]	Myrtaceae
Eupatorium cannabinum	[HEMP AGRIMONY]	Asteraceae
Euphrasia officinalis	[EYEBRIGHT]	Scrophulariaceae
Filipendula ulmaria (Spirea ulmaria)	[MEADOWSWEET]	Rosaceae
Fragaria vesca	[STRAWBERRY]	Rosaceae
Foeniculum vulgare var. *dulce* (sem.)	[FENNEL]	Apiaceae
Fucus vesiculosus	[BLADDERWRACK]	Fucaceae
Fumaria officinalis	[FUMITORY]	Fumariaceae
Galega officinalis	[GOAT'S RUE]	Leguminosae/ Papilionaceae
Gentiana lutea	[YELLOW GENTIAN]	Gentianaceae
Glechoma hederacea	[GROUND IVY, FIELD BALM]	Lamiaceae
Hamamelis virginiana	[WITCH-HAZEL]	Hamamelidaceae
Harpagophytum procumbens	[DEVIL'S CLAW]	Pedaliaceae
Hedera helix	[IVY]	Araliaceae
Helichrysum italicum, H. angustifolium	[EVERLASTING]	Asteraceae
Hieracium pilosella	[MOUSE EAR, HAWKWEED]	Asteraceae
Hydrocotyle asiatica	[INDIAN PENNYWORT]	Apiaceae
Hypericum perforatum	[ST JOHN'S WORT]	Clusiaceae
Hyssopus officinalis	[HYSSOP]	Lamiaceae
Inula graveolens	[ELECAMPANE]	Asteraceae
Iris pseudacorus	[IRIS, YELLOW FLAG]	Iridaceae
Juglans regia	[COMMON WALNUT]	Juglandaceae
Juniperus communis	[COMMON JUNIPER]	Cupressaceae
Juniperus communis (fruct.)	[JUNIPER BERRY]	Cupressaceae
Lactuca hortensis, L. sativa	[LETTUCE]	Asteraceae
Lactuca virosa	[WILD LETTUCE]	Asteraceae
Lamium album	[DEAD NETTLE]	Lamiaceae
Laurus nobilis (fol.)	[BAY LAUREL, SWEET BAY]	Lauraceae
Lavandula angustifolia, (L. vera, L. officinalis)	[LAVENDER]	Lamiaceae
Lavandula × intermedia	[LAVANDIN]	Lamiaceae
Lavandula latifolia	[SPIKE LAVENDER]	Lamiaceae
Ledum groenlandicum	[GREENLAND MOSS, LABRADOR TEA]	Ericaceae
Levisticum officinale	[LOVAGE]	Apiaceae
Linaria vulgaris	[TOADFLAX]	Scrophulariaceae
Malva sylvestris	[MALLOW]	Malvaceae
Matricaria recutita	[GERMAN CHAMOMILE]	Asteraceae
Melaleuca alternifolia	[TEA TREE]	Myrtaceae
Melilotus officinalis	[COMMON MELILOT]	Fabaceae
Melissa officinalis	[LEMON BALM, BEE BALM]	Lamiaceae
Mentha × piperita	[PEPPERMINT]	Lamiaceae
Mentha pulegium	[PENNYROYAL]	Lamiaceae

Mentha spicata	[SPEARMINT]	Lamiaceae
Mentha sylvestris, M. longifolia	[HORSEMINT]	Lamiaceae
Myrtus communis	[COMMON MYRTLE]	Myrtaceae
Ocimum basilicum	[SWEET BASIL]	Lamiaceae
Olea europaea	[OLIVE]	Oleaceae
Origanum majorana	[SWEET MARJORAM]	Lamiaceae
Origanum onites	[FRENCH MARJORAM, POT MARJORAM]	Lamiaceae
Origanum vulgare ssp. *hirtum, O. heracleoticum*	[OREGANO, WILD MARJORAM]	Lamiaceae
Ormenis mixta	[MOROCCAN CHAMOMILE]	Asteraceae
Passiflora incarnata	[PASSIONFLOWER, MAYPOPS]	Passifloraceae
Pelargonium graveolens	[ROSE GERANIUM]	Geraniaceae
Petroselinum crispum (P. sativum)	[PARSLEY]	Apiaceae
Peumus boldus	[BOLDO LEAF]	Monimiaceae
Phytolacca decandra, P. americana	[POKE WEED]	Phytolaccaceae
Picea mariana	[BLACK SPRUCE]	Pinaceae
Pimento officinalis	[PIMENTO]	Myrtaceae
Pimpinella anisum	[ANISEED]	Apiaceae
Pimpinella magna	[SAXIFRAGE, GREATER BURNET]	Apiaceae
Pinus sylvestris	[SCOTS PINE]	Pinaceae
Piper nigrum	[PEPPER]	Piperaceae
Pistacia lentiscus	[LENTISK, MASTIC TREE]	Anacardiaceae
Plantago major	[PLANTAIN]	Plantaginaceae
Polygonatum multiflorum, P. biflorum	[SOLOMON'S SEAL]	Convallariaceae/ Liliaceae
Portulaca sativa	[GOLDEN PURSLANE]	Portulacaceae
Potentilla anserina	[SILVERWEED]	Rosaceae
Primula veris	[COWSLIP]	Primulaceae
Prunus laurocerasus	[CHERRY LAUREL]	Rosaceae
Robinia pseudoacacia	[FALSE ACACIA]	Papilionaceae
Rosa canina	[WILD ROSE]	Rosaceae
Rosa centifolia	[CABBAGE ROSE]	Rosaceae
Rosa damascena	[DAMASK ROSE]	Rosaceae
Rosmarinus officinalis ct. camphor/cineole	[ROSEMARY]	Lamiaceae
Rosmarinus officinalis ct. verbenone	[ROSEMARY VERBENONE]	Lamiaceae
Ruscus aculeatus	[BUTCHER'S BROOM]	Liliaceae/Ruscaceae
Ruta graveolens	[RUE]	Rutaceae
Salvia officinalis	[SAGE]	Lamiaceae
Salvia sclarea	[CLARY]	Lamiaceae
Sambucus nigra	[ELDERFLOWER]	Caprifoliaceae
Santalum album	[SANDALWOOD]	Santalaceae
Santolina chamaecyparissus	[COTTON LAVENDER]	Asteraceae
Saponaria officinalis	[SOAPWORT]	Caryophyllaceae
Sarothamnus scoparius (Cytisus scoparius)	[BROOM]	Papilionaceae
Satureia hortensis	[SUMMER SAVORY]	Lamiaceae
Satureia montana	[WINTER SAVORY]	Lamiaceae
Scabiosa succisa (Succisa pratensis)	[BLUE BUTTONS]	Dipsacaceae
Solidago virgaurea	[GOLDEN ROD, AARON'S ROD]	Asteraceae
Solidago canadensis	[GOLDEN ROD]	Asteraceae
Spirea ulmaria	[MEADOWSWEET]	Rosaceae
Stachys officinalis (Betonica officinalis)	[BETONY]	Lamiaceae
Syzygium aromaticum	[CLOVE BUD]	Myrtaceae
Tanacetum vulgare	[COMMON TANSY]	Asteraceae
Taraxacum officinale	[DANDELION]	Asteraceae
Thuja occidentalis	[WHITE CEDAR]	Cupressaceae
Thymbra spicata	[BLACK THYME]	Lamiaceae
Thymus serpyllum	[WILD THYME]	Lamiaceae
Thymus vulgaris ct. geraniol	[SWEET THYME]	Lamiaceae

Thymus vulgaris ct. linalool	[SWEET THYME]	Lamiaceae
Thymus vulgaris ct. thujanol-4	[SWEET THYME]	Lamiaceae
Thymus vulgaris ct. thymol	[THYME]	Lamiaceae
Tilia × *europaea*	[LIME FLOWER, LINDEN BLOSSOM]	Tiliaceae
Tilia sylvestris (lig.)	[LIME SAPWOOD]	Tiliaceae
Urtica dioica	[NETTLE]	Urticaceae
Valeriana officinalis	[VALERIAN, ALL HEAL]	Valerianaceae
Vetiver zizanioides	[VETIVER]	Graminae
Viola tricolor ssp *arvensis*	[HEARTSEASE, WILD PANSY]	Violaceae
Viscum album	[MISTLETOE]	Viscaceae/ Loranthaceae
Vitis vinifera	[GRAPEVINE]	Vitaceae
Zingiber officinale	[GINGER]	Zingiberaceae

APPENDIX D

Analyses of distilled plant waters

The percentages given for the compounds in the waters are calculated simply by adding together the peak areas and expressing each one as a percentage of this. Compositions given in **bold** are the **essential oil.** It would have been preferable to have data for samples of the oil and the hydrolat from the same distillation, but this was not always possible.

Sources of hydrolats tested

A Herbes de Chevenoz
B Distillerie de la Louine
C Pranarom
D Fytosan
E Distilled by the authors

Achillea millefolium [YARROW] Asteraceae

Source A

%	*Compound*
3.58	2-Methyl propanal
2.14	2-Methyl propenal
4.91	3-Methyl butanal
2.90	2-Methyl butanal
2.94	Hexanal
64.19	Eucalyptol
1.11	Linalool
2.90	Unidentified, possibly a terpinol or terpinyl acetate
1.58	Unidentified, possibly a terpinol or terpinyl acetate
1.06	Possibly α-pinocarveol
3.48	Pinocarvone + pinocamphone
3.60	Isopinocamphone
0.66	α-Terpineol
4.30	Myrtenol or myrtenal
0.66	Geraniol

Achillea millefolium [YARROW] Asteraceae

Source B

%	*Compound*
1.41	Dimethyl sulphide
0.11	Probably 2-methylpropanal
0.88	Probably 2-octen-1-ol or isomer
0.81	3-Octanone or isomer
0.32	Unidentified
1.11	Limonene
50.04	Eucalyptol

0.83	Probably 1-nonen-3-ol or isomer
8.83	Linalool
2.12	α-Thujone
11.73	Camphor
6.96	Unidentified
2.79	*endo*-Borneol
7.42	Terpinen-4-ol
2.77	α-Terpineol
1.85	Unidentified

Angelica archangelica (rad.) [ANGELICA ROOT] Apiaceae

Source B

%	*Compound*
17.38	Acetone
2.52	Dimethyl sulphide
0.72	2-Butanone
4.59	Methyl butenol isomer
0.26	Possibly a pentenol isomer
0.22	Hexanone isomer
0.65	Verbenene
0.91	3-Octanone or isomer
1.33	3-Octanol
0.78	α-Phellandrene
0.30	Cymene isomer
0.21	*p*-Cymene
1.3	β-Phellandrene
6.48	Eucalyptol
53.12	Linalool
0.86	p-Mentha-1,8-dien-6-ol or $C_{10}H_{16}O$ isomer
1.16	Probably camphor
1.19	Unidentified $C_{10}H_{16}O$
0.69	Borneol
2.69	Terpinen-4-ol
1.83	α-Terpineol
0.83	Bornyl acetate

Balsamita suaveolens [COSTMARY, HERBE STE MARIE] Asteraceae

Source: Gallori et al (2001)

%	*Compound*
tr	1,4-Cineole
tr	α-Terpinene
3.51	1,8-Cineole
0.10	Linalool
6.22	α-Thujone
0.55	β-Thujone
1.76	Chrysanthenone
0.74	*cis*-Verbenol
0.46	*trans*-Pinocarveol
tr	*trans*-Verbenol
0.64	Pinocarvone
0.35	Borneol
0.10	Isopinocamphone
0.29	Terpenen-4-ol
0.23	Myrtenal
0.97	*cis*-Dihydrocarvone
1.25	*trans*-Carveol

2.19	*cis*-Carveol
74.92	Carvone
0.10	*cis*-Chrysanthenyl acetate
0.10	*cis*-Carvone oxide
0.68	*trans*-Carvone oxide
0.10	Isobornyl acetate
0.10	Carvacrol
tr	β-Bisabolene
tr	δ-Cadinene
tr	Selin-11-en-4-α-ol

Calendula officinalis [MARIGOLD] Asteraceae

Source A

%	*Compound*
0.71	Acetone
3.17	Dimethyl sulphide
0.50	2-Methyl propanal
0.83	3-Methyl butanal
0.82	2-Methyl-butanal
0.45	2-Hexenal
1.99	3-Hexen-1-ol probably *cis* by retention time
1.47	1-Hexanol
0.43	$C_{10}H_{14}$
0.56	Possibly β-myrcene
5.47	Eucalyptol
56.99	Linalool
0.95	Probably isomenthone
2.14	Terpinen-4-ol
3.03	α-Terpineol
1.40	Probably neral
1.39	Geraniol
2.80	Geranial
3.10	Lavandulyl acetate
4.09	Neryl acetate
7.71	Geranyl acetate

Centaurea cyanus [CORNFLOWER] Asteraceae

Source B

%	*Compound*
5.61	Acetone
1.33	Isobutanol (2-Methyl-1-propanol)
0.92	Butanol, probably *n*-
6.00	Siloxane (probably column bleed)
1.37	3-Methyl-1-butanol or isomer
1.08	Benzaldehyde
1.82	Siloxane (probably column bleed)
2.30	Octanal
9.24	Eucalyptol
15.64	Linalool
4.52	Nonanal
4.67	Camphor
3.77	Unidentified
4.54	Borneol
5.29	Terpinen-4-ol
7.24	α-Terpineol
4.07	Decanal

2.45	Undecanal
2.75	Dodecanal
2.40	Probably tridecanal
2.75	Probably tetradecanal
2.84	Probably pentadecanal
7.39	Probably hexadecanal

Note: The overall intensity of this chromatogram suggests the hydrolat to be low in organics.

Centaurea cyanus [CORNFLOWER] Asteraceae

Source C

%	*Compound*
18.32	6-Methyl-5-hepten-2-one
4.02	Eucalyptol
61.29	Linalool
5.33	Terpinen-4-ol
11.02	α-Terpineol

Note: The overall intensity of this chromatogram suggests the hydrolat to be low in organics.

Chamaemelum nobile (ROMAN CHAMOMILE) Asteraceae

Information given by Paris (2000)

0.998–1002	Density
0.34	α-Pinene
0.20	*n*-Isobutyl butyrate
6.50	Pinocarvone + pinocamphone
21	Transpinocarveol
	Isobutyl-3-hydroxy-2-methylene
10.38	Butanoate
2.02	Myrtenol
	2-Hydroxy-2-methyl-3-butenyl(Z)-
22.01	2-methyl-2-butenoate

The essential oil/water ratio is 310 mg/l (0.03%) (there are other compounds in the water not identified here).

Chamaemelum nobile [ROMAN CHAMOMILE] Asteraceae

Source B

%	*Compound*
0.46	Ethanol
1.44	Acetone
1.28	Methyl acetate
2.74	2-Methyl propanal
5.56	2-Methyl-2-propenal or isomer
2.36	2,3-Butanedione or ethenyl acetate
1.34	2-Butanone
5.08	3-Methyl butanal or isomer
2.96	2-Methyl butanal or isomer
1.52	Pentanal
0.33	2-Methyl-butanenitrile
0.31	Methylbutanol isomer (pentanol isomer)
0.64	3-Penten-2-one or isomer
4.73	Hexanal
0.65	Methyl pentanol (hexanol isomer)
1.52	Hexanal + probably phenol
2.22	3-Hexen-1-ol

0.65	2-Cyclopentene-1,4-dione or isomer
2.07	Probably a heptadieneal
0.72	Heptanal
0.20	Probably 2-heptenal or isomer
0.31	Benzaldehyde
0.30	Probably heptanol
2.94	2-Octen-1-ol
15.4	6-Methyl-5-hepten-2-one (possibly 3-octanone)
1.30	3-Octanol
1.32	Probably 3-hexenyl acetate
15.75	Eucalyptol
0.70	1-Octanol
13.59	Linalool
1.53	Camphor
1.34	*endo*-Borneol
4.97	Terpinen-4-ol
0.92	α-Terpineol
0.80	Unidentified

***Citrus aurantium* (flos)** [ORANGE FLOWER] Rutaceae

Source unknown

%	*Compound*
9.66	NI 1
2.15	*cis*-Linalyl oxide
1.29	*trans*-Linalyl oxide
9.36	Linalool
9.44	α-Terpineol
1.90	Phenylethyl alcohol
1.68	NI 2
1.14	NI 3
2.60	NI 4
3.01	*cis*-Phytol

Crataegus oxyacantha [HAWTHORN] Rosaceae

Source B

%	*Compound*
3.76	Acetone
42.54	Dimethyl sulphide
0.79	Probably 2-methyl propanal
0.84	Probably butanone
0.52	Pentanone
1.59	6-Methyl-5-hepten-2-one or isomer
0.64	Eucalyptol
45.26	Linalool
2.81	Terpinen-4-ol
1.24	α-Terpineol

Equisetum arvense [HORSETAIL] Equisetaceae

Source B

%	*Compound*
3.09	Acetone
25.70	Dimethyl sulphide
0.99	3-Octanone or isomer

0.34	Eucalyptol
53.29	Linalool
0.23	Camphor
0.48	4-Isopropylcyclohexanone or isomer
2.65	Unidentified
0.49	*endo*-Borneol
5.66	Terpinen-4-ol
3.55	α-Terpineol
0.50	Nerol
0.11	Carvone
1.28	Geraniol
0.30	Bornyl acetate
0.68	Probably 8,9-dehydrocycloisolongifolene
0.68	Caryophyllene oxide

Daucus carota [CARROT] Apiaceae

%	*Compound*
2.19	Acetone
7.10	Dimethyl sulphide
3.45	2-Methyl propanal
1.65	Butenal isomer
1.44	2-Butanone
0.61	Methyl butenol isomer
0.31	Methyl furan, probabl 2-isomer
19.88	3-Methyl butanal
9.94	2-Methyl butanal
0.54	Pentanal
0.50	Possibly 2-methyl butanenitrile
0.35	3-Methyl-1-butanol or isomer
0.61	Dimethyl disulphide
4.45	Hexanal
0.65	Heptanal
3.57	α-Pinene
0.46	Camphene
1.32	β-Myrcene
1.94	β-Pinene
2.07	α-Terpinene + *p*-cymene
1.92	Limonene
3.88	Eucalyptol
3.15	γ-Terpinene
28.02	Linalool

Daucus carota [CARROT] Apiaceae

%	*Compound*
2.16	Unidentified
1.28	Unidentified
1.22	Unidentified
46.94	Terpinen-4-ol
2.52	α-Terpineol
2.45	Chrysanthanyl acetate or isomer (2,7,7-Trimethyl-bicyclo[3.1.1]hept-2-en-6-yl acetate)
12.63	*endo*-Bornyl acetate
9.13	Unidentified
21.67	Geranyl acetate

Daucus carota (sem.) [CARROT SEED] Apiaceae

Source D

%	*Compound*
1.51	Acetone
1.20	Dimethyl sulphide
0.45	2-Butanone
0.42	2-Methyl-3-pentanone or isomer (hexanone isomer)
0.32	Eucalyptol
31.83	Linalool
45.86	Terpinen-4-ol
3.08	α-Terpineol
1.91	Geraniol
2.62	*endo*-Bornyl acetate
0.18	Unidentified
10.62	Geranyl acetate

Echinacea purpurea [PURPLE CONEFLOWER] Echinaceae

Source D

%	*Compound*
17.42	Acetone
5.49	Dimethyl sulphide + methyl acetate
18.36	2-Methyl propanal
1.31	2-Methyl-2-propenal or isomer
3.77	Butanedione isomer or ethenyl acetate
10.42	3-Methyl butanal or other pentanal isomer
7.59	2-Methyl butanal or other pentanal isomer
2.65	Pentanal
1.58	Toluene
15.58	Hexanal
0.55	Unidentified
0.53	Heptanal
0.23	6-Methyl-5-hepten-2-one
1.05	*p*-Cymene
4.43	Eucalyptol
2.31	Linalool
0.25	α-Campholene aldehyde
0.43	Camphor
0.70	Pinocarvone
1.47	Terpinen-4-ol
0.84	α-Terpineol
0.79	Myrtenal or myrtenol
1.50	Possibly a *p*-Mentha-1,8-dien-6-ol isomer
0.55	Probably pulegone isomer
0.21	Probably thymol

Filipendula ulmaria (*Spirea ulmaria*) [MEADOW SWEET] Rosaceae

Source B

%	*Compound*
6.39	Ethanol
6.75	Acetone
69.88	Dimethyl sulphide
1.49	2-Butanone

0.92	Probably isobutanol (2-methyl-1-propanol)
0.70	Benzene
0.59	Possibly a pentanone isomer
1.07	3-Methyl-1-butanol or isomer
1.11	2-Methyl-1-butanol or isomer
0.55	Probably ethanethiol
3.27	Eucalyptol
7.04	Camphor
0.24	Possibly bornyl formate

Fucus vesiculosus [BLADDERWRACK] Fucaceae

Source D

%	*Compound*
27.75	Acetone
60.05	Dimethyl sulphide
1.26	Butanedione isomer or ethenyl acetate
0.58	Dimethyl disulphide
0.98	Eucalyptol
6.05	Linalool
1.88	Terpinen-4-ol
1.46	α-Terpineol

Helichrysum angustifolium (H. italicum) [EVERLASTING] Asteraceae

Source D

The essential oil of *Helichrysum stoechas* resembles the oil of *H. angustifolium* and the two plants may be processed together as the various species of *Helichrysum* are very polymorphous and thus cannot easily be distinguished (Guenther 1952, vol. 5, p. 471).

%	*Compound*
0.68	Acetone
0.32	Dimethyl sulphide
2.67	2-Methyl propanal
0.69	2-Methyl-2-propenal
0.47	2-Butanone
0.66	3-Methyl butanal or isomer
5.53	2-Methyl butanal or isomer
11.07	3-Pentanone
20.05	3-Methyl-pentanone or isomer (hexanone isomer)
10.29	4-Methyl-3-hexanone
0.19	Linaloyl oxide
0.15	6-Methyl-5-hepten-2-one
14.41	Eucalyptol
1.73	2,4-Dimethyl-heptane-3,5-dione
11.17	Linalool
0.41	Fenchyl alcohol
0.37	Camphor
2.11	Possibly nerol oxide
0.57	Borneol
3.19	Terpinen-4-ol
4.59	Unidentified, possibly a ketone
6.51	α-Terpineol
0.73	Nerol
1.17	Possibly an isomer of unidentified ketone above
0.16	Bornyl acetate
0.13	Neryl acetate

Helichrysum italicum [EVERLASTING] Asteraceae

Source C

%	*Compound*
0.34	Acetaldehyde
2.31	Ethanol
5.75	Acetone
1.34	C_5H_8 pentadiene isomer
0.85	2-Methyl propanal
1.72	2-Methyl-2-propenal
4.06	2-Butanone
1.23	3-Methyl butanal or isomer
1.32	2-Methyl butanal or isomer
21.03	3-Pentanone
29.30	2-Methyl-3-pentanone or isomer (hexanone isomer)
3.21	2-Methyl-1-penten-3-one
0.87	3-Hexanone or isomer
16.58	4-Methyl-3-hexanone (heptanone isomer)
3.07	Decane
4.53	Eucalyptol
0.79	Probably a butyl cyclohexanol
1.49	Undecane
0.22	Camphor

Note: This chromatogram is overloaded indicating high levels of organics in the hydrolat. Repeated at a lower sampling level below.

Helichrysum italicum [EVERLASTING] Asteraceae

Source C

%	*Compound*
0.68	Ethanol
3.70	Acetone
1.80	Pentadiene isomer
1.65	2-Butanone
26.07	3-Pentanone
17.76	2-Methyl-3-pentanone or isomer (hexanone isomer)
3.46	2-Methyl-1-penten-3-one
17.98	4-Methyl-3-hexanone
1.10	C_8H_{16} ethyl-cyclohexane
1.79	4-Isopropyl-1-methylcyclohexane
6.68	Decane
1.52	$C_{10}H_{22}$ hydrocarbon
3.28	Cymene isomer
1.43	Probably limonene
3.52	$C_{10}H_{20}$ butylcyclohexane
1.58	Butylcyclohexanol isomer
0.73	$C_{11}H_{24}$ hydrocarbon
4.85	Undecane
0.41	Camphor

Hypericum perforatum [ST JOHN'S WORT] Hypericaceae

%	*Compound*
0.50	Acetaldehyde
5.04	Ethanol
13.51	Acetone
3.36	Pentadiene isomer
25.68	Dimethyl sulphide

2.69	2-Methyl propanal
14.83	Butenal isomer (2-Methyl-2-propenal)
1.31	Butanedione, probably 2,2-
3.21	Probably 2-butanone
1.60	Probably a methyl butenol
8.26	3-Methyl butanal or isomer
1.72	3-Methyl-2-butanone or isomer
1.80	2-Methyl butanal or isomer
1.83	2-Methyl-2-butenal or isomer
0.81	3-Penten-2-one or isomer
0.60	Probably 1-penten-3-ol
0.83	Unidentified
1.51	Possibly cyclopentanol
0.41	2,4-Hexadienal, or isomer
2.43	2-Methyl-3-butenal or isomer
2.51	Hexanal
3.59	Hexenal
1.21	3-Hexen-1-ol
0.75	Eucalyptol

Hyssopus officinalis [HYSSOP] Lamiaceae

%	*Compound*
3.69	Dimethyl sulphide
0.48	3-Methyl butanal
0.31	2-Methyl butanal
0.33	Probably methyl 2-methylbutanoate
0.36	7-Octen-4-ol or isomer
0.28	3-Octanone
0.47	β-Pinene
1.58	Eucalyptol
1.25	Linalool
0.36	*cis*-Thujone
0.31	*trans*-Thujone
29.13	Pinocamphone
60.03	Isopinocamphone
0.88	Myrtenol
0.29	Myrtenyl acetate
0.25	Geranyl acetate

Hyssopus officinalis [HYSSOP] Lamiaceae

Source A

%	*Compound*
0.46	2-Methyl propanal
0.77	3-Methyl butanal
0.39	2-Methyl butanal
0.79	β-Pinene
1.38	Eucalyptol
1.51	Linalool
0.46	*cis*-Thujone
0.36	*trans*-Thujone
1.99	Unidentified
30.40	Pinocamphone
57.76	Isopinocamphone
1.74	Unidentified
1.18	Geraniol
0.79	Probably isoledene

Hyssopus officinalis [HYSSOP] Lamiaceae

Source E

%	*Compound*
3.82	Probably linalool
4.74	Pinocamphone
91.44	Isopinocamphone

Juniperus communis (fruct.) [JUNIPER BERRY] Cupressaceae

Source B

%	*Compound*
1.76	Acetone
0.32	Probably 2-butanone
0.32	3-Octanone or isomer
0.14	Ethenylmethyl-benzene isomer
0.04	α-Phellandrene
0.72	Cymene isomer + possibly α-terpinene
0.15	*p*-Cymene
1.59	β-Phellandrene
0.48	Eucalyptol
2.19	$C_{10}H_{12}$ probably an ethenyl-ethyl-benzene
0.44	$C_{10}H_{12}$ probably *p*-cymenene
0.77	$C_{10}H_{12}$ probably an ethenyl-ethyl-benzene
3.66	Linalool
0.31	*cis*-Thujone
1.46	*trans*-Thujone
3.85	4-Isopropylcyclohexanone
74.95	Terpinen-4-ol
5.12	α-Terpineol
0.44	Carvone
0.29	3-Carvomenthone

Lavandula angustifolia [LAVENDER] Lamiaceae

Four lavender waters (sampled by immersing SPME fibre during 5 min).
Source: Plotto et al (2001).

%	*Compound*
0–tr	Camphene
0–0.3	β-Pinene
0–0.2	Myrcene
0.10–1.70	Limonene
1.1–6.4	Cineole
0–0.80	3-Octanone
0–0.30	*p*-Cymene
0–0.20	Terpinolene
0–0.12	1-Hexanol
0.14–0.32	3-Octanol
0.42–0.76	*cis*-Linalool oxide
0.38–0.61	*trans*-Linalool oxide
1.00–2.15	Camphor
47.90–58.86	Linalool
0.07–0.19	Linalyl acetate
0.06–0.40	α-Santalene
0.20–0.64	Bornyl acetate
0.04–0.21	Caryophyllene
1.92–11.78	Terpenen-4-ol

0.35–2.41	*trans*-β-Farnesene
1.10–3.45	Lavandulol
4.26–7.36	α- and β-Terpineol
1.03–4.32	Borneol
0–1.06	Neryl acetate
0–0.10	Geranyl acetate
1.05–1.79	Nerol
3.21–5.97	Geraniol
0–3.05	Caryophyllene oxide
0–2.22	Coumarin

Lavandula angustifolia [LAVENDER] Lamiaceae

Source B

%	*Compound*
2.23	Acetone
0.97	Dimethyl sulphide
0.63	2-Methyl propanal
1.20	3-Methyl butanal or isomer
0.50	2-Methyl butanal or isomer
0.18	Hexanal
0.10	1-Hexanol
0.35	Benzaldehyde
0.35	Linaloyl oxide
0.49	2-Octen-1-ol or isomer
1.06	3-Octanone
0.31	3-Octanol
4.09	Eucalyptol
68.31	Linalool
1.49	Camphor
1.45	*endo*-Borneol
7.51	Terpinen-4-ol
0.81	Crypton
4.36	α-Terpineol
0.52	Decanal
0.53	Nerol
0.91	Geraniol
0.43	Lavandulyl acetate
0.27	Undecanal
0.22	Dodecanal
0.24	Tridecanal
0.27	Tetradecanal
0.22	Pentadecanal

Lavandula angustifolia [LAVENDER] Lamiaceae

Source C

%	*Compound*
10.11	Acetone
0.92	Probably a methyl-butenol isomer
0.47	Pentanone isomer
0.86	Linaloyl oxide
4.80	3-Octanone
1.31	Isocineol
2.43	Eucalyptol
19.86	Linalool
2.38	Camphor

1.45	Possibly nerol oxide
2.71	4-Isopropylcyclohexanone or isomer
1.21	Unidentified
1.07	Probably *endo*-borneol
26.95	Terpinen-4-ol
23.48	α-Terpineol

Lavandula* × *intermedia 'Grosso' [LAVANDIN] Lamiaceae

Source: Plotto et al (2001), California, two samples.

	% Compound
tr	Camphene
0.10	β-Pinene
0.09–0.32	Myrcene
0.57–4.66	Limonene
1.57–4.45	Cineole
0.05–0.28	γ-Terpinene
0.08–0.28	3-Octanone
0–0.10	1-Hexanol
tr	3-Octanol
0.32–0.80	*cis*-Linalool oxide
0.16–0.64	*trans*-Linalool oxide
0.81–10.96	Camphor
55.70–68.49	Linalool
0–0.12	Linalyl acetate
0–tr	α-Santalene
0.08–0.09	Bornyl acetate
0.09–0.10	Caryophyllene
4.26–4.39	Terpenen-4-ol
tr	Cryptone
0.17–0.27	trans-β-Farnesene
0.94–1.36	Lavandulol
7.27–8.98	α- and β-Terpineol
1.35–2.33	Borneol
0–tr	Neryl acetate
0–tr	Geranyl acetate
1.13–1.69	Nerol
3.34–5.25	Geraniol
tr	Coumarin

Lavandula latifolia [SPIKE LAVENDER] Lamiaceae

Source: Plotto et al (2001).

%	*Compound*
0.32	β-Pinene
tr	Myrcene
29.13	Cineole
tr	γ-Terpinene
tr	3-Octanone
tr	TerpinoLene
tr	1-Hexanol
0.13	*cis*-Linalool oxide
tr	*trans*-Linalool oxide
32.29	Camphor
22.65	Linalool
tr	Linalyl acetate
tr	Bornyl acetate

tr	Caryophyllene
0.71	Terpenen-4-ol
0.79	*trans*-β-Farnesene
tr	Lavandulol
4.95	α- and β-Terpineol
2.26	Borneol
tr	Neryl acetate
0.56	Nerol
1.80	Geraniol
tr	Coumarin

[tr = <0.1]

Marjoram (Wild) unspecified

Source A

%	*Compound*
2.95	Acetone
9.81	2-Methyl propanal
14.22	3-Methyl butanal
7.38	2-Methyl butanal
0.52	Pentanal
2.05	Probably methyl 2-methylbutanoate
1.40	Hexanal
2.36	2-Hexenal
9.75	7-Octen-4-ol or isomer
4.49	3-Octanone
2.03	3-Octanol
3.05	*p*-Cymene
3.76	Eucalyptol
2.73	Linalool
5.28	Pinocamphone
24.61	Terpinen-4-ol + isopinocamphone
1.03	β-Citronellol
0.88	Geraniol
0.64	Probably isoledene
1.05	Probably caryophyllene oxide

Marjoram (Wild) unspecified

Source A

%	*Compound*
0.23	α-Thujene
0.35	α-Pinene
0.26	7-Octen-4-ol or isomer + 3-octanone
27.13	Sabinene
0.29	β-Pinene
8.22	β-*trans*-Ocimene
6.42	β-*cis*-Ocimene
0.42	β-Phellandrene + trace eucalyptol
0.69	γ-Terpinene
0.19	Linalool
0.12	Unidentified, possibly an acetate
0.18	Terpinen-4-ol
2.02	β-Bourbonene
18.75	Caryophyllene
5.52	α-Farnesene
5.71	α-Caryophyllene

14.84	Germacrene D
2.27	Possibly a muurolene isomer
2.64	*d*-Cadinene
2.66	Unidentified
1.08	Caryophyllene oxide

Malva sylvestris [COMMON MALLOW] Malvaceae

Source B

%	*Compound*
1.55	Ethanol
10.19	Acetone
68.83	Dimethy sulphide
5.06	2-Butanone
0.33	Probably 2-methyl-propanenitrile
0.36	Isobutanol (2-methyl-1-propanol)
0.23	3-Methyl-2-butanone or isomer (an isomer of pentanone)
0.44	2-Pentanone or isomer
0.45	3-Pentanone or isomer
0.28	Probably methyl tetrahydrofuran or isomer
0.26	2-Methylbutanenitrile
1.04	3-Methylbutanenitrile
0.27	1-Pentanol or isomer
0.67	Dimethyl disulphide
0.86	Hexanone isomer
0.56	Ethanethiol
0.34	6-Methyl-5-hepten-2-one or isomer
1.36	Eucalyptol
5.45	Linalool
0.26	Camphor
0.35	Terpinen-4-ol
0.21	α-Terpineol
0.67	Unidentified $C_{10}H_{16}O$

Matricaria recutita [GERMAN CHAMOMILE] Asteraceae

Source A

%	*Compound*
1.00	Acetone
2.08	2-Methyl propanal
0.90	2-Butanone
1.19	3-Methyl-1-butanol
0.95	2-Methyl-1-butanol
0.43	Dimethyl disulphide
0.55	Probably 2-hexanone
2.32	3-Octanone
2.23	Eucalyptol
4.88	1-Octenyl acetate
12.77	Linalool
2.03	Probably *p*-menthone + camphor
3.05	Pinocamphone + unidentified
1.01	Neral
1.44	Probably geraniol
2.27	Probably geranial
43.89	Lavandulyl acetate
5.13	Neryl acetate
10.48	Geranyl acetate
1.39	Probably β-farnesene

Melaleuca alternifolia [TEA TREE] Myrtaceae

Source D (distilled in Australia)

%	*Compound*
0.3	Unknown
2.9	1,8-Cineole
86.0	Terpinen-4-ol
0.1	Unknown
0.2	Unknown
8.6	α-Terpineol
0.69	A phenol
0.2	Unknown
0.1	Unknown

Melaleuca alternifolia [TEA TREE] Myrtaceae

Source D (distilled in France)

%	*Compound*
4.4	1,8-Cineole
0.1	Linalool
0.5	*trans-p*-Menth-2-en-1-ol
86.0	Terpinen-4-ol
0.25	Unknown
0.1	*trans*-Piperitol
0.19	Unknown
7.3	α-Terpineol
0.17	*cis*-Piperitol
0.39	A phenol

Melilotus officinalis [COMMON MELILOT] Fabaceae

Source B

%	*Compound*
0.29	Acetone
9.08	Dimethyl sulphide
25.87	Eucalyptol
0.34	$C_{10}H_{12}$
2.56	Linalool
9.86	*cis*-Thujone
2.78	*trans*-Thujone
15.65	Camphor
21.67	*p*-Menthone
2.54	Isomenthone
1.88	*endo*-Borneol
3.39	Menthol
1.40	Terpinen-4-ol
1.19	α-Terpineol
0.31	Probably 2,6,6-trimethyl-1,3-cyclohexadiene-1-carboxaldehyde or isomer
1.20	Bornyl acetate

Melissa officinalis [LEMON BALM] Lamiaceae

Source B

%	*Compound*
19.78	Acetone
75.43	Dimethyl sulphide

2.09	2-Butanone
2.69	Dimethyl disulphide

Melissa officinalis [LEMON BALM] Lamiaceae

%	*Compound*
1.83	Acetone
4.98	Dimethyl sulphide
19.27	2-Methyl propanal
19.83	3-Methyl butanal
12.87	2-Methyl butanal
0.28	Dimethyl disulphide
1.11	Hexanal
4.36	2-Hexenal
0.82	2,5-Diethyltetrahydrofuran or isomer
5.31	6-Methyl-5-hepten-2-one
1.14	3-Octanone
0.71	3-Octanol
5.17	Linalool
0.46	*cis*-Rose oxide
0.28	*trans*-Rose oxide
0.66	2,2-Dimethylocta-3,4-dienal or isomer
1.34	Isomenthone
0.63	Isopinocamphone
5.38	Neral
4.06	Probably methyl 3,7-dimethyl-6-octenoate or isomer
8.54	Geranial
0.20	Neryl acetate
0.76	Geranyl acetate

Melissa officinalis [LEMON BALM] Lamiaceae

Source A

%	*Compound*
4.19	Acetone
0.65	2-Methyl propanal
4.12	3-Methyl butanal
1.44	2-Methyl-butanal
0.54	2,5-diethyltetrahydro-furan or isomer
25.54	6-Methyl-5-hepten-2-one
0.80	3-Octanol
5.84	Linalool
0.28	*cis*-Rose oxide
0.24	*trans*-Rose oxide
0.79	2,2-Dimethylocta-3,4-dienal or isomer
27.09	Neral
28.48	Geranial

Mentha × *piperita* [PEPPERMINT] Lamiaceae

Source C

%	*Compound*
1.43	Eucalyptol
0.12	Probably linalool
43.98	*p*-Menthone
19.56	Isomenthone
31.33	Menthol
0.14	Probably nerol

2.34	Probably menthofuran or isomer
1.11	Menthyl acetate

Mentha × piperita [PEPPERMINT] Lamiaceae

Source: AGORA website (Aromatherapy Global Online Research Archives).
Aromatic compounds contained in the water ***(there are other compounds in the water not identified here).***

Primary oil	*Water oil*	
0.41	-	α-Pinene
0.47	-	β-Pinene
0.17	-	Sabinene
0.95	-	Limonene
2.82	4.62	1,8-Cineole
0.41	-	Paracymene
0.23	0.71	Octanol 3
0.14	0.28	Octen-1-ol-3
20.24	18.89	Menthone
0.13	-	Menthofurane
5.00	5.15	Isomenthone
0.25	-	Neomenthyl acetate
0.11	0.81	Linalool
5.12	0.36	Menthyl acetate
5.17	4.75	Neomenthol
0.70	3.72	β-Caryophyllene
49.03	44.81	Menthol
1.12	3.42	Isomenthol
0.37	0.51	α-Terpineol
0.49	6.40	Piperitone
	0.39	Caryophyllene oxide
0.14		Viridiflorol

This peppermint hydrolat is the product of a specific distillation of fresh plants. The volatile organic compounds in the water was extracted using pentane. The essential oil/water ratio is 320 mg/l (0.03%).

Pelargonium graveolens [GERANIUM] Geranaceae

Source: Rajeswara Rao et al (2002). Comparison of essential oil and water from three batches.

Primary oil	*Water oil*	*Compound*
0.2–0.4	-	α-Pinene
0.1	0.4–6.2	Sabinene
0.1–0.2	-	Myrcene
0.1	-	α-Phellandrene
tr–0.1	-	*p*-Cymene
0.2	0.1	Limonene
0.2	-	(*Z*)-β-Ocimene
0.2	tr–0.1	(*E*)-β-Ocimene
0.1	0.7–1.2	*cis*-Linalool oxide (furanoid)
tr–0.1	0.1–0.4	*trans*-Linalool oxide (furanoid)
tr–0.1	tr–0.1	Terpinolene
6.7–8.1	14.7–19.6	Linalool
0.5–0.8	0.2–0.3	*cis*-Rose oxide
0.2–0.3	0.1–0.2	*trans*-Rose oxide
0.2–0.6	0.3–0.4	Menthone
5.3–7.3	4.5–5.9	Isomenthone
0.1–0.2	0.1–0.4	Terpinen-4-ol
0.2–1.4	3.3–4.8	α-Terpineol
0.1	0.1–0.2	Nerol
27.5–28.2	26.8–33.4	Citronellol

19.4–22.1	21.3–38.4	Geraniol
0.8–1.0	0.5–1.7	Geranial
6.2–7.5	0.2–0.3	Citronellyl formate
4.1–4.7	0.2–0.4	Geranyl formate
tr	tr–0.1	β-Phenylethyl acetate
tr–0.4	0–0.2	Citronellyl acetate
0.3–0.5	0–0.3	Neryl acetate
0.1–0.4	0–0.1	α-Cubebene
0.3–0.4	0–0.1	α-Ylangene
0.2–0.5	0.1–1.6	α-Copaene
0.3–0.6	-	β-Bourbonene
0.1–0.2	-	β-Caryophyllene
1.0–1.2	0–0.1	Citronellyl propionate
tr–0.1	-	Guaia-6,9-diene
0.1–0.2	-	Geranyl propionate
0.3–0.6	-	α-HumuLene
0.1–0.2	-	Germacrene D
1.8–2.2	0–tr	α-Salinene
0.1	-	Geranyl isobutyrate
tr–0.1	0–0.1	α-MuuroLene
1.4–1.7	0–0.1	Citronellyl butyrate
tr–0.1	-	γ-Cadinene
0.1–0.3	tr–0.1	Calamene
tr–0.1	-	Geranyl butyrate
1.0	0.3–0.4	β-Phenylethyl tiglate
0.1	0–0.1	Geranyl isovalerate
0.2	0–tr	Citronellyl valerate
4.9–5.5	0.7–0.9	10-*epi*-γ-Eudesmol
0–tr	-	Geranyl valerate
0.1–0.3	0–0.1	β-Eudesmol
0.6–0.7	1.0–1.2	Citronellyl tiglate
1.8–2.1	0.1	Geranyl tiglate

Pelargonium graveolens [GERANIUM] Geranaceae

%	*Compound*
1.18	Acetone
1.60	Dimethyl sulphide
0.23	2-Methyl propanal
0.33	Butenal isomer
0.33	3-Methyl butanal
0.23	2-Methyl butanal
0.34	Probably C7/8 ketone
0.49	α–Pinene
2.59	Linaloyl oxide
0.87	Probably sabinene
0.60	β-Pinene
0.62	Limonene
0.52	Eucalyptol
0.47	γ–Terpinene
33.45	Linalool
1.23	*p*-Menthone
38.73	Isomenthone
2.61	β-Citronellol
0.88	Neral
8.65	Geraniol
1.73	Geranial

0.63	Geranyl acetate
1.73	Possibly isoledene

Pelargonium graveolens [GERANIUM] Geranaceae

Source A

%	*Compound*
0.38	Acetone
1.00	Dimethyl sulphide
1.28	Hexanal
1.60	α-Pinene
0.98	Linaloyl oxide
3.94	β-Myrcene
4.56	α-Phellandrene
4.64	*p*-Cymene
3.36	Limonene
2.83	β-Phellandrene + eucalyptol
13.12	Linalool
1.06	*p*-Menthone
38.63	Isomenthone
4.83	β-Citronellol
12.31	Geraniol
0.75	Geranial
4.72	Probably isoledene

Pelargonium graveolens [GERANIUM] Geranaceae

Source C

%	*Compound*
0.92	Acetone
13.12	6-Methyl-5-hepten-2-one
36.53	Linalool
3.12	*cis*-Rose oxide
0.44	*trans*-Rose oxide
5.20	*p*-Menthone
29.83	Isomenthone
1.83	α-Terpineol
7.97	β-Citronellol
1.03	Geraniol

Pinus sylvestris [SCOTS PINE] Abietaceae

Source B

%	*Compound*
9.61	Acetone
0.67	Dimethyl sulphide
1.92	2-Butanone
2.59	Probably a methyl butenol isomer
0.55	3-Methyl-2-butanone or isomer
0.61	2-Pentanone
0.33	2-Methyl-3-pentanone (a hexanone isomer)
0.59	Toluene
1.28	3-Octanone
0.28	Limonene
36.49	Eucalyptol
7.77	Linalool
2.17	Fenchyl alcohol

2.46	*p*-Mentha-1,8-dien-6-ol or isomer
6.58	Camphor
1.55	Pinocamphone isomer, *cis*- or *trans*-
2.14	*endo*-Borneol
1.48	Pinocamphone isomer, *cis*- or *trans*-
4.89	Terpinen-4-ol
14.12	α-Terpineol
0.87	Bornyl acetate
1.78	Menth-8-en-1-yl acetate (β-terpinyl acetate)
0.44	Methyl eugenol

Pinus sylvestris [SCOTS PINE] Pinaceae

Source E

%	*Compound*
11.32	Probably linalool
36.44	Unidentified
52.24	Possibly α-Terpineol

Note: The overall intensity of this chromatogram suggests the hydrolat to be low in organics.

Plantago major [GREATER PLANTAIN] Plantaginaceae

Source B

	% *Compound*
0.54	Acetone
23.37	Dimethyl sulphide
0.56	Dimethyl disulphide
2.09	2-Octen-1-ol
1.16	$C_8H_{12}O$ possibly an aldehyde
4.90	3-Octanone
0.66	3-Octanol
4.95	Eucalyptol
1.43	$C_{10}H_{12}$ probably an ethyl ethenyl benzene
0.64	$C_{10}H_{12}$ probably an ethyl ethenyl benzene
43.88	Linalool
1.59	*cis*-Thujone
1.00	$C_{10}H_{10}$ probably a diethenyl benzene
0.31	*trans*-Thujone
0.58	$C_{10}H_{10}$ probably a diethenyl benzene
1.64	Camphor
2.56	1,3,4-Trimethyl-3-cyclohexene-1-carboxaldehyde or isomer
1.82	Terpinen-4-ol
1.07	α-Terpineol
0.56	Nerol
1.61	Geraniol
3.10	Probably thymol

Rosa damascena [DAMASK ROSE] Rosaceae

%	*Compound*
10.20	Ethanol
1.47	Acetone
0.68	Methyl acetate
0.62	2,3-Butadione
7.57	Ethyl acetate
0.45	Isovaleraldehyde
2.49	Valeraldehyde (pentanal)

0.57	2-Methyl butanol
0.48	Hexanol
0.84	Heptanal
0.68	Benzaldehyde
0.68	Prob 6-methyl-5-hepten-2-one
7.79	β-Myrcene
3.51	α-Phellandrene
6.38	*p*-Cymene + β-*trans*-ocimene
0.97	$C_{10}H_{14}$
21.89	Limonene + β-phellandrene
1.57	γ-Terpinene
3.32	Linalool
4.10	α-TerpinoLene
2.63	*cis*-Rose oxide
1.38	Phenyl ethyl alcohol + unknown
2.83	*trans*-Rose oxide + unknown
1.29	Terpinen-4-ol
1.30	α-Terpineol
14.29	Citronellol + probably neral

Specifications for a **NATURAL ROSE WATER**

Distillation water: Bulgarska Rosa Plovdiv

Appearance:	Clear liquid
Colour:	Colourless
Odour:	Typical of roses

Physico-chemical indices

Essential oil content %:	Min 0.025
Ethanol content %:	Max 4
pH:	4–7.5
Composition:	Contains the basic ingredients of rose oil: geraniol, citronellol, nerol, phenyl alcohol, ethyl alcohol
Packing:	200 dm^3 barrels with a protective inner coating
Storage:	In dark and cool
Expiry term:	One year

%	*Compound*
0.11	*cis*- and *trans*-Linalyl oxide
4.9	Linalool
0.2	Terpineol-4
0.05	Neral
1.8	α-Terpineol
0.18	Geranial
28.5	Citronellol
7.15	Nerol
0.52	β-phenylethyl acetate
27.9	Geraniol
7.4	β-phenylethyl alcohol
0.19	Methyl eugenol
0.2	Eudesmol
0.9	Eugenol
0.55*	Carvacrol
0.23	Citronellic acid
0.69	Neric acid
8.7	Geranic acid

* [possible contamination from thyme water]

Essential oil/water ratio <0.02%.

Rosa damascena [DAMASK ROSE] Rosaceae

Source C

%	*Compound*
5.29	Ethanol
1.93	Acetone
2.44	Benzaldehyde
21.84	Linalool
2.68	*cis*-Rose oxide
0.56	*trans*-Rose oxide
1.98	Camphor
0.82	Probably nerol oxide
1.98	Terpinen-4-ol
2.80	α-Terpineol
9.24	β-Citronellol
26.78	Nerol
3.48	Neral
14.11	Geraniol
3.19	Probably 2-phenylethyl acetate
0.90	Methyl eugenol

Rosmarinus officinalis ct. verbenone [ROSEMARY VERBENONE] Lamiaceae

Source C

%	*Compound*
0.66	3-Octanone
5.07	Eucalyptol
4.22	Linalool
2.24	Unidentified, possibly a $C_{10}H_{14}O$ ketone
44.14	Camphor
5.47	*endo*-Borneol
1.09	Pinocamphone + unidentified co-eluting component
3.13	Terpinen-4-ol
1.97	α-Terpineol
17.53	Verbenone (2-pinen-4-one)
2.05	Geraniol
12.43	*endo*-Bornyl acetate

Salvia officinalis [SAGE] Lamiaceae

Source B

%	*Compound*
0.12	Ethanol
1.50	Acetone
1.19	Dimethyl sulphide
0.40	2-Methyl propanal
0.29	2-Butanone
0.39	Isobutanol (2-methyl-1-propanol)
0.17	3-Methyl-2-butanone or isomer
0.20	3-Methyl-2-butanone or isomer
0.29	3-Methyl-1-butanol or isomer
0.13	2-Hexen-1-al
0.25	3-Hexen-1-ol
0.18	1-Hexanol
0.65	2-Octen-1-ol
0.15	3-Octanone
50.60	Eucalyptol

1.18	Linalool
8.40	*cis*-Thujone
1.76	*trans*-Thujone
28.65	Camphor
1.26	*endo*-Borneol
1.17	Terpinen-4-ol
1.06	α-Terpineol

Note: This chromatogram is overloaded indicating high levels of organics in the hydrolat. Repeated at a lower sampling level below.

Salvia officinalis [SAGE] Lamiaceae

Source B

%	*Compound*
0.11	Acetone
0.32	Dimethyl sulphide
0.60	2-Octen-1-ol
0.13	3-Octanone
55.39	Eucalyptol
1.18	Linalool
8.62	*cis*-Thujone
2.17	*trans*-Thujone
27.46	Camphor
1.53	*endo*-Borneol
1.22	Terpinen-4-ol
0.98	α-Terpineol
0.29	Bornyl acetate

Salvia sclarea [CLARY] Lamiaceae

%	*Compound*
0.55	Acetone
43.12	Dimethyl sulphide
0.55	2-Methyl propanal or isomer
1.14	3-Methyl butanal
1.02	2-Methyl butanal
0.56	Probably linaloyl oxide
0.34	Possibly a C_8/C_{10} alcohol
0.18	Possibly a C_8/C_{10} alcohol
0.22	Eucalyptol
0.07	1-Octenyl acetate
44.70	Linalool
3.62	α-Terpineol
0.29	Nerol
0.61	Geraniol
0.45	Lavandulyl acetate
1.06	Neryl acetate
1.54	Geranyl acetate

Thymus vulgaris ct. linalool [SWEET THYME] Lamiaceae

Source C

%	*Compound*
1.57	Acetone
0.41	2-Methyl propanal
0.36	2-Methyl-2-propenal
0.36	3-Methyl butanal or isomer
0.23	Possibly methyl 2-methylbutanoate

0.95	Linaloyl oxide
1.48	Eucalyptol
71.38	Linalool
3.12	Camphor
0.50	Borneol
0.48	Terpinen-4-ol
14.48	α-Terpineol
1.24	Nerol
2.52	Geraniol
0.93	Bornyl acetate

Urtica dioica [NETTLE] Urticaceae

Source B

%	*Compound*
0.55	Ethanol
0.46	Acetone
71.50	Dimethyl sulphide
0.80	2-Butanone
0.48	2-Pentanone or isomer
0.71	3-Pentanone or isomer
0.45	2-Methyl-1-butanol or isomer
2.34	Dimethyl disulphide
0.19	Possibly ethanthiol
3.71	Eucalyptol
0.16	*cis*-Thujone
7.53	Camphor
0.11	Probably *endo*-borneol

Viola tricolor ssp. ***arvensis*** [HEARTSEASE] Violaceae

Source B

%	*Compound*
1.70	Dimethyl sulphide
19.44	Eucalyptol
1.47	$C_{10}H_{12}$ Probably an ethyl ethenyl benzene
23.46	Linalool
4.01	*cis*-Thujone
0.81	$C_{10}H_{10}$ probably a diethenyl benzene
0.31	*trans*-Thujone
29.99	Camphor
3.89	*endo*-Borneol
2.95	Probably terpinen-4-ol
3.21	α-Terpineol
1.16	Probably dodecane
1.69	Probably tetradecane
3.27	Probably hexadecane
2.64	Probably octadecane

Note: The overall intensity of the spectra suggest the presence of only low levels of organics present in the hydrolat.

APPENDIX E
Hydrolat gas chromatographs

Gas chromatographs of some of the hydrolats discussed in this book are shown below. See Appendix D for the detailed lists of volatile organic compounds found in the hydrolats tested.

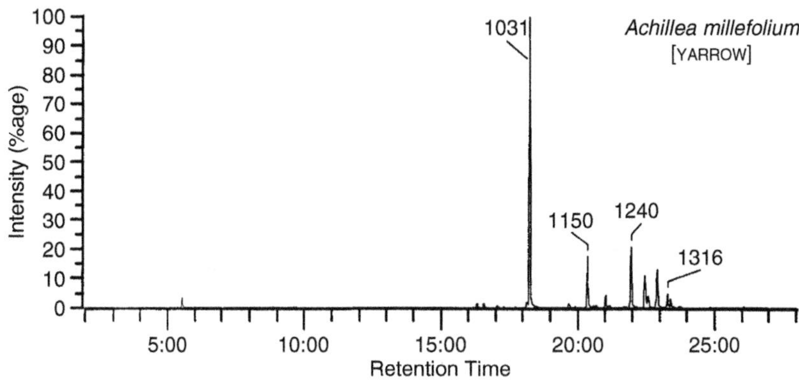

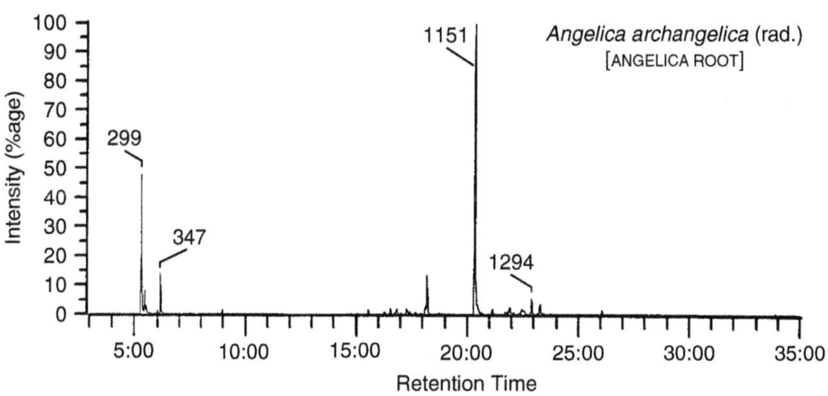

These chromotographs are included by kind permission of Dr Bill Morden, Senior Mass Spectrometrist at LGC Laboratories, Runcorn.

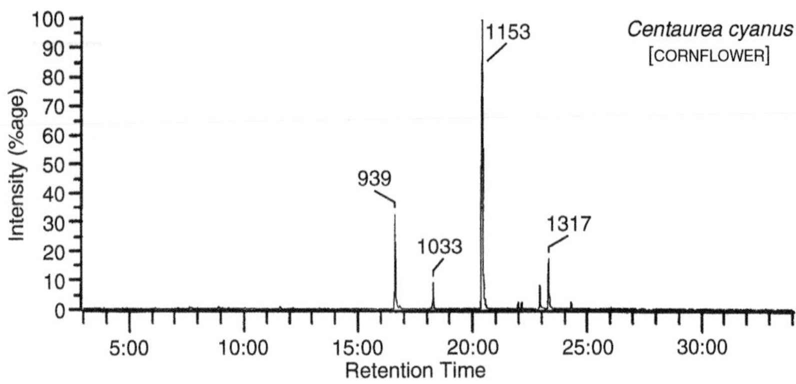
Centaurea cyanus
[CORNFLOWER]
Intensity (%age)
Retention Time
939
1033
1153
1317

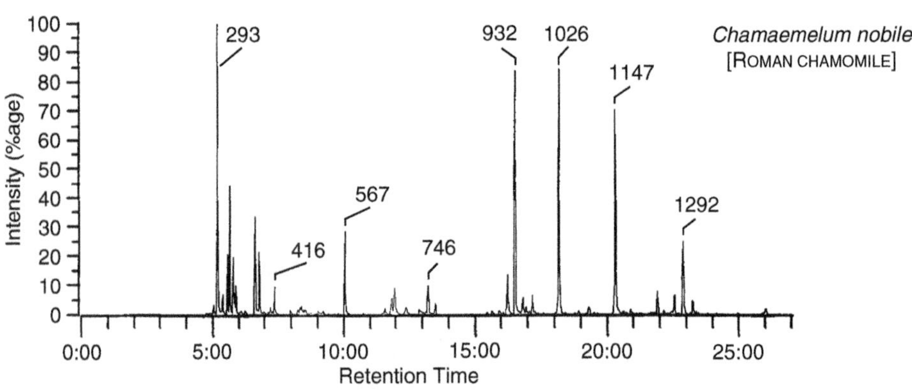
Chamaemelum nobile
[ROMAN CHAMOMILE]
Intensity (%age)
Retention Time
293
416
567
746
932
1026
1147
1292

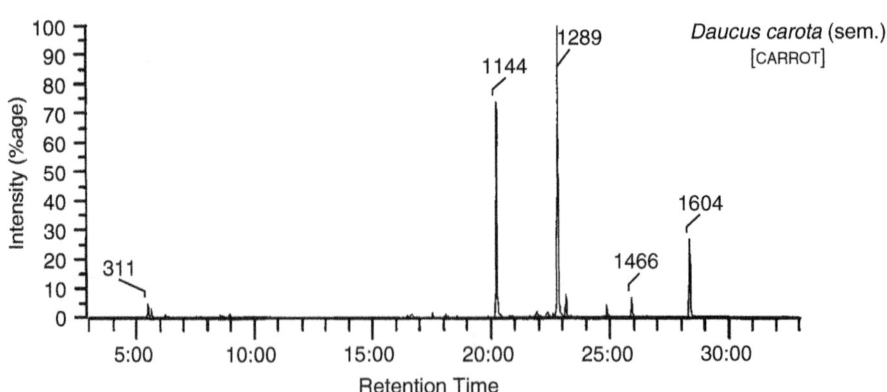
Daucus carota (sem.)
[CARROT]
Intensity (%age)
Retention Time
311
1144
1289
1466
1604

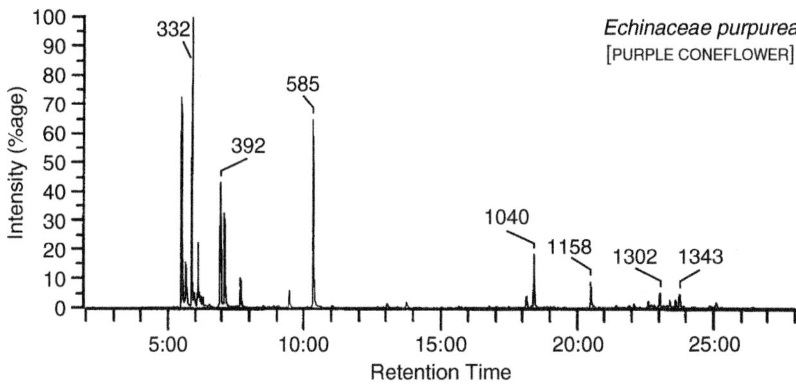
Echinaceae purpurea
[PURPLE CONEFLOWER]
Intensity (%age)
100
90
80
70
60
50
40
30
20
10
0
332
585
392
1040
1158
1302
1343
5:00
10:00
15:00
20:00
25:00
Retention Time

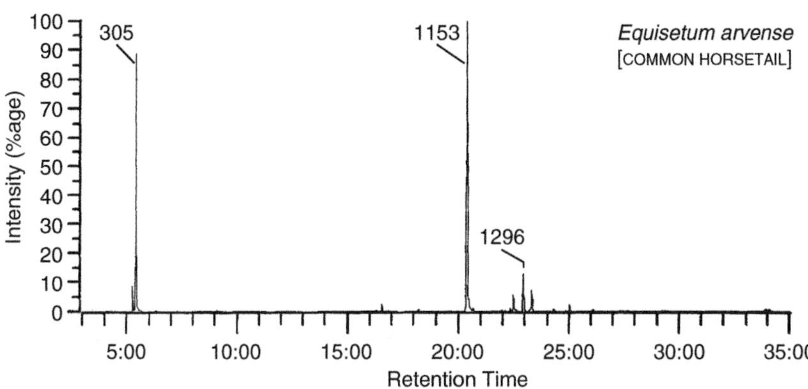
Equisetum arvense
[COMMON HORSETAIL]
Intensity (%age)
100
90
80
70
60
50
40
30
20
10
0
305
1153
1296
5:00
10:00
15:00
20:00
25:00
30:00
35:00
Retention Time

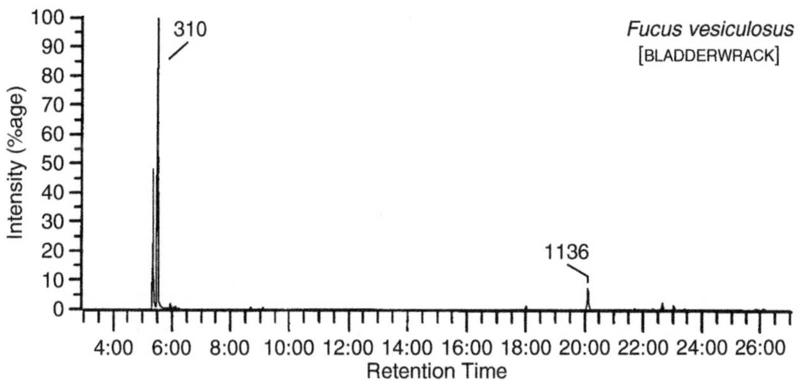
Fucus vesiculosus
[BLADDERWRACK]
Intensity (%age)
100
90
80
70
60
50
40
30
20
10
0
310
1136
4:00
6:00
8:00
10:00
12:00
14:00
16:00
18:00
20:00
22:00
24:00
26:00
Retention Time

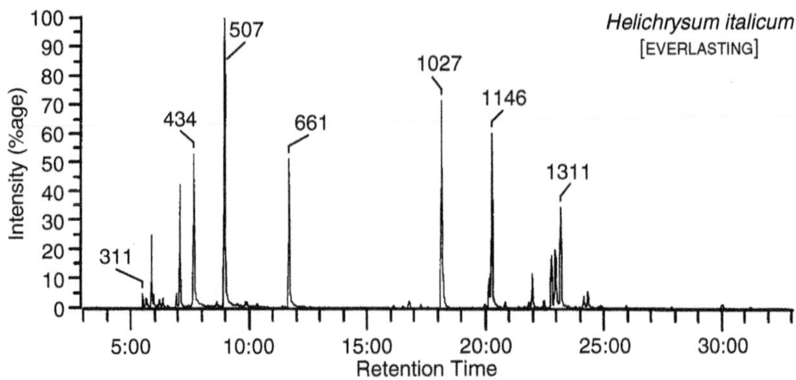
Helichrysum italicum
[EVERLASTING]
Intensity (%age)
100
90
80
70
60
50
40
30
20
10
0
311
434
507
661
1027
1146
1311
5:00
10:00
15:00
20:00
25:00
30:00
Retention Time

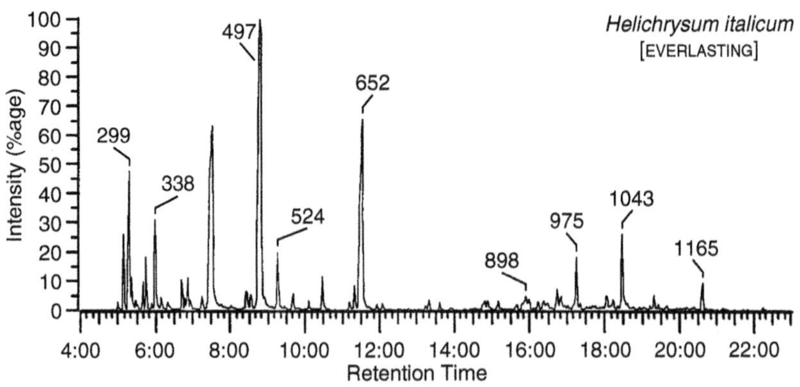
Helichrysum italicum
[EVERLASTING]
Intensity (%age)
100
90
80
70
60
50
40
30
20
10
0
299
338
497
524
652
898
975
1043
1165
4:00
6:00
8:00
10:00
12:00
14:00
16:00
18:00
20:00
22:00
Retention Time

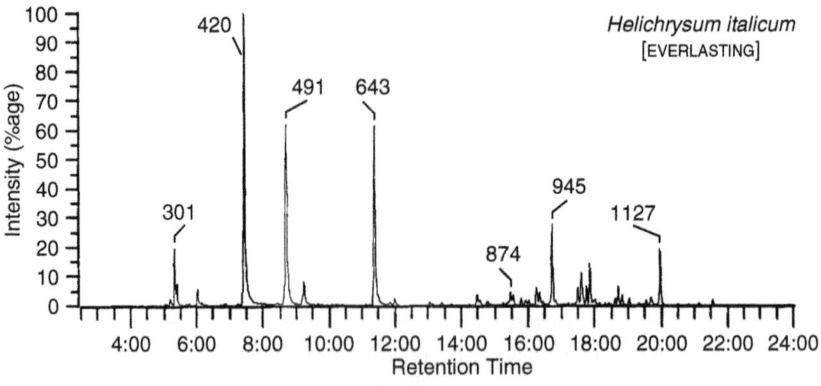
Helichrysum italicum
[EVERLASTING]
Intensity (%age)
100
90
80
70
60
50
40
30
20
10
0
301
420
491
643
874
945
1127
4:00
6:00
8:00
10:00
12:00
14:00
16:00
18:00
20:00
22:00
24:00
Retention Time

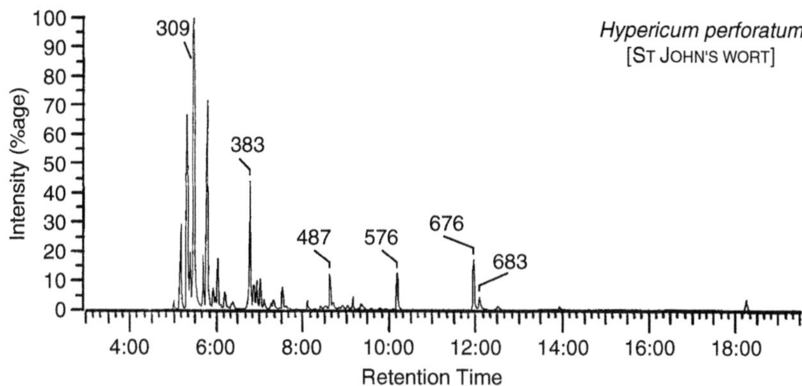
Hypericum perforatum
[ST JOHN'S WORT]
309
383
487
576
676
683
Intensity (%age)
100
90
80
70
60
50
40
30
20
10
0
4:00
6:00
8:00
10:00
12:00
14:00
16:00
18:00
Retention Time

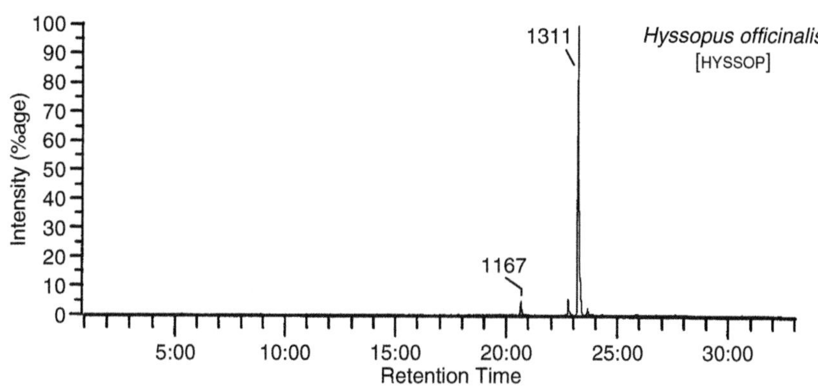
Hyssopus officinalis
[HYSSOP]
1311
1167
Intensity (%age)
100
90
80
70
60
50
40
30
20
10
0
5:00
10:00
15:00
20:00
25:00
30:00
Retention Time

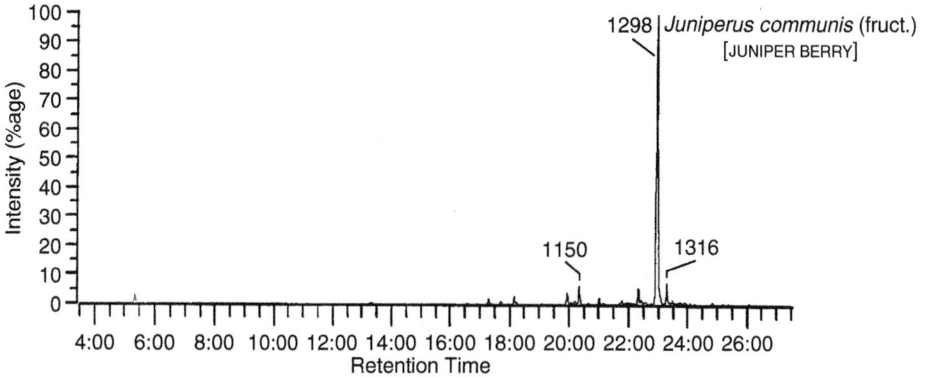
Juniperus communis (fruct.)
[JUNIPER BERRY]
1298
1150
1316
Intensity (%age)
100
90
80
70
60
50
40
30
20
10
0
4:00
6:00
8:00
10:00
12:00
14:00
16:00
18:00
20:00
22:00
24:00
26:00
Retention Time

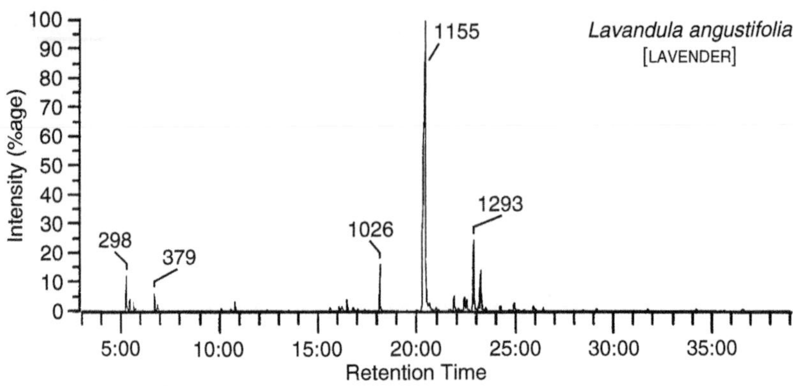
Lavandula angustifolia
[LAVENDER]
Intensity (%age)
Retention Time
100
90
80
70
60
50
40
30
20
10
0
5:00
10:00
15:00
20:00
25:00
30:00
35:00
1155
1293
1026
298
379

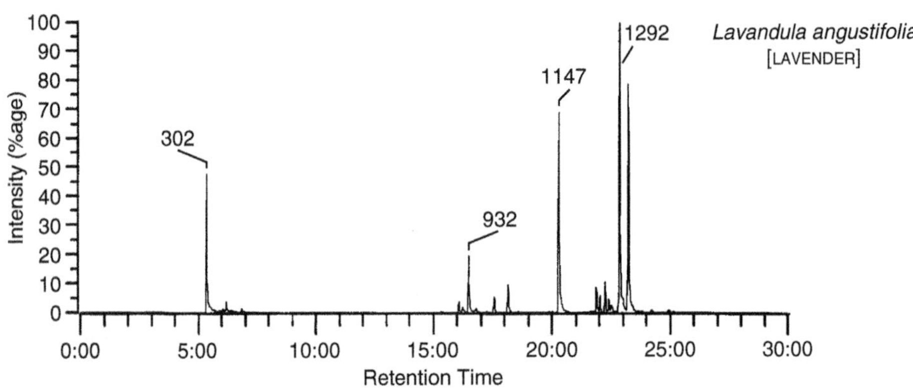
Lavandula angustifolia
[LAVENDER]
Intensity (%age)
Retention Time
100
90
80
70
60
50
40
30
20
10
0
0:00
5:00
10:00
15:00
20:00
25:00
30:00
1292
1147
302
932

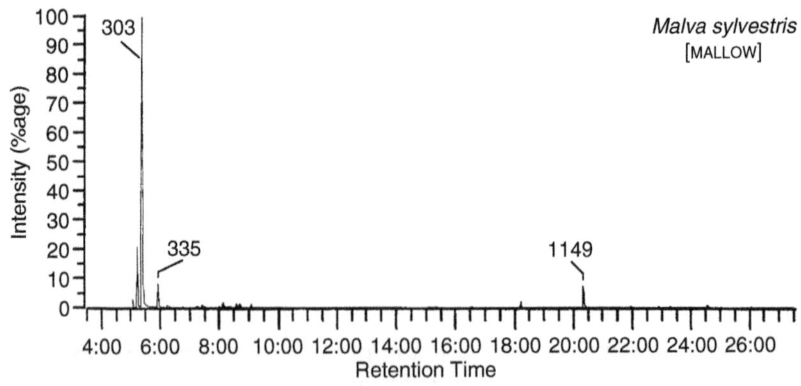
Malva sylvestris
[MALLOW]
Intensity (%age)
Retention Time
100
90
80
70
60
50
40
30
20
10
0
4:00
6:00
8:00
10:00
12:00
14:00
16:00
18:00
20:00
22:00
24:00
26:00
303
335
1149

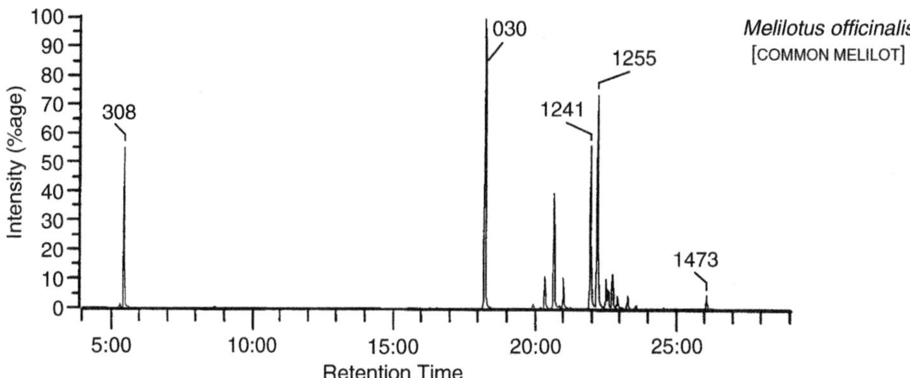

Melilotus officinalis
[COMMON MELILOT]
Intensity (%age)
Retention Time
308
030
1241
1255
1473

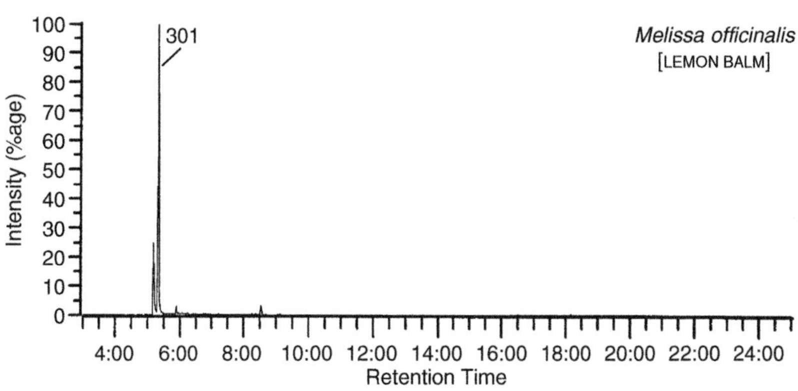

Melissa officinalis
[LEMON BALM]
Intensity (%age)
Retention Time
301

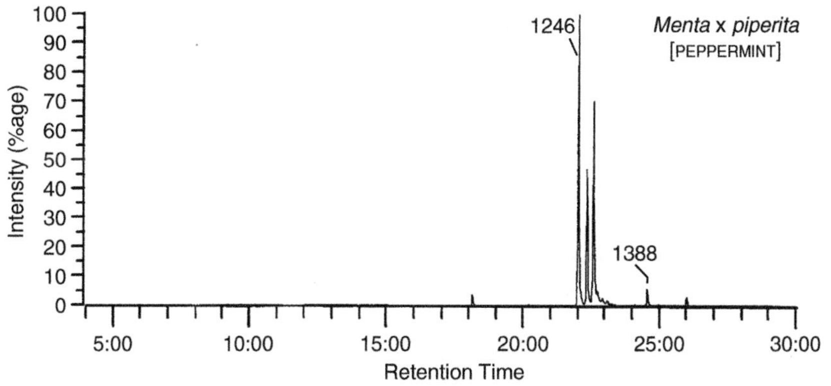

Menta x piperita
[PEPPERMINT]
Intensity (%age)
Retention Time
1246
1388

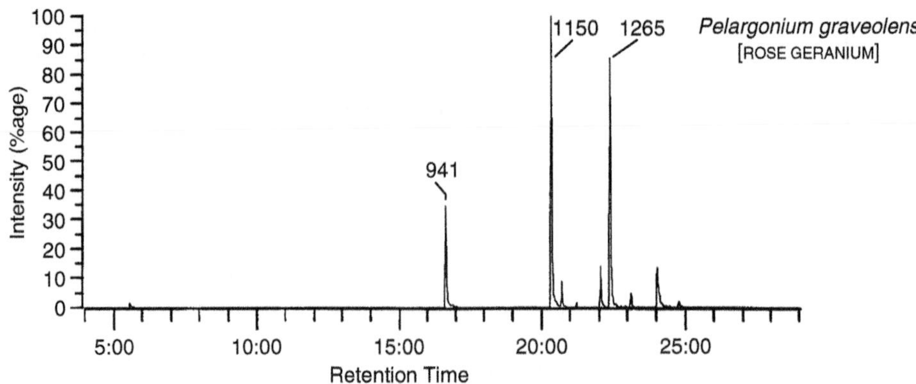
Pelargonium graveolens
[ROSE GERANIUM]
Intensity (%age)
Retention Time
941
1150
1265
100
90
80
70
60
50
40
30
20
10
0
5:00
10:00
15:00
20:00
25:00

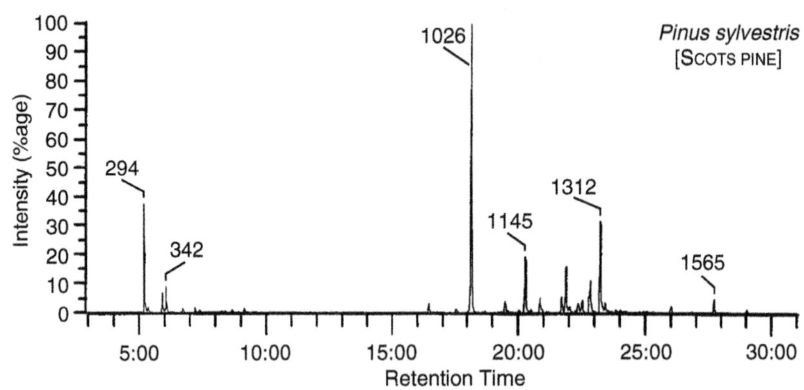
Pinus sylvestris
[SCOTS PINE]
Intensity (%age)
Retention Time
294
342
1026
1145
1312
1565
100
90
80
70
60
50
40
30
20
10
0
5:00
10:00
15:00
20:00
25:00
30:00

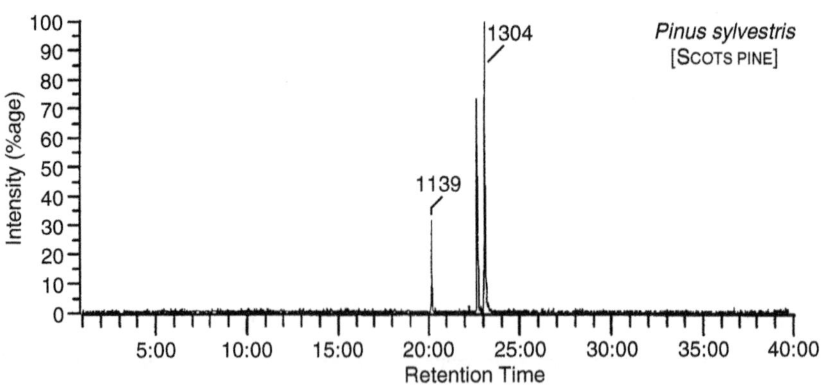
Pinus sylvestris
[SCOTS PINE]
Intensity (%age)
Retention Time
1139
1304
100
90
80
70
60
50
40
30
20
10
0
5:00
10:00
15:00
20:00
25:00
30:00
35:00
40:00

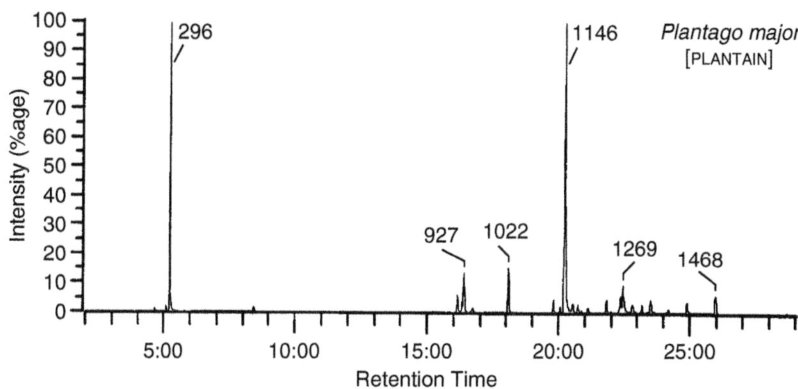
100
90
80
70
60
50
40
30
20
10
0
Intensity (%age)
296
927
1022
1146
1269
1468
Plantago major
[PLANTAIN]
5:00
10:00
15:00
20:00
25:00
Retention Time

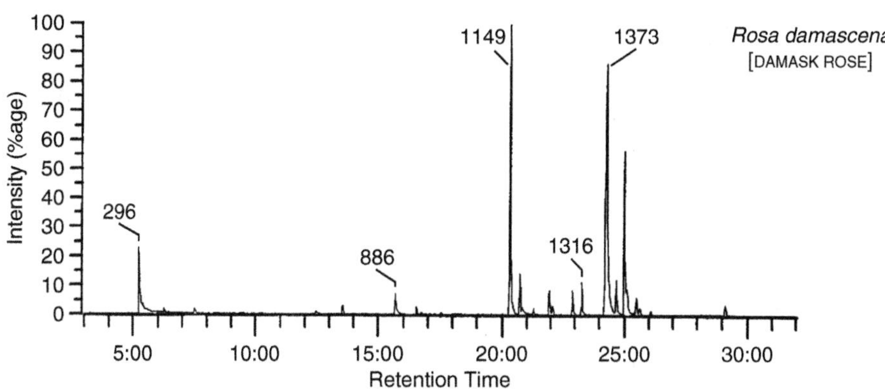
100
90
80
70
60
50
40
30
20
10
0
Intensity (%age)
296
886
1149
1316
1373
Rosa damascena
[DAMASK ROSE]
5:00
10:00
15:00
20:00
25:00
30:00
Retention Time

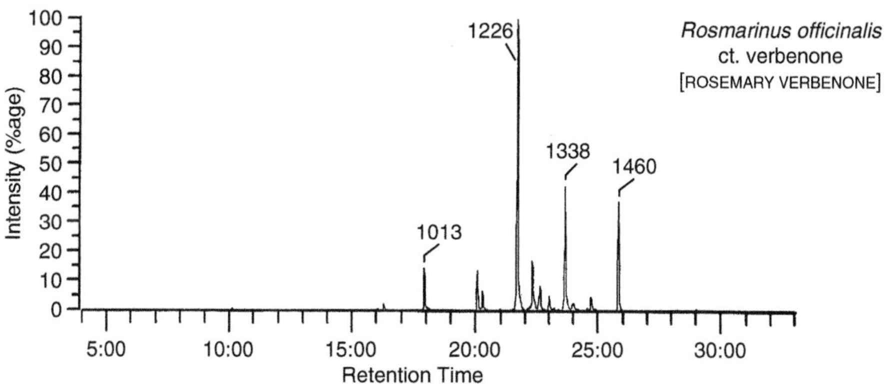
100
90
80
70
60
50
40
30
20
10
0
Intensity (%age)
1013
1226
1338
1460
Rosmarinus officinalis
ct. verbenone
[ROSEMARY VERBENONE]
5:00
10:00
15:00
20:00
25:00
30:00
Retention Time

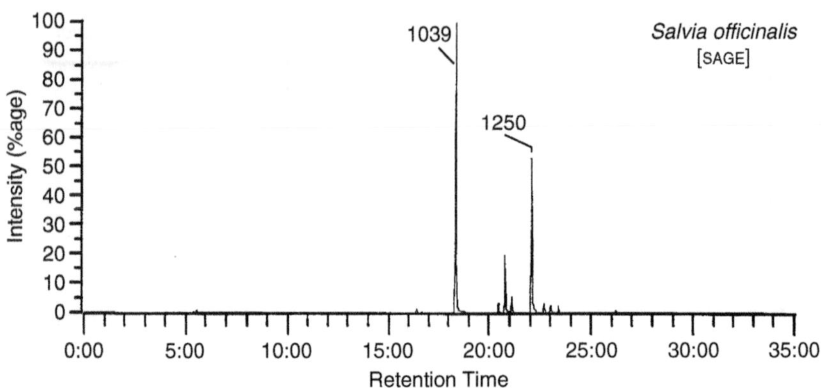

Salvia officinalis
[SAGE]
1039
1250
Intensity (%age)
100
90
80
70
60
50
40
30
20
10
0
0:00
5:00
10:00
15:00
20:00
25:00
30:00
35:00
Retention Time

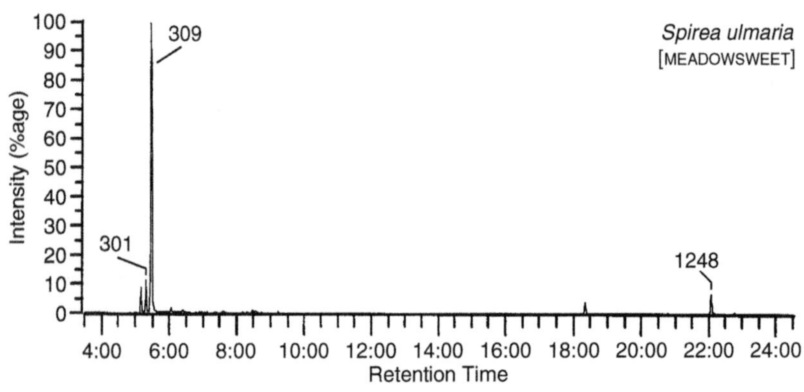

Spirea ulmaria
[MEADOWSWEET]
309
301
1248
Intensity (%age)
100
90
80
70
60
50
40
30
20
10
0
4:00
6:00
8:00
10:00
12:00
14:00
16:00
18:00
20:00
22:00
24:00
Retention Time

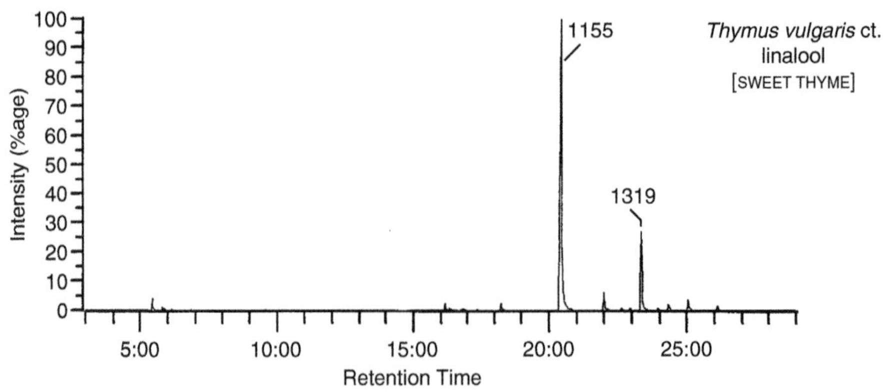

Thymus vulgaris ct. linalool
[SWEET THYME]
1155
1319
Intensity (%age)
100
90
80
70
60
50
40
30
20
10
0
5:00
10:00
15:00
20:00
25:00
Retention Time

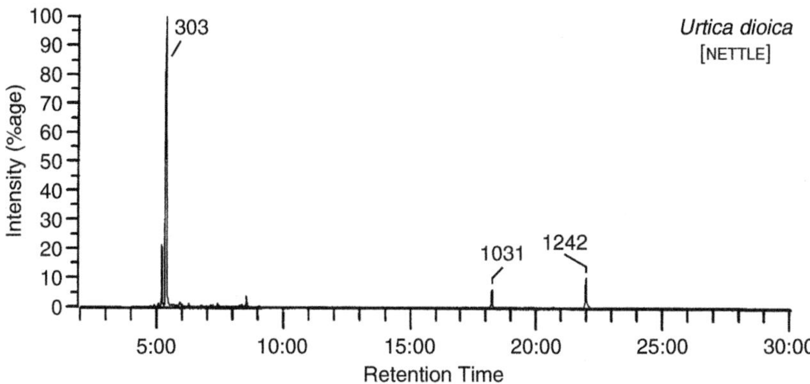
Urtica dioica
[NETTLE]
Intensity (%age)
100
90
80
70
60
50
40
30
20
10
0
303
1031
1242
5:00
10:00
15:00
20:00
25:00
30:00
Retention Time

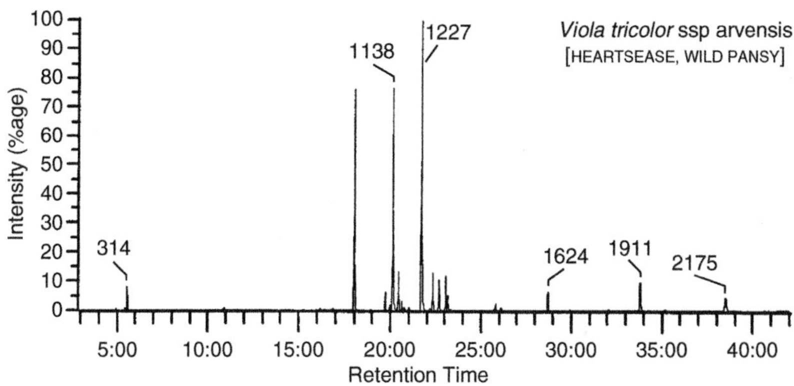
Viola tricolor ssp arvensis
[HEARTSEASE, WILD PANSY]
Intensity (%age)
100
90
80
70
60
50
40
30
20
10
0
314
1138
1227
1624
1911
2175
5:00
10:00
15:00
20:00
25:00
30:00
35:00
40:00
Retention Time

Glossary

Active principle: constituent having a medicinal action
Adaptogenic: having a positive general effect on the body irrespective of disease condition, especially under stress
Alcohols: group of hydrocarbon compounds frequently found in essential oils and distilled waters
Aldehydes: class of organic compounds standing between alcohols and acids
Alexipharmic: neutralizing a poison
Allelopathy: inhibiting influence exerted by one plant over others by the production of a chemical inhibitor, usually a terpenoid or phenolic
Allopathy: system of medicine which uses drugs with effects opposite to the symptoms produced by the disease (in contrast to homoeopathy)
Alveolitis: inflammation of tooth socket
Amenorrhoea: absence of menstruation outside pregnancy in premenopausal women
Anaesthetic: eliminating or reducing feeling, consciousness
Analeptic: fortifying, restorative
Analgesic: relieving or eliminating pain
Anodyne: relieving pain; analgesic
Anthelmintic: destructive of intestinal worms
Anticoagulant: impeding the clotting of blood
Antifungal: counteracting a fungus
Antiinflammatory: reducing or suppressing inflammation
Antiphlogistic: preventing or curing inflammation; antipyretic
Antipyretic: counteracting inflammation or fever; febrifuge
Antiseptic: inhibiting proliferation of microbes, safe to use on the body; bacteriostatic
Antispasmodic: preventing spasms, convulsions
Antitussive: relieving or preventing coughing
Antiviral: counteracting a virus
Anxiolytic: relieving anxiety and tension
Aperient: mildly laxative
Aperitive: stimulating the appetite
Aromatic compound: organic chemical compound derived from benzene
Astringent: causing contraction of living tissues (often mucous membranes); reducing haemorrhages, secretions, diarrhoea, etc.
Bactericidal: destroys microbes
Balneotherapy: treatment by medicinal baths
Balsamic: soothing mucous inflammation especially of respiratory and urinary tracts
Calmative: mildly sedative

Cardiotonic: having a tonic effect on the heart

Cariogenic: causing caries

Carminative: relieving flatulence, intestinal gases

Cathartic: purgative

Chemotype: visually identical plants with significantly different chemical components, resulting in different therapeutic properties; abbreviated to ct. as in *Thymus vulgaris* ct. alcohol

Cholagogic: stimulating gall bladder contraction to promote the flow of bile; choleretic

Choleretic: stimulating the production of bile; cholagogic

Cicatrizant: promoting formation of scar tissue and healing

Cohobation: the recycling of the water used in the distillation process; no water is discarded and the water is enriched (saturated) with water-soluble molecules from the plant material

Colloid: a mixture in which one substance is divided into minute particles (called colloidal particles) and dispersed throughout a second substance, and when this is water the colloid is called a hydrosol; when it is air it is called an aerosol. Colloidal particles are larger than molecules but too small to be observed with a microscope; however, their shape and size (usually between 10^{-7} and 10^{-5} cm, approximately 5–5000 angstroms) can be determined by electron microscopy (Bookshelf 1994)

The physical nature of a solution is easy to understand, for example a sugar solution where the molecules of sugar are evenly dispersed throughout the water giving a homogeneous system. This is not the case when larger molecules are added to water; then we do not have homogeneity but a system made up of two parts, called phases. The water forms what is known as the continuous phase and the large molecules make up the other phase, known as the disperse phase and this whole system is known as being colloidal. In this example we have a colloidal solution and this is usually called a sol. Sols contain particles which are larger than small molecules but smaller than visible particles; these may be larger molecules or clumps of smaller molecules clinging together (Fox & Cameron 1975)

Cordial: a stimulant

Coumarin: a chemical compound, $C_9H_6O_2$, with a high boiling point (290°C) found within the lactones; hardly volatile with steam thus found mainly in expressed oils and sparingly in some distilled essential oils and theoretically not at all in the distilled waters

Cultivar: cultivated variety; a plant produced by horticulture or agriculture not normally occurring naturally; labelled by adding a 'name' to the species as in *Lavandula angustifolia* 'Maillette'

Decoction: preparation made by placing the plant material in cold water, bringing to the boil and simmering. Made in a covered pan to prevent escape of the volatile compounds

Decongestant: relieving congestion (respiratory diseases), dispelling excess local blood supply
Demulcent: soothing, protecting mucous membranes
Depurative: purifying or cleansing the blood and internal organs (e.g. diuretics, diaphoretics)
Diaphoretic: causing or increasing perspiration; sudorific
Digestive: aiding, stimulating digestion
Diuretic: aiding production of urine
Dysmenorrhoea: painful or difficult menstruation
Dyspepsia: disturbed digestion, indigestion
Electrolyte: chemical or its solution in water which conducts current through ionization; a compound that in solution dissociates into ions
Emetic: causing vomiting
Emmenagogic: inducing or regularizing menstruation; euphemism for abortifacient
Emollient: soothing, softening the skin
Empyreumatic: having an unpleasant or uncharacteristic taste or odour which arises when some organic substances are subject to the distillation process; sometimes a burnt note due to poor distillation
Erethism: abnormal irritability or sensitivity
Essential oil: plant volatile oil obtained by distillation; ethereal oil
Eubiotic: brings about conditions favourable to life and healing
Eupeptic: aiding digestion
Expectorant: promoting the removal of mucus, phlegm
Febrifuge: agent which reduces temperature; antipyretic
Fruit: the ripe seeds and their surrounding structures; Latin *fructum* (abbreviated to fruct.)
Fungistatic: arresting the growth of fungi
Galactogogic: promoting the secretion of milk; lactogen, galactogen
GC, GLC: an analytical process to separate individual components from a volatile mixture; the sample to be analysed is vaporized before introduction into a column which has a stationary liquid phase and is carried through the column by an inert gas. As components emerge they are recorded on a chromatograph as a series of peaks, the area under the peak giving an indication of the quantity and their position on the graph giving a clue to their identity
Genus: important botanical classification of related but distinct species given a common name; genera (pl.) are in turn grouped into families; the first word of the binomial botanical name denotes the genus
Haemostatic: checking blood flow
Herb: non-woody soft leafy plant; plant used in medicine and cooking
Hepatic: pertaining to the liver, beneficial to the liver
Hepatotoxic: toxic to the liver
Homoeopathy: system of medicine using tiny amounts of drugs which would produce in a healthy body symptoms similar to those of the disease (as distinct from allopathy)
Hybrid: natural or man-made plant produced by the fertilization of one species by another; indicated by × as in *Mentha × piperita*
Hydrolat: the French word *hydrolat* describes the condensed steam which has passed through the plant material. Guérain

(1886) gave hydrolat as a pharmaceutical term, being 'a colourless liquid which is obtained by distilling water with odorous flowers or with some other aromatic substances'; Mansion (1971) translates hydrolat as medicated water

Hydrosol: consists of very fine particles of a solid substance dispersed throughout water. A hydrosol stands between a suspension (a coarse mixture where the particles are much larger than colloidal particles) and a solution; in a true solution the particles of dissolved substance are of molecular size and thus smaller than colloidal particles

Hypertensor: agent increasing blood pressure; pressor

Hypnotic: inducing sleep

Hypotensor: agent reducing blood pressure

Immunostimulant: stimulating the immune system

Infusion: an extract of plant material made by pouring boiling water on herb (usually dried) and allowing to infuse to produce a solution of the soluble constituents; tea, herbal tea, tisane

Insectifuge: repels insects

Irritant: excessively stimulating causing inflammation

Lactogenic: promoting the secretion of milk; galactogogue

Laxative: loosening the bowel contents, promoting evacuation

Lipolytic: breaks down fatty substance

Lipophilic: having strong affinity for lipids

Litholytic: breaks down stones (e.g. kidney stones)

MS: mass spectrometer; an instrument for determining the composition of a compound; it is often coupled to a GC output to identify the volatile components of essential oils and hydrolats as they emerge

Mucolytic: breaks down mucus

Narcotic: inducing sleep, drowsiness

Nematicide: kills roundworms

Nervine: affecting the nervous system; soothing nervous excitement

Oestrogenic: simulating the action of female hormones

Officinalis: used in medicine; recognized in the pharmacopoeia

Oligomenorrhoea: a condition of infrequent menstruation

Organic: grown without the use of chemical fertilizers, pesticides, etc.; biologic

Organoleptic: concerned with testing the effects of a substance on the senses, particularly taste and smell

Oxymel: honey and vinegar mixture

Parabens: proprietary name of a preservative, normaly low molecular weight esters of 4-hydroxybenzoic acid

Percutaneous: applied through the skin

Pharmacokinetics: study of absorption, distribution, metabolism and elimination of drugs

Phlebotonic: having a toning action on the veins

Phlegm: mucus from the bronchial tubes

Phytotherapy: treatment of disease by the use of plants and plant extracts; herbalism

Probiotic: favouring the beneficial bacteria in the body, while inhibiting harmful microbes; literally 'for life' as distinct from antibiotic, 'against life'

Prophylactic: preventing disease

Pruritis: itchiness
Purgative: strongly laxative
Refreshing: reducing overheating; mildly laxative
Resolvent: reducing inflammation and swelling
Rubefacient: increasing local blood circulation causing redness of the skin
Sclerosis: hardening of tissue
Sedative: soothing, making drowsy
Simple: herb used medicinally; medicine made from a herb
Soporific: causing sleep
Spasmolytic: relieving convulsions, spasmodic pains and cramp
Stimulant: exciting the functions of various organs
Stomachic: agent which stimulates the secretory activity of the stomach
Stone: hard stone-like concretion in the urinary tract or gall bladder
Styptic: arresting haemorrhage by means of an astringent quality; haemostatic
Subspecies: subdivision of a species, often denoting a geographic variation; structure or colour are peculiar to subspecies and are more definite than characteristics identifying varieties; subspecies can interbreed; abbreviated to ssp.
Sudorific: inducing sweating; diaphoretic
Synergy: increased effect of two or more medicinal substances working together
Taenifuge: expelling worms
Taxonomy: scientific classification of living things
Termitifuge: expelling termites
Thalassotherapy: treatment by sea water to improve health and well-being
Theriac: antidote to bites of poisonous animals, especially snakes
Tisane: plant infusion; tea
Tonic: producing or restoring normal vigour or tension (tone)
Tranquillizer: relieves anxiety, calms down
Triturated: ground to a powder
Variety: indicates a botanical rank between subspecies and forma; abbreviated to var. as in *Citrus aurantium* var. *amara*
Vasoconstrictive: contracting blood vessels, raising blood pressure; hypertensor
Vasodilatory: enlarging blood vessels, reducing blood pressure; hypotensor
Vermifuge: expelling intestinal worms; anthelmintic
Vesicant: producing skin blisters (therapeutically to induce counter-irritant serum)
Viricide: kills a virus
Vulnerary: promoting healing of wounds

References

Acta Botanica 32: 49. Cited in: Beckstrom-Sternberg S M, Duke J A 1996 Handbook of medicinal mints (aromathematics): phytochemicals and biological activities. CRC Press, Boca Raton, p. 397

AGORA 2001 Aromatherapy Global Online Research Archives (website)

Aydin S, Baer K H C, Öztürk Y 1996 The chemistry and pharmacology of origanum (kekik) water. 27th International Symposium on Essential Oils, September, Wien

Balz R 1986 Les huiles essentielles et comment les utiliser. Self-published, Crest

Bartram T 1995 Encyclopaedia of herbal medicine. Grace Publishers, Christchurch

Battaglia S 1995 The complete guide to aromatherapy. Perfect Potion, Virginia

Baudoux D 1996a 2000 Ans de découvertes aromathérapiques pour une médecine d'avenir. Self-published

Baudoux D 1996b Formulaire d'aromathérapie pratique. Self-published

BBC News 2001 Fresh clue to homoeopath mystery. (7 November 2001) news.bbc.co.uk/hi/english/health/newsid_1643000/1643364.stm

Beckstrom-Sternberg S M, Duke J A 1996 Handbook of medicinal mints (aromathematics): phytochemicals and biological activities. CRC Press, Boca Raton

Bego G-V 1995 Discover what's essential about essential oils. Jakin, Lausanne

Beneviste J. See Davenas E, Beauvais F, Amarsa J et al 1988 Human basophil degranulation triggered by very dilute serum against IgE. 1988 Nature 333: 816–818

Bernadet M 1983 La phyto-aromathérapie pratique. Dangles, St Jean-de-Braye

Bohra P, Vaze A S, Pangarkar V G, Taskar A 1994 Adsorptive recovery of water soluble essential oil components. Journal of Chemical Technology and Biotechnology 66: 97–102

Bonnelle C 1993 Des hommes et des plantes. Editions du Parc Naturel Régional du Vercors, Lens-en-Vercors

Borchard R E, Barnes C D, Eltherton L G 1991 Drug dosage in laboratory animals: a handbook, 3rd edn. Telford Press, Caldwell, NJ

Boukef M K 1986 Médecine traditionelle et pharmacopée: les plantes dans la médecine traditionelle tunisienne. Agence de Coopération Culturelle et Technique

Bouzid N, Toulgouate K, Villarem G, Gaset A 1997 Analyse quantitative des fractions d'huile essentielle pouvant co-exister lors d'hydrodistillation de plantes aromatiques. Rivista Italiana Eppos 79: 15–25

Bowles E J 1995 The essential oil chemistry workbook: teacher's guide. Self-published, Hawthorn

Bown D 1995 Encyclopedia of herbs and their uses. BCA, London

Buchbauer G, Jirovetz L, Nikiforova A, Remberg G, Raverdino V 1990 Headspace analysis and aroma compounds of Austrian hay-blossoms (Flores graminis, Graminis flos) used in aromatherapy. Journal of Essential Oil Research 2: 185–191

Buchbauer G, Jirovetz L, Jäger W, Plank C, Dietrich H 1993 Fragrance compounds and essential oils with sedative effects upon inhalation. Journal of Pharmaceutical Sciences 82(6): 660–664

Budavari S (ed) 1996 The Merck index, 12th edn. Merck Research Laboratories, Whitehouse Station, NJ

Castleman M 1991 The healing herbs. Rodale Press, Emmaus, PA

Catty S 1998a Hydrosols. Pacific Institute of Aromatherapy Conference, San Francisco

Catty S 1998b Poster. P and C Acqua Vita.

Catty S 2000 Hydrosols. International Federation of Professional Aromatherapists Conference, Harrogate (October)

Catty S 2001 Hydrosols: the next aromatherapy. Healing Arts Press, Rochester

Claeys G 1992 Précis d'aromathérapie familiale. Equilibres, Flers

Clair C 1961 Of herbs and spices. Abelard-Schuman, London

Clarke S 2002 Essential chemistry for safe aromatherapy. Churchill Livingstone, Edinburgh

Clarkson R E 1972 The golden age of herbs and herbalists. Dover, New York

Concise Columbia Encyclopedia 1991 Columbia University Press, New York

Culpeper N (n.d.) Culpeper's complete herbal. Foulsham, Slough

Davies J 1985 A garden of miracles. Muller, London

Davis P 1988 Aromatherapy: an A–Z. Daniel, Saffron Walden

de Bonneval P 1992 Votre santé par les plantes. Equilibres, Flers

Decobecq D, Lavina P 2000 L'eau. Petit Guide no. 62. Aedis, Vichy

Distillerie de la Louine 2001 Brochure. Barnarve

Dodoens R 1554 Cruydeboek. [English translation 1578]

Dodt C K 1996 The essential oils book. Storey Communications, Pownal, VT

Duraffourd P 1987 Les huiles essentielles et la santé. La Maison de Bien-Etre, Montreuil-sous-Bois

Economic and Medicinal Plant Research 5: 195

enfleurage.com 2001

Farley J 1783 The London art of cookery and housekeeper's complete assistant by John Farley, principal cook at the London Tavern, Dublin. Price, Dublin, p. 208

Fischer-Rizzi S 1990 Complete aromatherapy handbook: essential oils for radiant health. Sterling Press, New York

Fleisher A 1991 Water soluble fractions of the essential oils. Perfumer and Flavorist 16(3): 37–41

Fleisher A, Fleisher Z 1985 Yield and quality of essential oil from *Pelargonium graveolens* cultivated in Israel. Journal of Science, Food Agriculture 36: 1047–1050

Fölsch 1930a Die Fabrikation und Verarbeitung von ätherischen Ölen. Wien, p. 47. Cited in: Guenther E 1948 The essential oils. Van Nostrand, New York, vol. 1, p. 155

Fölsch 1930b Die Fabrikation und Verarbeitung von ätherischen Ölen. Wien. Cited in: Foster S 1996 Chamomile: *Matricaria recutita* and *Chamaemelum nobile*. Botanical Series no. 307. American Botanical Council, Austin, p. 6

Forbes R J 1948 (reprint 1970) A short history of the art of distillation. E J Brill, Leiden

Foster S 1996 Chamomile: *Matricaria recutita* and *Chamaemelum nobile*. Botanical Series no. 307. American Botanical Council, Austin, p. 6

Fowler P, Wall M 1997 COSHH and CHIPS: ensuring the safety of aromatherapy. Complementary Therapies in Medicine 5: 112–115

Fox B A, Cameron A G 1975 Food science: a chemical approach. English Universities Press, London, p. 104

Franchomme P, Pénoël D 1990 L'aromathérapie exactement. Jollois, Limoges

Franchomme P, Pénoël D 1996 L'aromathérapie exactement, 2nd edn. Jollois, Limoges

Gallori S, Flamini G, Bilia A R, Morelli I, Landini A, Vincieri F F 2001 Chemical composition of some herbal drug preparations: essential oil and aromatic water of costmary (*Balsamita suaveolens* Pers.). Journal of Agriculture and Food Chemistry 49(12): 5907–5910

Gattefossé R-M 1993 [translation of 1937 publication] Gattefossé's aromatherapy. Daniel, Saffron Walden

Genders R 1972 A history of scent. Hamish Hamilton, London

Genders R 1977 A book of aromatics. Darton, Longman and Todd, London

Genders R 1986a Cosmetics from the earth. Alfred van der Marck, New York

Genders R 1986b Natural beauty: the practical guide to wildflower cosmetics. Webb and Bower, Exeter

Gerard J 1964 Gerard's herbal (1636). Spring Books, London

Goëb P H 1998 Aromathérapie pratique et familiale: connaître l'essentiel sur les huiles essentielles. IAPM, Chenai, Tamil Nadu

Gokhale N N 1959 The distillation waters. Indian Perfumery 3(2): 95–97

Grace U-M 1996 Aromatherapy for practitioners. Daniel, Saffron Walden, pp. 84–85

Grieve M 1992 A modern herbal. Tiger Books, London

Grieve M 1998 A modern herbal. Tiger Books, London

Griggs B 1997 New green pharmacy. Vermilion, London, p. 293

Grosjean N (n.d.) Aromatherapy: essential oils for your health. Vie Arôme, Graveson

Grosjean N 1993a L'aromathérapie: santé et bien être par les huiles essentielles. Albin Michel, Paris

Grosjean N 1993b Aromatherapy from Provence. Daniel, Saffron Walden

Guenther E 1948 The essential oils. Van Nostrand, New York, vol. 1

Guenther E 1949 The essential oils. Van Nostrand, New York, vol. 2

Guenther E 1952 The essential oils. Van Nostrand, New York, vol. 5

Guérain P (ed) 1886 Dictionnaire des dictionnaires. Librairie des Imprimeries Réunis, tome 3

Harborne J B, Baxter H 1983 Phytochemical dictionary: a handbook of bioactive compounds from plants. Taylor and Frost, London

Harmsworth c.1924 Harmsworth's business encyclopaedia. Educational Book Co., London, vol. 1, p. 418

Helliwell K 1989 Manufacture and use of plant extracts. In: Grievson M, Barber J, Hunting A L L (eds) Natural ingredients in cosmetics. Micelle, Weymouth, pp. 26–27

Hephrun B 2000a Toilet waters. Aromatica. Butterburr and Sage, Reading (Winter): 18–19

Hephrun B 2000b Aromatica. Butterburr and Sage, Reading (Autumn): 7

Higher Nature 2002 Silver: the remedy for health that modern medicine almost forgot. Higher Nature (7): 14

Holy Bible 1978 New International Version. Hodder and Stoughton, London

Huang K C 1993 The pharmacology of Chinese herbs. CRC Press, Boca Raton

Huxtable R J 1992 This and that: the essential pharmacology of herbs and spices. Tips 13: 15–20

Hyde C, Hyde L 1985 Favorite recipes. Cookbook Publishers, Olathe, KS, p. C

innerself.com/magazine/herbs/essential_oils 2001

International Journal of Oriental Medicine 1990 International Journal of Oriental Medicine 15(4): 194

Jacobson M 1990 Glossary of plant derived insect deterrents. CRC Press, Boca Raton

Journal of Essential Oil Research 7: 271

J Food Hyg Soc Jap 33(6): 569

JSPR 22 1986 Journal Stored Products Research 22:141. In: Beckstrom-Sternberg S M, Duke J A 1996 Handbook of Medicinal Mints (Aromathematics): phytochemicals and biological activities. CRC, Boca Raton p. 397

Kang R, Helms R, Stout M J, Jaber H, Chen Z, Nakatsu T 1992 Antimicrobial activity of volatile constituents of *Perilla frutescens* and its synergistic effects with polygodial. Journal of Agricultural and Food Chemistry 40: 2328–2330

Keeler R F, Tu A T 1991 Toxicology of plant and fungal compounds. Handbook of natural toxins. Marcel Dekker, New York, vol. 6, p. 665

Keller E 1991 Aromatherapy handbook for beauty hair and skin care. Healing Arts Press, Vermont

Kettenring M M 1994 Aromaküche: Gesund und Phantasievoll Kochen mit ätherischen Ölen. Joy Verlag, Sulzberg

Keville K, Green M 1995 Aromatherapy: a complete guide to the healing art. Crossing Press, Freedom

Korting H C, Schafer-Korting M, Hart H, Laux P, Schmid M 1993 Anti-inflammatory activity of hamamelis distillate applied topically to the skin. European Journal of Clinical Pharmacology (Spring)

Kresanek J 1982 Healing plants. Byeway Books, Slovart, Bratislava

Kubo A, Kubo I 1995 Antimicrobial agents from *Tanacetum balsamita.* Journal of Natural Products. 58: 1565–1569

Larkey SV, Pyles T (eds) 1941 An herbal (from the press of Richard Banckes), 1525. Scholars' Facsimile and Reprints, New York

Lautié R, Passebecq A 1979 Aromatherapy: the use of plant essences in healing. Thorsons, Wellingborough

Lee W H, Lee L 1992 The book of practical aromatherapy. Keats, New Canaan

Liébaert J 1975 Catholicisme: hier, aujourd'hui, demain. Letouzey et Ané, Paris, p. 1194

Life Application Study Bible 1996 Tyndale, Illinois, vol. 8–9, 1 Kings 5

Loeper M, Lesure A 1948 Formulaire pratique de thérapeutique et de pharmacologie, 36th edn. Doin, Paris

Lonicer A 1578 Kräuterbuch. Frankfurt.

Lower E S 1999 Shrub in a cold climate. Soap, Perfumery and Cosmetics (October): 65

Luu D V, Luu C 1993 Connaissance de l'eau. IMDERPLAM, Candillargues

Lydon J, Duke S 1989 The potential of pesticides from plants. In: Craker L, Simon J (eds) Herbs, spices and medicinal plants: recent advances in botany, horticulture and pharmacology. Oryx Press, Phoenix, vol. 4, pp. 1–41

Mabey R 1988 The complete new herbal. Elm Tree Books, London, p. 61

Machale K W, Nirinjan K, Pangarkar V G 1997 Recovery of dissolved essential oils from condensate waters of basil and *Mentha arvensis* distillation. Journal of Chemical Technology and Biotechnology 69: 362–366

Maneuvrier 2003 Personal communication

Mansion J E 1971 Harrap's new standard French and English dictionary. Harrap, London

Mathiolus P A 1554 Commentarii in VI libros Pedacii Dioscorides Anazarbei de materia medica. Venice. (Contains an appendix De ratione distillandi aquas ex omnibus plantis et quomodo genuini odores in ipse aquis conservari possint). Cited in: Forbes R J 1948 (reprint 1970) A short history of the art of distillation. E J Brill, Leiden

Menache A, Greek R 1999 Letter. Express (4 March 1999): 37

Mesue 1471 De medicinis universalibus et particularibus. Venice. Cited in : Forbes R J 1948 (reprint 1970) A short history of the art of distillation. E J Brill, Leiden

Mills S Y 1985 The dictionary of modern herbalism. Thorsons, Wellingborough, p. 219

Mise en Scène 2002a La thalassothérapie: la santé par la mer. Mise en Scène (printemps): 20

Mise en Scène 2002b L'eau au robinet: une histoire qui coule de source. Mise en Scène (printemps): 8

Mitchell J, Rook A J 1979 Botanical dermatology: plants and plant products injurious to the skin. Greenglass, Vancouver, xiii, p. 787

Mojay G 1996 Aromatherapy for healing the spirit. Gaia, London, p. 12

Montesinos C 1991 Eléments de réflexion sur quelques hydrolats. Ecole Lyonnaise de Plantes Médicinales, Lyons

Muroi H, Kubo I 1993 Combination effects of antibacterial compounds in green tea flavor against *Streptococcus mutans*. Journal of Agricultural and Food Chemistry 41: 1102–1105

Nasr J 2000 Aromatic waters – the missing link. Aromatherapist 7(4): 24–27

naturesgift.com/hydrosols

Newcastle Chronicle 1896 Encyclopaedic dictionary. Newcastle Chronicle, Newcastle upon Tyne, vol. 3, p. 508

New Scientist 2001 Homoeopathy isn't all hokum. New Scientist (10 November 2001): 4

Nigg H N, Seigler D S (eds) 1992 Phytochemical resources for medicine and agriculture. Plenum Press, New York, p. 455

Nowak R 2003 Oil and water do mix. New Scientist (22 February 2003): 17

nutrition.org.uk

Ody P 1997 100 Great natural remedies. Kyle Cathie, London, p. 44

Ohloff G 1994 Scent and fragrances. Springer-Verlag, New York. pp. viii–ix

Ortiz de Urbina A V, Martin M L, Montero M J, Moran A, San Roman L 1989 Sedating and antipyretic activity of the essential oil of *Calamintha sylvatica* ssp. *ascendens*. Journal of Ethnopharmacology 25: 165–171

Palma L 1964 Le piante medicinali. Società Editrice Internazionale, Milan

Paris M 2000 Hydrolats. 2nd Medical Aromatherapy Conference, Nice

Pashley R 2003 Journal of Physical Chemistry B 107: 1714. Reported in: Nowak R 2003 Oil and water do mix. New Scientist (22 February 2003): 17

Payne B 1999 Hydrolats for therapeutic use. Positive Health (September): 19–21

Pennington H 1999 Lessons from GM potatoes. Biologist 46(2): 51

Peyron L 1962 Etude de l'essence de géranium des eaux obtenue dans l'hydrodistillation du geranium rosat du Maroc. Comptes Rendues, Académie des Sciences 255: 2981–2982

Plotto A, Roberts D, Kim H, McDaniel M 2001 Aroma quality of lavender water: a comparative study. Perfumer and Flavorist 26 (May/June): 44–64

Poucher W A 1936 Perfumes, cosmetics and soaps. Chapman and Hall, London, vol. 2, pp. 34–35

Price D K 1962 Government and science. Oxford University Press, New York

Price L 1990 The history of aromatic medicine. Cosmetics Toiletries Manufacturers Supplies

Price L 1993 Aromatic waters. Riverhead, Hinckley

Price S 1995 Aromatherapy workbook. Thorsons, London, p. 222

Price S 1997 Aromatic water. The Aromatherapist 3(2): 44–47

Price L, Price S 1998 Essential waters. Pretium, Hinckley

Price S, Price L 1999 Aromatherapy for health professionals. Churchill Livingstone, Edinburgh

Prima Fleur Information leaflet. Prima Fleur, San Rafael

Proserpio G, Dorato S 1983 Officinal plants forbidden or not advisable for cosmetic products. Relata Technica 34: 63–69

Rajeswara Rao B R, Kaul P N, Syamasundar K V, Ramesh S 2002 Water soluble fractions of rose-scented geranium (Pelargonium species) essential oil. Bioresource Technology 84: 243–246

Ramsey C 2001 Message in a molecule. Health Matters 3(9) (Nov/Dec): 1

Revillion N 2003 Personal communication

Reynolds E F 1993 Martindale: the extra pharmacopoeia, 29th edn. Pharmaceutical Press, London, pp. 783, 784

Rivista Italiana Eppos 1994 12: 5

Rooibos Tea Control Board, South Africa

Rose J 1992 The aromatherapy book. North Atlantic Books, Berkeley

Rose J 1994 Hydrosols: the other product of distillation. Aromatherapy Correspondence course, Jeanne Rose Aromatherapy, San Francisco, California

Rose J 1999 375 Essential oils and hydrosols. Frog, Berkeley

Roulier G 1990 Les huiles essentielles pour votre santé. Dangles, St Jean-de-Braye

Rouvière A, Meyer M-C 1989 La santé par les huiles essentielles. M. A. Editions, Paris

Russell G B 1986 Phytochemical resources for crop protection. New Zealand Journal of Technology 127–134

Ryrie C 1998 The healing energies of water. Gaia, London, p. 102

Sağdiç O, Özcan M 2003 Antibacterial activity of Turkish spice hydrosols. Food Control 14: 141–143

sabia.com 1997-1999

Sairn A, Meloan C E 1986 Compounds from leaves of bay (*L. nobilis*) as repellents for *Tribolium castraneum* (Herbst) when added to wheat flour. Journal of Stored Products Research 22: 141. Cited in: Beckstrom-Sternberg S M, Duke J A 1996 Handbook of medicinal mints (aromathematics): phytochemicals and biological activities. CRC Press, Boca Raton, p. 397

Salmon, W 1710 Cited in Grieve M 1998 A modern herbal. Tiger Books, London, p. 226

Samal S, Choi B-J, Geckeler K E 2001 The first water-soluble main-chain polyfullerene. Chemical Communications 1373

Sanoflore 2000 Sanoflore catalogue. Organic care. Route de Lozeron par Beaufort, 26400 Gigors et Lozeron, France.

Schauenberg P, Paris F 1990 Guide to medicinal plants. Lutterworth Press, Cambridge

Schnaubelt K 1999 Medical aromatherapy. Frog, Berkeley

Sherwood Taylor F 1938 A short history of science. Heinemann, London

Shimizu M, Matsuzawa T, Yonezewa S et al 1990 Antiinflammatory constituents of topically applied crude drugs. IV. Constituents and antiinflammatory effect of Paraguayan crude drug

'alhucema' (*Lavandula latifolia* Vill.). Chemical and Pharmaceutical Bulletin (Tokyo) 38(8): 2283–2284
Shoyakugaku Zasshi 1996 In: Beckstrom-Stenberg SM, Duke J A (eds) Handbook of medicinal mints (aromathematics): phytochemicals and biological activities. CRC Press, Boca Raton, p. 402
Siegel B S 1988 Love, medicine and miracles. Arrow Books, London
6scent www.aromatherapycenter.com/sixth_spr98.htm
Smith T 1989 The side effects book. Insight Editions, Worthing
Spring M A 1988 Ethnopharmacologic analysis of medicinal plants used by Laotian Hmong refugees in Minnesota. Journal of Ethnopharmacology 26: 65–91
Stevenson C 1994 The use of aromatherapy massage on post cardiac surgery patients. Complementary Therapies in Medicine 2: 27–35
Stitt P A 1990 Why George should eat broccoli. Dougherty, Milwaukee
Streicher C 1996 Hydrosols: the subtle complement to essential oils. plexus 1:22
Stuart M (ed) 1982 VNR colour dictionary of herbs and herbalism. Van Nostrand Reinhold, New York
Stuart M (ed) 1987 The encyclopedia of herbs and herbalism. Black Cat, London
Svoboda I 2002 Personal communication
Svoboda K 2002 Personal communication
Taddei I, Giachetti D, Taddei E, Mantovani P, Bianchi E 1988 Spasmolytic activity of peppermint, sage and rosemary essences and their major constituents. Fitoterapia 59(6): 463–468
Thonnat N 2001 Le bon mangeur. Editions de la Federation de Cardiologie, Paris:, pp. 218–219
Tyler V E 1993 The honest herbal. Pharmaceutical Products Press, New York
Tyman J H P 1990 Research on constituent components of essential oils. Essential Oil Trade Symposium, Brunel University, London, June
Urdang G 1948 The origin and development of the essential oil industry. In: Guenther E 1948 The essential oils. Van Nostrand, New York, vol. 1, p. 3
Valnet J 1964 Aromathérapie. Maloine, Paris
Valnet J 1980 The practice of aromatherapy. Daniel, Saffron Walden
Vevy 1989 Correct use of hydroessentials. Instant Skin Care Reports. Lexicon Vevy 3: 53
Viaud H 1983 Huiles essentielles – hydrolats. Présence, Sisteron
von Rechenberg 1910 Theorie der Gewinnung und Trennung der ätherischen Öle. Leipzig, p. 362. In: Guenther E 1948 The essential oils. Van Nostrand, New York, vol. 1, p. 159
Wagner, Wolf (eds) 1977 New natural products (RS164.156.176). In: Beckstrom-Sternberg S M, Duke J A 1996 Handbook of medicinal mints (aromathematics): phytochemicals and biological activities. CRC Press, Boca Raton, p. 397
Walker P B M 1991 Chambers science and technology dictionary. Chambers, Edinburgh
Watt M 2000 Rose distillation in Turkey. Aromatica. Butterburr and Sage, Reading (Winter): 12
Wesley J 1792 Primitive physic, 24th edn. Whitfield, London
Whitton P 2003 Personal communication
Winter R 1984 A consumer's dictionary of cosmetic ingredients. Crown Publishers, New York
Winter R 1999 A consumer's dictionary of cosmetic ingredients. Three Rivers Press, New York
Woodward M 1964 Gerard's herbal. Spring Books, London
Wren R C 1975 Potter's new cyclopaedia of botanical drugs and preparations. Health Science Press, Bradford nr Holsworthy
Yamamoto A, Umemori S, Muranishi S 1994 Absorption enhancement of intrapulmonary administered insulin by various absorption enhancers and protease inhibitors in rats. Journal of Pharmacy and Pharmacology 46: 14–18
Youth Bible 1993 New Century Version. Nelson Word, Milton Keynes
Yu S G, Anderson P J, Elson C E 1995 Efficacy of B-ionone in the chemoprevention of rat mammary carcinogenesis. Journal of Agricultural and Food Chemistry 43: 2144–2147
Zheng G-Q, Kenney P M, Lam L K T 1992 Sesquiterpenes from clove (*Eugenia caryophyllata*) as potential anticarcinogenic agents. Journal of Natural Products 55(7): 999–1003
Ziman J 1968 Public knowledge. Cambridge University Press, Cambridge

Index

Aaron's rod *(Solidago virgaurea)*, 143, 224, 229
Abies balsamea (Balm of Gilead, Balsam fir, Canada balsam), 95, 215, 227
Abscesses, breast, 112
Abumeron, 13
Acacia decurrens (Green Wattle, Mimosa), 95, 215, 227
Acetates, 75
Acetic acid, 63
Acetone, 63, 67, 71
Aches, 159
Achillea millefolium see Yarrow *(Achillea millefolium)*
Acids, 63, 86–7
  see also specific acid
Acne
  geranium, 182–4
  lavender, 120
  Roman chamomile, 103
  rose, 137
  thyme, 145
  use of hydrolats for, 154, 209
  yarrow, 96
Advantages of distilled plant waters, 4
Aftershave, 209
Agaricus campestris (Field mushroom), 96, 197, 215, 227
Ajowan seed, 52
Alchemy, 11–12, 14
Alcohol
  addition to hydrolats, 38, 158–9
  analysis of hydrolats, 48, 83–4
  molecules in water, 64, 72–3
  pimento water, 37
  properties of, 94
Aldehydes, 29, 65, 74, 85
Alecost *see* Costmary
Algae, 56, 57
Alkali, 64
Allergic reactions, 128
All heal *(Valeriana officinalis)*, 43, 63, 147, 225, 230
Aloe vera, 37, 154
Aloysia triphylla (Lemon verbena), 96, 122, 215, 227
Alphabetical list of hydrolats, 95–148
Alpha-phellandrene, 63, 66, 74, 82
Alpha-pinene, 66–7, 74, 82
Alpha-terpineol, 73
American liverwort *(Anemone hepatica)*, 96, 215, 227
Amines, 64
Ammonia, 64
Anaemia, 116
Anagallis arvensis (Scarlet pimpernel), 96, 215, 227
Analgesics, 197
Analysis of hydrolats
  chemistry of aromatic molecules, 76–91
  methods of extraction, 61–3
  molecules found in water, 63–70, 71–5
Anemone hepatica (American liverwort), 96, 215, 227
Anethum graveolens (Dill), 51, 97, 215, 227
Angelica *(Angelica archangelica)*
  analysis of, 63, 67, 71–5
  angelica root, 14, 52, 232
  angelica seed, 52
  therapeutic properties of, 97, 215
Animal testing, 6
Aniseed *(Pimpinella anisum)*, 36, 52, 70, 116, 132, 222
Anthelmintics, 197
Antiallergics, 197
Antibacterials, 197
Anticancers, 198
Antidiabetics, 198
Antifungals, 198
Antihaemorrhagics, 212
Antiinfectious, 198
Antiinflammatories, 198
Antioxidants, 198
Antiparasitics, 199
Antirheumatics, 199
Antiseptics, 199

Antispasmodics, 199
Antitoxics, 199
Antivirals, 200
Aphrodisiacs, 98, 136
Apium graveolens (Smallage, Wild celery), 97, 215, 227
Appearance of hydrolats, 58
Arab influences, 11–13
Arbutus uva ursi (Bearberry, Mountain Box), 97, 216, 227
Arctium lappa (Beggar's buttons, Greater Burdock), 98, 227
Aristotle, 25
Arnica *(Arnica montana)*, 52, 98, 227
Aromatherapy, origins of, 1–2
Aromatic molecules, chemistry of, 76–91
Aromatic oils, 16
Aromatic ring, 83
Aromatic water *see* Hydrolats
Aromatic whipped cream, 174–5
Artemesia abrotanum (Lad's love, Southernwood), 98, 216, 227
Artemesia absinthium (Wormwood), 13, 98, 227
Artemesia arborescens (Great mugwort, Tree wormwood), 98, 216, 227
Artemesia dracunculus (Tarragon), 36, 99, 163, 216, 227
Artemesia vulgaris (Felon herb, Mugwort), 99, 217, 227
Arthritis, 5, 24, 141, 146, 200
Artificial waters, 3
Ascariasis, 213
Aspirin, 16
Asthma, 128, 134, 192, 200
Astringents, 200
Atlas cedarwood *(Cedrus atlantica)*, 101, 199, 216, 227
Atoms, 76–80
Avenzoar, 13
Avicenna, 12

Baby care, 160–1
Bach flower remedies, 7
Bacteria, 23, 56, 57
Bactericides, 9
Bad breath, 127
Balm *see* Lemon Balm
Balm of Gilead *(Abies balsamea)*, 95, 227
Balsam herb *see* Costmary
Balsamita suaveolens see Costmary
Balsams, 10, 16
Baptism, 22
Basil *(Ocimum basilicum)*, 36, 66, 128, 164, 184, 221
Batchelor's button *see* Cornflower
Baths, 152, 160
Bay *(Laurus nobilis)*
  digestive problems, 164
  history of aromatic medicine, 10
  lice, 168
  oil content, 52
  therapeutic properties of, 118–19, 197, 198, 219
  vaccination side effects, 157
Bearberry *(Arbutus uva ursi)*, 97, 216, 227
Bedsores, 209
Bee balm *see* Lemon Balm
Beggar's buttons *(Arctium lappa)*, 98, 227
Beliefs, 21
Benedictine monks, 13
Benzene ring, 83
Benzoin, 14
Berbers, 12
Bergamot, 16, 65, 66
Beta-caryophyllene, 82
Beta-phellandrene, 63, 66, 74
Beta-pinene, 66, 67, 74, 82
Beta-terpineol, 73
Beta-thujone, 68
Betony *(Stachys officinalis)*, 100, 143, 229
Betula (Birch), 100, 227
Beverages, 156–7
  see also Decoctions; Teas; Tisanes
Birch *(Betula)*, 100, 227
Bismuth subnitrate, 56
Bites, insect, 114, 120, 130, 144
Bitter orange flower *see* Neroli; Petitgrain
Black alder tree, 195
Black spruce *(Picea mariana)*, 131, 222, 229
Black tea, 190
Black thyme *(Thymbra spicata)*, 144, 224, 229
Bladder infections, 101
  see also Urinary tract problems
Bladderwrack *(Fucus vesiculosus)*, 67, 71–5, 111–12, 218, 238
Bleeding gums, 172
Blepharitis, 125
Blessed thistle *(Cnicus benedictus)*, 42, 106, 227
Bloating, 106
Bluebottle *see* Cornflower
Blue buttons *(Scabiosa succisa)*, 143, 224, 229
Blue leaved mallee *(Eucalyptus polybractea)*, 218, 228
Body, water in the, 23
Boils, 200
Boldo leaf *(Peumus boldus)*, 131, 164, 195, 222, 229
Bonding of atoms, 77–80
Borage *(Borago officinalis)*, 11, 100, 227
Borneol, 36, 72, 84
Bornyl acetate, 66, 75, 87
Boswellia carteri (Frankincense), 9, 14, 161
Bottled water, 23

Box, 41, 100, 216, 227
Breast abscesses, 112
British Dietetic Association, 23
Broad leaved peppermint *(Eucalyptus dives)*, 218, 228
Bronchitis, 117, 128, 169, 200
Broom *(Sarothamnus scoparius)*, 142, 224, 229
Bruises, 200
Burning bush *(Dictamnus albus)*, 108, 218, 228
Burns, 120
Butanone, 71
Butcher's broom *(Ruscus aculeatus)*, 162, 223, 229

Cabbage, 11
Cadinene, 73
Caffeine, 188–9
Calamus, 14, 52
Calendula officinalis see Marigold; Pot marigold
Calming effects of plants, 200
Camphone, 67
Camphor, 63, 67, 68, 71, 86
Canada balsam *(Abies balsamea)*, 215
Canella bark, 15
Capillaries, broken, 170
Caraway *(Carum carvi)*
  analysis of, 70
  essential oil, 36
  history of herbs, 10
  seed, 52
  slimming recipe, 171
  therapeutic properties of, 101, 216
Cardamom *(Eletteria cardamomum)*, 109, 218, 228
Carmelite water, 14
Carminatives, 201
Carrot *(Daucus carota)*
  analysis of, 63, 71–5, 236
  carrot seed, 107–8, 218, 236–7
  therapeutic properties of, 162, 171
Carum carvi see Caraway
Carvacrol, 84
Carveol, 72
Carvone, 63, 67, 68, 86
Caryophyllene, 63, 66, 67, 73
Case studies, 181–6
Cataracts, 148
Catarrh, 145, 201
Catty, Suzanne, 94
Cautions, 158, 195
Cavendish, Henry, 25
Cayenne, 65
Cedar, 10, 45, 167, 171
Cedrus atlantica (Atlas cedar), 101, 199, 216, 227
Celery seed, 52
Cellulite, 95, 161, 209
Centaurea cyanus see Cornflower
Centaury, 36
Chamaemelum nobile see Roman chamomile
Chamomile flowers, 51, 52
Chamomile (not specified), 36, 39, 170
  see also German chamomile; Moroccan chamomile; Roman chamomile
Chelidonium majus (Greater celandine), 166, 217, 227
Chemical changes during distillation, 45
Chemical sprays, 20
Chemistry, 6, 15–16, 76–91
Chenopodium album (Fat hen, White goosefoot), 103, 217, 227
Cherry laurel *(Prunus laurocerasus)*, 37, 134, 222, 229
Chickenpox, 101, 162, 201
Child care, 150, 160–1
Cicatrizants, 201–2
Cineole, 69
Cinnamic acid, 63
Cinnamon *(Cinnamomum verum)*
  analysis of, 63
  cinnamon ceylon, 52
  cinnamon leaf, 173
  essential oil, 36
  history of aromatic plant medicine, 9, 14
  therapeutic properties of, 103–4, 125
Circulation, 95, 99, 138, 162, 202
Cistus ladaniferus (Laudanum, Rock rose), 105, 170, 217, 227
Citron, 36
Citronella, 64
Citrus aurantium see Neroli; Orange flower; Petitgrain
Citrus limon see Lemon
Clary sage *(Salvia sclarea)*
  analysis of, 63, 66, 69, 71–5, 254
  therapeutic properties of, 140–1, 168, 169, 184, 224
Cleanser, water as a, 22
Cloves *(Syzygium aromaticum)*
  clove bud, 143–4, 229
  clove stems, 52
  history of aromatic medicine, 14
  oil content, 52
  therapeutic properties of, 125, 185–6
Cnicus benedictus (Blessed thistle, Holy thistle), 42, 106, 227
Cohobation, 45, 46, 49–50, 49–54
Colds, 112, 116, 162, 202
Colic, 101, 106, 145, 202
Colitis, 125, 151
Colours of hydrolats, 58
Common horsetail *see* Horsetail
Composition of water, 25
Compresses, 152–3, 160, 165

Conjunctivitis, 113, 125, 136, 165
Constipation, 136, 163, 195
Contraceptive pill, 20
Convallaria majalis (Lily of the valley), 106, 227
Cooking, 173–7
Copper, 57
Coriander *(Coriandrum sativum)*
  analysis of, 65
  coriander seed, 14, 51, 52
  drying plants, 43
  essential oil, 36
  history of aromatic medicine, 10
  therapeutic properties of, 106–7, 125, 160, 217
Cornflower *(Centaurea cyanus)*
  analysis of, 63, 71–5, 233–4
  appearance of, 58
  compresses, 152–3
  for eye conditions, 166
  for skin care, 170
  for sore throats, 172
  therapeutic properties of, 101–2, 216
Costmary *(Balsamita suaveolens)*
  analysis of, 69, 71–5, 232
  costmary water, 63, 67
  therapeutic properties of, 99
Cost of hydrolats, 59–60
Costus root, 52
Cotinus coggyria (Smoke tree), 107, 227
Cotyledon umbilicus (Kidneywort), 107, 217, 227
Coughs
  cherry laurel, 134
  elecampane, 117
  ground ivy, 112
  hyssop, 116
  myrtle, 128
  tea tree, 123
  witch hazel, 202
Coumarin, 74
Covalent bond, 79–80
Cowslip, 134, 229
Crataegus laevigata (Hawthorn), 71–5, 107, 217, 228, 235
Creams, 154
Crocus sativus (Saffron), 107, 228
Crohn's disease, 125
Croup, 117
Crusades, the, 14
Cubebs, 52
Culinary uses/recipes, 157, 173–7
Culpeper, Nicholas, 15–16, 18
Cumin, 107, 217, 228
Cypress *(Cupressus sempervirens)*
  for bleeding gums, 172
  for broken capillaries, 170
  for cellulite, 161
  for circulation, 162
  essential oil, 36
  history of aromatic medicine, 10
  Italian cypress, 107
  oil content of distillates, 52
  recipe, 185–6
  for slimming, 171
  still hardware, 45
  therapeutic properties of, 107, 217
Cystitis, 101, 109, 155, 202

Damask rose *(Rosa damascena)*, 169, 170
Dandelion *(Taraxacum officinale)*, 144, 229
Dandruff, 101, 127, 153
Date and orange-blossom baklava, 176–7
Daucus carota see Carrot
Dead nettle *(Lamium album)*, 118, 220, 228
Death, life and, 21
Decanted essential oil, 49
Decoctions, 187, 194–5
Decomposition, 45
Density of hydrolats, 58
Depression, 182
Dermatitis, 96, 137, 145, 154
Detoxification, 163
Devil's claw *(Harpagophytum procumbens)*, 114, 218, 219, 228
Diabetes, 118, 142
Diarrhoea, 163
Dictamnus albus (Burning bush, Dittany), 108, 218, 228
Diethyl ether, 50–1
Digestion
  kidneywort, 107
  orange-blossom water, 173
  peppermint, 126
  rooibos tea, 192
  rosemary, 138
  use of hydrolats for, 25, 151, 155, 164, 202–3
  wormwood, 98
Dill *(Anethum graveolens)*, 51, 97, 215, 227
Dilution, increased, 30
Dimethyl sulphide, 63, 70, 74
Discovery of new plants, 15
Dispersants, 157–8
Distillates, 41–2, 48, 51
  see also Hydrolats
Distillation
  development of, 11, 12
  general, 43–4
  methods, 20, 37, 46, 177–8
  prepared waters, 35–6
  water oil, 50–1
  water used, 44–5
Dittany *(Dictamnus albus)*, 108, 218, 228
Diuretics, 203
Doctrine of signatures, 14
Double blind trials, 5

Douches, 153
Dried herbs, 191
Drinks, 23
  see also Decoctions; Teas; Tisanes
Drying, 42–3
Dry skin, 209
Dysmenorrhoea, 124, 184

Ear, nose and throat problems, 157
  see also specific problem
Eau-de-Cologne, 16, 39, 180
Echinacea purpurea (Purple coneflower), 67, 71–5, 108, 218, 228, 237
Eczema
  carrot seed, 108
  general use of hydrolats, 151, 210
  lavender, 120
  lime leaf, 146
  Roman chamomile, 103
  rooibos tea, 192
  safety of hydrolats, 182
  sage, 140
  sandalwood, 142
  thyme, 145
  yarrow, 96
Egypt, 9–10
Elderflower *(Sambucus nigra)*, 39, 43, 141–2, 200, 224, 229
Elecampane *(Inula graveolens)*, 52, 117, 200, 219, 228
Electronegativity, 26–8
Electrons, 76–8
Electrovalent bond, 78
Eletteria cardamomum (Cardamom), 109, 218, 228
Emmenagogues, 203
Endometriosis, 203
Energising plants, 203–4
Enteritis, viral, 185–6
Enterobiasis, 213
Epilepsy, 116
Equisetum arvense see Horsetail
Erigeron canadensis (Fleabane), 109, 162, 218, 228
Essencier (Florentine vase), 45, 49, 50
Essential oils
  combining with hydrolats, 4
  obtaining, 49 (*see also* Distillation)
  preparation of hydrolats, 31–2
  primary and secondary, 49
  quality of, 35
  recovered, 49, 50–1
  safety, 2
  shelf-life, 57–8
  solubility, 36, 47
  sourcing materials, 3
  treating arthritis, 5
Essential water *see* Hydrolats
Esters, 29, 65–6, 87, 94
  see also specific ester
Ethanol
  eau-de-Cologne, 16
  extraction, 50–1
  presence in hydrolats, 72, 153, 165
  properties, 64
  solubility, 28
Ethers, 29, 48
Eucalyptol, 63, 69, 73
Eucalyptus globulus (Tasmanian blue gum), 109, 198, 218, 228
Eucalyptus polybractea (Blue leaved mallee), 218, 228
Eucalyptus smithii (Gully gum), 163
Eucalyptus (unspecified), 11, 36, 58, 166, 169
Eugenol, 84
Eupatorium cannabinum (Hemp agrimony), 109, 218, 228
Euphrasia officinalis (Eyebright), 109–10, 165, 218, 228
Evaporation, 43
Eucalyptus dives (Broad leaved peppermint), 218, 228
Everlasting
  analysis of, 71–5, 238–9
  appearance of, 58
  skin care, 170
  therapeutic properties of, 114–15, 218–19, 219
Evidence, 5–7
Expectorants, 204
External use, 152–5
Extraction methods, 61–3
  see also specific method
Eyebright *(Euphrasia officinalis)*, 109–10, 165, 218, 228
Eyes
  care of, 153
  conditions/irritation, 128, 165–6 (*see also specific condition*)
  drops for, 165
  hydrolats for use on, 204
  information about, 124
  lotion for, 13

False acacia *(Robinia pseudacacia)*, 134, 222, 229
False hydrolats *see* Prepared waters
False waters, 3
Farina, J. M., 16
Farming, 20
Fat hen *(Chenopodium album)*, 103, 217, 227
Feet, 205
Felon herb *(Artemesia vulgaris)*, 99, 216, 227
Feminis, Paul, 16
Fenchyl alcohol, 64, 84

Fennel *(Foeniculum vulgare)*
- analysis of, 61
- essential oil, 36
- fennel seed, 51, 52
- fennel tea, 111
- history of aromatic medicine, 11
- regulations for preparation of, 37
- therapeutic properties of, 110–11, 164, 165, 171, 173, 218

Ferns, 41, 195
Fever, 127, 145, 205
Fever few *(Chrysanthemum parthenium)*, 103, 227
Field balm *(Glechoma hrederacea)*, 112, 228
Field horsetail *see* Horsetail
Field mushroom *(Agaricus campestris)*, 96, 197, 215, 227
Filipendula ulmaria see Meadowsweet
Filtration, 56
Flatulence, 101, 111, 127, 144
Flavour, 15
Fleabane *(Erigeron canadensis)*, 109, 162, 218, 228
Flocculation, 56, 57
Flooding, 21
Floral water *see* Hydrolats
Florentine vase, 45, 49, 50
Flu, 104, 124, 141, 162, 202
Food poisoning, 143
Fragaria vesca (Strawberry), 111, 218, 228
Fragrance, 4
Fragrant water *see* Hydrolats
Frankincense *(Boswellia carteri)*, 9, 14, 161
Freckles, 96, 133, 210
French marjoram *(Origanum onites)*, 129, 222, 229
- *see also* Marjoram

Fresh herbs, 190–1
Frigidity, 136, 205
Fucus vesiculosus see Bladderwrack
Fumitory *(Fumaria officinalis)*, 112, 228
Fungal infections, 104, 123, 152
Fungi, 56

Galactogens, 205
Galangal, 52, 56
Galega officinalis (Goat's rue), 112, 218, 228
Gall bladder, 147
Gardenia, 65, 66
Gargles, 157
Garlic, 36, 70
Gas chromatography (GC), 61, 257–67
Gas chromatography-mass spectrometry (GC-MS), 61–2
Geber, 12
Gentiana lutea (Yellow gentian), 112, 218, 228
Gentian (unspecified), 36, 58
Geraniol, 64, 72, 84
Geranium *(Pelargonium graveolens)*
- for acne, 183
- analysis of, 63, 65, 69, 70, 71–5, 248–50
- for bleeding gums, 172
- for cellulite, 161
- for chickenpox, 162
- essential oil, 36, 64
- for hypertension, 167
- for PMS, 168
- for skin problems, 171, 182–4
- for stomach upsets, 164
- therapeutic properties of, 130–1, 222

Geranyl acetate, 87
Germacrene D, 63, 66, 67, 74, 82
German chamomile *(Matricaria recutita)*, 71–5, 122–3, 170, 220, 245
- *see also* Chamomile; Roman chamomile

Giardiasis, 213
Gingergrass, 64
Ginger *(Zingiber officinale)*, 52, 116, 147–8, 225, 230
Gingivitis, 115, 205
Glechoma hrederacea (Ground ivy, Field balm), 112, 228
Glossary, 269–73
Goat's rue *(Galega officinalis)*, 112, 218, 228
Golden purslane *(Portulaca sativa)*, 133, 222, 229
Golden rod *(Solidago virgaurea)*, 143, 224, 229
Gout, 100, 107, 146, 205
Grains of paradise, 15
Grape spirit, 13
Graphic representation of molecules, 80–1
Greater burdock *(Arctium lappa)*, 98, 227
Greater burnet *(Pimpinella magna)*, 132, 222, 229
Greater celandine *(Chelidonium majus)*, 165, 217, 227
Great mugwort *(Artemesia arborescens)*, 98, 216, 227
Greenland moss *(Ledum groenlandicum)*, 121, 220, 228
Green wattle *(Acacia decurrens)*, 95, 215, 227
Grieve, Maud, 18, 37
Ground ivy *(Glechoma hrederacea)*, 112, 228
Gully gum *(Eucalyptus smithii)*, 163
Gynaecological problems, 25, 205

Haemorrhage, 135
Haemorrhoids, 104, 107, 113, 133
Hair care, 151–2, 153, 167, 205–6
Hair loss, 128
Hamamelis virginiana see Witch hazel
Hardware, still, 45
Harpagophytum procumbens (Devil's claw), 114, 218, 219, 228
Hawkweed *(Hieracium pilosella)*, 115, 219, 228
Hawthorn *(Crataegus laevigata)*, 71–5, 107, 217, 228, 235

Hay fever, 192
Headaches
  common melilot, 124
  compresses, 152–3
  lavender, 119, 121
  lime leaf, 146
  recipe for relief of, 167
  rose, 136
  wild thyme, 144
Healing treatments with water, 24–5
Heart, 201, 206
Heartburn, 105, 134
Heartsease *(Viola tricolor)*, 147, 230, 255
Hedera helix (Ivy), 114, 228
Helichrysum, 63, 69
Hemp agrimony *(Eupatorium cannabinum)*, 109, 218, 228
Hepatics, 206
Herbalism, 5
Herbs, fresh, 190–1
Herpes, 125, 210
Hexanal, 65, 74
Hexane extraction, 50–1
Hieracium pilosella (Hawkweed, Mouse ear), 115, 219, 228
High blood pressure, 109, 138, 167, 185–6, 206
Hippocrates, 10
History of aromatic medicine, 9–18
Holy thistle *(Cnicus benedictus)*, 42, 106, 227
Holy wars, the, 13
Homoeopathy, 4
Honey, 192
Honeysuckle, 39, 65
Hormonal imbalances, 131, 206
Horsemint *(Mentha sylvestris)*, 127, 197, 221, 228
Horsetail *(Equisetum arvense)*, 42, 69, 71–5, 109, 228, 235–6
Hungary water, 13–14
Hydrocarbons, 48, 63, 66–7, 73–4, 82
  see also specific hydrocarbon
Hydrocortisone cream, 113
Hydrocotyle asiatica (Indian pennywort), 115, 228
Hydrodiffusion, 43, 45
Hydroessentials, 38–9
Hydrogen bonding, 26
Hydrolats
  advantages of, 4, 149–50
  appearance of, 58
  cautions when using, 158
  composition of, 4–5
  cost of, 59–60
  definition of, 2
  density of, 58
  external use of, 152–5
  gas chromatography, 257–67
  internal use of, 155–8
  making your own, 177–80
  obtaining, 31–2
  odour of, 58–9
  pH of, 58
  plant types, 41–2
  preservatives, 57–8
  quality of, 59
  storage, 55–6, 56–7
  terminology, 33
  therapeutic properties of, 215–25
  uses of, 150–1, 151–2
  yield of, 46–7
Hydrolysis, 45
Hydrophobic, 28
Hydrophilic compounds, 4
Hydrosols *see* Hydrolats
Hygiene, 9
Hypericum perforatum see St John's wort
Hypertension, 110, 137, 167, 185–6, 206
Hypotensors, 206
Hyssop *(Hyssopus officinalis)*
  analysis of, 63, 71–5, 86, 240
  cautions, 195
  essential oil, 36
  storage of, 56
  therapeutic properties of, 116, 219
Hysteria, 146

Immunostimulants, 206
Increased dilution, 30
Indian pennywort *(Hydrocotyle asiatica)*, 115, 228
Indian valerian *(Valeriana wallichii)*, 225
Indigestion, 134, 140, 148, 192
  see also Digestion
Inflammation, reducing, 10
Influenza, 104, 125, 141, 162, 202
Infusions, 7, 188–90, 192–4
Inorganic chemistry, 76
Insect bites, 114, 120, 131, 145
Insomnia, 125, 130, 206
Internal use, 2, 4, 36, 150, 155–8
Inula graveolens (Elecampane), 52, 117, 200, 219, 228
Ionic bond, 78
Iris *(Iris pseudacorus)*, 117, 219, 228
Irritation of the skin, 211
Isomenthone, 86
Isomers, 88
Isopinocamphone, 63
Isoprene units, 81–2
Isovaleranic acid, 63
Italian cypress *(Cupressus sempervirens)*, 107
Ivy *(Hedera helix)*, 114, 228

Jasmin, 39, 66
Judging by water, 22

Juniper *(Juniperus communis)*
essential oil, 36
juniper berry
analysis of, 71–5, 241
oil content, 52
therapeutic properties of, 117–18, 161, 171, 219
juniper branch, 117–18
still hardware, 45
therapeutic properties of, 166, 169, 171, 219
Ketones, 48, 63, 67–8, 71–2, 85–6, 94
see also specific ketone

Kidneys, 101, 141, 143
Kidney stones, 100, 173
Kidneywort *(Cotyledon umbilicus)*, 107, 217, 227
Knowledge, 6, 17
Kyphi, 10

Labdanum, 9
Labrador tea *(Ledum groenlandicum)*, 121, 220, 228
Lactuca hortensis (Lettuce), 42, 118, 219, 228
Lactuca virosa (Wild lettuce), 118, 219, 228
Lad's love *(Artemesia abrotanum)*, 98, 216, 227
Lambliasis, 213
Lamium album (Dead nettle), 118, 220, 228
Laudanum *(Cistus ladaniferus)*, 105, 170, 217, 227
Laurus nobilis see Bay
Lavandin *(Lavandula* x *intermedia)*, 71–5, 120, 200, 220, 228, 243
Lavandula angustifolia see Lavender
Lavandula latifolia (Spike lavender), 71–5, 120–1, 228, 243
Lavandulol, 64, 72, 84
Lavandulyl, 66, 75, 87
Lavender cotton, 142, 224
Lavender *(Lavandula angustifolia)*
analysis of, 66, 67, 69, 71–5, 241–2
for babies and children, 161
for chickenpox, 162
for digestion problems, 163
drying, 43
essential oil, 36
flocculation, 56
for haircare, 167, 168
history of aromatic medicine, 13, 15, 16
hydroessentials, 39
lavender flowers, 51
for mild depression, 182
odour, 59
for skin conditions, 170, 171, 182
therapeutic properties of, 119–20, 220
for thrush, 172
Lavoisier, Antoine Laurent, 25

Ledum groenlandicum (Greenland Moss, Labrador tea), 121, 220, 228
Legs, 167, 207
Lemon balm *see* Melissa
Lemon *(Citrus limon)*
eau-de-Cologne, 16
essential oil, 36
hydroessentials, 39
lemon peel, 13, 14, 125
therapeutic properties of, 106, 162, 173
Lemon verbena *(Aloysia triphylla)*, 96, 122, 215, 227
Lentisk *(Pistacia lentiscus)*, 133, 162, 222, 229
Lettuce *(Lactuca hortensis)*, 42, 118, 219, 228
Levisticum officinale (Lovage), 52, 121, 164, 220, 228
Lice, 168
Life and death, 21
Lilac, 65
Lily, 65
Lily of the valley *(Convallaria majalis)*, 106, 227
Lime *(Tilia)*
lime blossom, 66, 191
lime flower, 170, 230
lime leaf, 146, 225
lime sapwood, 146–7, 225, 230
storage, 56
see also Linden blossom
Limonene, 74, 82
Linaloe, 65
Linalool, 63, 64, 65, 73, 84
Linalyl, 66, 75, 87
Linaria vulgaris (Toadflax), 122, 220, 228
Linden blossom *(Tilia europaea)*, 56, 146, 169, 230
Lipolytics, 207
Lipophilic substances, 4
Liquid-liquid extraction, 61–2
Liquid-solid partitioning, 62
Litholytics, 207
Liver detoxification, 121
Lotions, 154
Lourdes, 24
Lovage *(Levisticum officinale)*, 52, 121, 164, 220, 228
Lumbago, 143
Lustration, 22
Lymph glands/nodes, 168, 172, 207, 212

Macerated plant waters, 178–9
Maceration, 187
Magnolia, 65
Mallow *(Malva sylvestris)*, 42, 71–5, 122, 228, 245
Marigold *(Calendula officinalis)*, 15, 71–5, 100–1, 227, 233

Marjoram *(Origanum majorana)*
analysis of, 63, 66, 69, 71–5, 244
essential oil, 36
for headaches, 167
for menstruation cramps, 184
therapeutic properties of, 129–30, 164, 168, 222
Mars, Jean, 90
Mastic tree *(Pistacia lentiscus)*, 133, 162, 222, 229
Matricaria recutita see German chamomile
Mature skin, 211–12
Maypops *(Passiflora incarnata)*, 130, 229
Meadowsweet *(Filipendula ulmaria, Spirea ulmaria)*
analysis of, 71–5, 237
appearance of, 58
therapeutic properties of, 110, 143, 218
Measles, 101
Medicated water *see* Hydrolats
Medicine, 6, 10–11, 16
Megaleion, 10
Melaleuca alternifolia see Tea tree
Melilot *(Melilotus officinalis)*
analysis of, 71–5
appearance of, 58
drying, 43
therapeutic properties of, 123–4, 162, 166, 220, 246
Melissa *(Melissa officinalis)*
analysis of, 63, 67, 69, 71–5, 246–7
cohobation, 53
distillation process, 45
drying, 43
essential oil, 36
history of aromatic medicine, 11, 13, 14, 15
teas, 191–2
therapeutic properties of, 124–5, 184, 221
Menopause, 136, 139, 168, 207
Menstruation cramps, 125, 184
Mentha pulegium (Pennyroyal), 86, 127, 221, 228
Mentha spicata (Spearmint), 127, 221, 228
Mentha sylvestris (Horsemint), 127, 197, 221, 228
Mentha x *piperita see* Peppermint
Menthone, 86
Methyl alcohol, 64
Methyl-butanal, 75
Methyl iodide, 58
Migraines, 125, 146, 151, 207
see also Headaches
Mimosa *(Acacia decurrens)*, 95, 215, 227
Minerals, 24
Mint, 13, 37, 166
Mistletoe *(Viscum album)*, 56, 147, 225, 230
Molecules, 47–8, 63–91
Moroccan chamomile *(Ormenis mixta)*, 130, 222, 229
see also Chamomile
Mould, 57
Mountain box *(Arbutus uva ursi)*, 97, 216, 227
Mouse ear *(Hieracium pilosella)*, 115, 219, 228
Mouth ulcers, 136
Mouthwashes, 152, 157, 207
Mucolytics, 207
Mucous membranes, 152
Mugwort *(Artemesia vulgaris)*, 99, 216, 227
Mushroom *see* Field Mushroom
Myrrh, 9, 10, 14
Myrtenyl acetate, 66
Myrtle *(Myrtus communis)*, 69, 127–8, 163, 166, 221, 229
Myths, 21

Natural products, 2–3
Nature of water
a basic necessity, 20
bottled water, 23
healing treatments with water, 24–5
increased dilutions, 30
introduction, 19
judging by water, 22
life and death, 21
physical power of water, 21
polar solvent-solubility in water, 28–30
scientists who investigated water, 25
structure of liquid water, 26–8
universal distillation process, 20
visual aspects, 22
water as a solvent and cleanser, 22
water in the body, 23
Nausea, 128, 136, 148, 164
Nebulizers, 153
Negative molecules, 89–91
Neroli *(Citrus aurantium* var. *amara)*, 16, 65, 66, 73, 171
Nerve pain, 25
Nervousness, 129
Nervous system, 168
Nettle *(Urtica dioica)*, 42, 71–5, 147, 225, 230, 255
Neurons, 76–8
Niaouli, 36
Nomenclature, 31–4, 35
Nose bleeds, 113
Nutmeg, 14, 36, 125

Oak, 41
Obesity, 25, 112
Obtaining hydrolats, 31–2
Ocimum basilicum (Basil), 36, 66, 164, 184, 221
Odour of hydrolats, 58–9
Oily skin, 210

Ointments, 16
Olive *(Olea europaea)*, 128–9, 221, 229
Onion, 36, 70
Orange bigarade *see* Neroli
Orange-blossom water, 173
Orange flower *(Citrus aurantium)*
  analysis of, 71–5
  cohobation, 53
  essential oil, 36
  history of aromatic medicine, 12, 13, 14, 16, 17
  hydroessentials, 39
  for menopausal symptoms, 168
  orange flower water, 69, 157, 235
  regulations for the preparation of, 37
  storage, 56
  therapeutic properties of, 104–6, 197, 217
  see also Neroli; Petitgrain
Orange rosemary sorbet, 175
Oregano *(Origanum vulgare)*
  essential oil, 36
  for severe stomach poisoning, 185–6
  storage of, 56
  therapeutic properties of, 129–30, 166, 168, 172, 173, 222
Organic chemistry, 76
Origanum majorana see Marjoram
Origanum onites (French marjoram, Pot marjoram), 129, 222, 229
  see also Marjoram
Origanum vulgare see Oregano
Origins of aromatherapy, 1–2
Ormenis mixta (Moroccan chamomile), 130, 222, 229
Osmosis, 45
Osteoarthritis, 25
Oxides, 29, 69, 73, 88
  see also specific oxide
Oxygen, 83
Oxyuriasis, 213

Pain relief, 25, 152, 156, 159
Palmarosa, 39, 64
Palpitations, 146
Panaceas, 2, 12
Pancreas, 207
Paracelsus, 14
Parasites, 151, 168
Parsley *(Petroselinum crispum)*, 11, 131, 222, 229
Passionflower *(Passiflora incarnata)*, 130, 229
Patchouli, 43, 52
Pelargonium graveolens see Geranium
Penicillin, 16
Pennyroyal *(Mentha pulegium)*, 86, 127, 221, 228
Peppermint *(Mentha* x *piperita)*
  analysis of, 63, 71–5, 247–8
  for chickenpox, 162
  cohobated, 51
  for digestive problems, 164, 185–6
  essential oil, 36
  for general health, 166
  for headaches, 167
  hydroessentials, 39
  mouthwash, 172
  therapeutic properties of, 125–7, 218, 221
  for thrush, 172
  for urinary infections, 173
Pepper *(Piper nigrum)*, 64, 116, 133, 229
Perfume, 179
Perfumed oils, 10
Perfumery, 16
Period pains, 125, 184
Personal hygiene, 15
Petitgrain *(Citrus aurantium* var. *amara)*, 65, 66, 105, 157, 217
Petroselinum crispum (Parsley), 11, 131, 222, 229
Peumus boldus (Boldo leaf), 131, 164, 195, 222, 229
Pharyngitis, 207
Phenols, 69, 83–4
Phenyl ring, 83
PH of hydrolats, 58
Physical aspects of hydrolats, 55–60
Physical power of water, 21
Physics, 6
Phytolacca decandra (Poke root), 131, 222
Picea mariana (Black spruce), 131, 222, 229
Pimento *(Pimento officinalis)*, 37, 52, 132, 222, 229
Pimpinella anisum see Aniseed
Pimpinella magna (Greater burnet, Saxifrage), 132, 222, 229
Pinene, 66
Pine *(Pinus sylvestris)*
  analysis of, 71–5, 250–1
  appearance of, 58
  distillation, 45
  pine needles, 66
  therapeutic properties of, 132, 160, 161, 185–6, 222
Pinocamphone, 63
Pinus sylvestris see Pine
Piper nigrum (Pepper), 64, 116, 133, 229
Pistachio *(Pistacia lentiscus)*, 133, 162, 222, 229
Plantain *(Plantago major)*, 41, 42, 133, 165, 222, 251
Plant medicine, 16–17
Plants used for distillation of hydrolats, 42
Pleurisy, 121, 141
Poke root *(Phytolacca decandra)*, 131, 222
Polar solvent, 28–30
Pollution, 20
Polygonatum multiflorum (Solomon's seal), 133, 222, 229
Poor man's weatherglass, 96

Poppy, 42
Poroplast technique, 50–1
Portulaca sativa (Golden purslane), 133, 222, 229
Positive molecules, 89–91
Potassium sorbate, 57
Potentilla anserina (Silverweed), 133–4, 222, 229
Pot marigold *(Calendula officinalis)*, 15, 71–5, 100–1, 227, 233
Pot marjoram *(Origanum onites)*, 129, 222, 229
  see also Marjoram
Premenstrual syndrome (PMS)
  clary, 141
  lemon balm, 125
  lemon verbena, 96
  recipe for relief of, 168
  rose, 136
  sage, 139
  yarrow, 95
Preparation of hydrolats, 31–2
Prepared water *see* Hydrolats
Prepared waters (false hydrolats)
  addition of alcohol, 38
  conclusion, 40
  eau-de-Cologne, 39–40
  hydroessentials, 38–9
  identifying, 35
  internal use of, 36
  methods of production and uses, 37–8
  not distilled, 35–6
  recipe, 179–180
  witch hazel, 39
Preservatives, 38, 57–8, 158–9
Priestley, Joseph, 25
Primary essential oil, 49
Propyl iodide, 58
Protons, 76–8
Prunus laurocerasus (Cherry laurel), 37, 134, 222, 229
Psoriasis, 103, 108, 142, 154, 210
Public fountains, 21
Purge and trap, 62
Purple coneflower *(Echinacea purpurea)*, 67, 71–5, 108, 218, 228, 237
Purslane, 42

Quality of distilled plant waters, 35, 59
Quality of hydrolats, 59
Quality of water, 44
Quinsy, 121

Recipes
  for common ailments, 159–71
  culinary, 173–7
  making your own hydrolats, 177–80
Recirculation of water, 53
Recovered essential oil, 49, 50–1
Rectal use of hydrolats, 157
Redness of the skin, 211
Red poppy, 191
Relaxation, 24, 200
Religion, 21
Renaissance herbals, 15–16
Renal cleanser, 208
Research, 17
Resins, 10
Respiratory problems, 25, 169, 208
  see also specific problem
Rheumatism
  baths, 152
  bladderwrack, 112
  elderflower, 141
  general use of hydrolats, 151, 169, 208
  juniper, 118
  sage, 140
  spa treatments, 25
  thalassotherapy, 24
  white and silver birch, 100
Rheumatoid arthritis, 112, 118, 146
Robinia pseudacacia (Acacia), 134, 222, 229
Rock rose *(Cistus ladaniferus)*, 105, 170, 217, 227
Roman chamomile *(Chamaemelum nobile)*
  analysis of, 63, 67, 71–5, 234–5
  for baby and childcare, 160
  for chickenpox, 162
  for eye problems, 166
  for headaches, 167
  for lice, 168
  for pain relief, 152
  for PMS, 168
  for sore throats, 172
  therapeutic properties of, 102–3, 216–17
  see also Chamomile; German chamomile
Rooibos tea, 192
Rosa canina (Wild rose), 134, 169, 222, 229
Rosacea, 154, 182–4
Rose, Jeanne, 94
Rose geranium *see* Geranium
Rosemary *(Rosmarinus officinalis)*
  for aches and pains, 160
  analysis of, 71–5, 253
  appearance of, 58
  for colds and flu, 162
  for digestive problems, 163
  essential oil, 36
  for general health, 166
  history of aromatic medicine, 11, 13–14, 14, 15, 16
  for infected gums, 172
  for legs, 167
  for the nervous system, 168
  for rheumatism, 169
  for severe stomach poisoning, 185–6
  for skin conditions, 170

Rosemary (*Contd.*)
therapeutic properties of, 137–8, 138, 223
for urinary infections, 173
Rosa damascena (damask rose), 169, 170
Rose *(Rosa)*
analysis of, 64, 65, 66, 69, 71–5, 251–3
cohobation, 53
culinary recipes, 173
for eye conditions, 165
as a facial tonic, 170
history of aromatic medicine, 11, 12–13, 13, 14
hydroessentials, 39
for menopause, 168
regulations for the preparation of, 37
rose water, 46, 63, 252
therapeutic properties of, 134–7, 181–2, 223
Rue *(Ruta graveolens)*, 138–9, 165, 229
Ruscus aculeatus (Butcher's broom), 162, 223, 229
Ruta graveolens (Rue), 138–9, 165, 229

Sabinene, 63, 66, 67, 74, 82
Safety, 2–3, 150
Saffron *(Crocus sativus)*, 107, 228
Sage *(Salvia officinalis)*
analysis of, 63, 69, 71–5, 253–4
appearance of, 58
cohobated, 51
for digestive problems, 163
essential oil, 36
for general health, 166
for hair problems, 167
history of aromatic medicine, 11, 14, 15
for legs, 167
for lice, 168
for rheumatism, 169
for skin, 170
therapeutic properties of, 139–40, 223
Salvia sclarea see Clary sage
Sambucus nigra (Elderflower), 39, 43, 141–2, 200, 224, 229
Sandalwood *(Santalum album)*, 52, 142, 229
Santolina, 36
Saponaria officinalis (Soapwort), 58, 142, 224, 229
Sarothamnus scoparius (Broom), 142, 224, 229
Sassafras, 36
Satureia see Savory
Saunas, 24
Savin, 52
Savory *(Satureia)*
appearance of, 58
essential oil, 36
therapeutic properties of, 142–3, 166, 168, 224
see also Summer savory; Winter savory
Saxifrage *(Pimpinella magna)*, 132, 222, 229
Scabious *(Scabiosa succisa)*, 143, 224, 229
Scalp, 205–6
Scarlet pimpernel *(Anagallis arvensis)*, 96, 215, 227
Scars, 171, 201–2, 209, 210–11
Scented barks, 10
Sciatica, 107
Science, rise of, 16
Scots pine *see* Pine
Seasonal affective disorder (SAD), 95
Sea water, 24
Seaweed, 24, 161
Secondary essential oil, 49
Sedatives, 208
Self-treatment, 2–3
Senna, 195
Sensitive skin, 211
Severe stomach poisoning, 185–6
Shapes of plants, 14
Shelf-life of hydrolats, 55
Shingles, 146, 208
Silver, 57
Silver Birch *(Betula pendula)*, 100, 227
Silverweed *(Potentilla anserina)*, 133–4, 222, 229
Skin
irritations/problems, 25, 103, 114, 123
mature, 211–12
oily, 210
sensitive, 211
skin care, 16, 151–2, 153–4, 169–71, 208–12
skin care products, 37
tonics, 32
Slimming, 171, 212
Smallage *(Apium graveolens)*, 97, 215, 227
Smoke tree *(Cotinus coggyria)*, 107, 227
Soapwort *(Saponaria officinalis)*, 58, 142, 224, 229
Social science, 6
Solidago virgaurea (Aaron's rod, Golden Rod), 143, 224, 229
Solid phase extraction, 62
Solomon's seal *(Polygonatum multiflorum)*, 133, 222, 229
Solubility, 4
Solvent, water as a, 22
Sore throats
clary, 141
ivy, 115
myrtle, 128
recipe for, 172
rose, 136
silverweed, 133
tea tree, 123
thyme, 145
Sourcing good materials, 3
Southernwood *(Artemesia abrotanum)*, 98, 216, 227

Spanish influences, 11–13
Spa treatments, 24–5
Spearmint *(Mentha spicata)*, 127, 221, 228
Spices, 10
Spike lavender *(Lavandula latifolia)*, 71–5, 120–1, 228, 243
Spikenard, 9, 14
Spirea ulmaria see Meadowsweet
Spleen, 98
Sports injuries, 25
Sprays, 154
Springs, 23, 24–5, 47
Stachys officinalis (Betony), 100, 143, 229
Stainless steel, 57
Static and dynamic head space extraction, 62–3
Steam baths, 24
Steam distillation, 44
  see also Distillation
Stills, 11, 12, 15, 45, 57
Stinging nettle *see* Nettle
St John's wort *(Hypericum perforatum)*, 71–5, 115–16, 154, 219, 239–40
Stomach, 212
Stomach upsets, 164, 173, 185–6
Storage of herbs, 189–90
Storage of hydrolats, 55–7
Strawberry *(Fragaria vesca)*, 111, 218, 228
Stress reduction, 24
Structure of liquid water, 26
Styptics, 212
Sulphides, 70, 74
Summer savory *(Satureia hortensis)*, 142, 229
  see also Savory
Sunburn, 96, 103, 131, 142, 211
Sunstroke, 130
Sweet basil *(Ocimum basilicum)*, 36, 66, 128, 164, 184, 221
Sweet bay *see* Bay
Sweet fennel *see* Fennel
Sweet marjoram *see* Marjoram
Sweet orange flower *see* Orange flower
Sweet pea, 65
Sweet thyme *(Thymus vulgaris)*, 145–6, 164, 185–6, 254–5
  see also Thyme
Synthetics, 16, 17

Tanacetum vulgare (Tansy), 15, 51, 58, 144, 224, 229
Tangerine, 36
Tannic acid, 4
Tannin, 188–9
Tansy *(Tanacetum vulgare)*, 15, 51, 58, 144, 224, 229
Tapeworms, 103
Tap water, 20
Tarragon *(Artemesia dracunculus)*, 36, 99, 163, 216, 227
Tasmanian blue gum *(Eucalyptus globulus)*, 109, 198, 218, 228
Taraxacum officinale (Dandelion), 144, 229
Teas, 7, 156–7, 160, 188, 190, 191–2
Tea tree *(Melaleuca alternifolia)*, 71–5, 123, 172, 220, 246
Teeth, 172
Teething, 160
Temperature of hydrolats, 55–6
Terminology, 31–4
Terpenes, 4, 28, 48, 93
Terpinen-4-ol, 64, 73, 84
Tetanus, 133
Thalassotherapy, 24
Therapeutic index, 197–213
Therapeutic value, 48–9
Threadworms, 213
Throat infections, 125
Thrush, 104, 117, 123, 172, 212
Thuja, 144, 224
Thujanol thyme *(Thymus vulgaris)*, 225
  see also Thyme
Thujone, 63, 67, 68, 86
Thymbra spicata (Black thyme), 144, 224, 229
Thyme linalool, 71–5
Thyme *(Thymus vulgaris)*
  analysis of, 69
  for digestive problems, 163
  for dry skin, 170
  for general health, 166
  history of aromatic medicine, 10, 11, 13, 16
  for infected gums, 172
  for lice, 168
  for rheumatism, 169
  still hardware, 45
  storage of, 56
  therapeutic properties of, 116, 144–6, 224–5
  for urinary infections, 173
Thymol, 84
Thymus serpyllum (Wild thyme), 144, 224, 229
Thyroid stimulants, 111–12, 212
Tidal waves, 21
Tilia see Lime
Time of distillation, 46
Tisanes, 7, 160, 188, 190–1
Tissington, 24
Toadflax *(Linaria vulgaris)*, 122, 220, 228
Toothache, 114
Trapped wind, 106
Travel sickness, 148
Treatments with water, healing, 24–5
Tree wormwood *(Artemesia arborescens)*, 98, 216, 227
Tuberculosis, 117
Turkish baths, 24

Turkish delight, 177
Turkish rose water, 46
  see also Rose water
Turmeric, 36
Turner, William, 15–16
Turpentine, 14, 65

Ulcers, 151
Universal distillation process, 20
Uplifting plants, 203–4
Urinary tract problems, 155, 173, 212
  see also specific problem
Urtica dioica (Nettle), 42, 71–5, 147, 225, 230

Vaccinations, 157, 172, 212
Vaginal douches, 152
Vaginitis, 117, 142
Valerian *(Valeriana officinalis)*, 43, 63, 147, 225, 230
Valnet, Jean, 18
Vaporizers, 155
Varicose veins
  compresses, 152–3
  general use of hydrolats, 213
  German chamomile, 104
  golden rod, 143
  Italian cypress, 107
  witch hazel, 113
  yarrow, 95
Vegetable soup, 174
Verbena, 36, 166
Vermifuges, 213
Vervain, 165
Vetiver*(Vetiver zizanioides)*, 52, 147, 230
Viaud, Henri, 94
Vinegars, 7, 10
Viola tricolor (Heartsease, Wild pansy), 147, 230, 255
Viola (unspecified), 63, 71–5
Viscum album (Mistletoe), 56, 147, 225, 230
Visual aspects of water, 22
Volatile molecules in the distilled waters, 47–8
Vomiting, 213

Wallflowers, 15
Walnut, 117, 219, 228
Water
  composition, 25
  drinking, 156–7
  oil, 49, 50–1
  pH value, 44
  retention, 107, 125
  see also Distillation; Nature of water
Watt, James, 25
Weight loss, 171
Wells, 21
White Birch *(Betula alba)*, 100, 227
White cedar *(Thuja occidentalis)*, 229
  see also Cedar
White goosefoot *(Chenopodium album)*, 103, 217, 227
Whitethorn, 107
Whooping cough, 117
Wild celery *(Apium graveolens)*, 97, 215, 227
Wild lettuce *(Lactuca virosa)*, 118, 219, 228
  see also Lettuce
Wild marjoram *see* Oregano
Wild pansy *(Viola tricolor)*, 147, 230, 255
Wild rose *(Rosa canina)*, 134, 170, 222, 229
  see also Rose
Wild thyme *(Thymus serpyllum)*, 144, 224, 229
  see also Thyme
Willow herb, 191
Wines, 7
Winterbloom, 113–14
Winter savory *(Satureia montana)*, 142–3, 224, 229
  see also Savory
Witch hazel *(Hamamelis virginiana)*, 39, 113–14, 154, 171, 218
World Health Organization (WHO), 23
Worms, 213
Wormwood *(Artemesia absinthium)*, 13, 98, 227
  see also Tree wormwood
Worship, 21
Wounds, 10, 143, 213
Wrinkled skin, 211–12

Yarrow *(Achillea millefolium)*
  analysis of, 67, 71–5, 231
  therapeutic properties of, 95, 170, 200, 215
Yellow flag *(Iris pseudacorus)*, 117, 219, 228
Yellow gentian *(Gentiana lutea)*, 112, 218, 228
  see also Gentian
Yield of hydrolats, 46–7
Ylang-ylang, 36, 66, 167

Zingiber officinale (Ginger), 52, 116, 147–8, 225, 230

Printed and bound by CPI Group (UK) Ltd, Croydon, CR0 4YY
03/10/2024
01040472-0004